THE ROUTLEDGE INTERNATIONAL HANDBOOK OF FAT STUDIES

The Routledge International Handbook of Fat Studies brings together a diverse body of work from around the globe and across a wide range of Fat Studies topics and perspectives. The first major collection of its kind, it explores the epistemology, ontology, and methodology of fatness, with attention to issues such as gender and sexuality, disability and embodiment, health, race, media, discrimination, and pedagogy. Presenting work from both scholarly writers and activists, this volume reflects a range of critical perspectives vital to the expansion of Fat Studies and thus constitutes an essential resource for researchers in the field.

Cat Pausé is Fat Studies scholar at the Institute of Education, Massey University, New Zealand, and the co-editor of *Queering Fat Embodiment*.

Sonya Renee Taylor is an international award-winning writer and performer, published author, and founder and Radical Executive Officer of The Body is Not An Apology, an international digital media and education company committed to radical self-love and body empowerment as the foundational tool of social justice.

THE ROUTLEDGE INTERNATIONAL HANDBOOK OF FAT STUDIES

*Edited by Cat Pausé and
Sonya Renee Taylor*

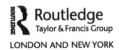

LONDON AND NEW YORK

First published 2021
by Routledge
2 Park Square, Milton Park, Abingdon, Oxon OX14 4RN

and by Routledge
605 Third Avenue, New York, NY 10158

Routledge is an imprint of the Taylor & Francis Group, an informa business

British Library Cataloguing-in-Publication Data
A catalogue record for this book is available from the British Library

Library of Congress Cataloging-in-Publication Data
Names: Pausé, Cat, editor. | Renee Taylor, Sonya, 1976– editor.
Title: The Routledge international handbook of fat studies / edited by Cat Pausé and Sonya Renee Taylor.
Description: Milton Park, Abingdon, Oxon ; New York, NY : Routledge, 2021. | Series: Routledge international handbooks | Includes bibliographical references and index.
Identifiers: LCCN 2020045970 (print) | LCCN 2020045971 (ebook) | ISBN 9780367502928 (hardback) | ISBN 9781003049401 (ebook)
Subjects: LCSH: Obesity—Case studies. | Obesity—Social aspects—Case studies. | Overweight persons—Case studies.
Classification: LCC RA645.O23 R68 2021 (print) | LCC RA645.O23 (ebook) | DDC 362.1963/98--dc23
LC record available at https://lccn.loc.gov/2020045970
LC ebook record available at https://lccn.loc.gov/2020045971

ISBN: 978-0-367-50292-8 (hbk)
ISBN: 978-0-367-50294-2 (pbk)
ISBN: 978-1-003-04940-1 (ebk)

Typeset in Bembo
by Apex CoVantage, LLC

This book is dedicated to the global fat community

CONTENTS

Contents

CONTRIBUTORS

Editors

Cat Pausé, PhD, is a Fat Studies scholar at Massey University in New Zealand. She is the lead editor of *Queering fat embodiment* (Ashgate), and has coordinated three international conferences – *Fat Studies: Reflective intersections* (2012), *Fat Studies: Identity, agency, embodiment* (2016), and *Fat Studies: Past, present, futures* (2020). Her research is focused on the effects of fat stigma on health and well-being on fat individuals and how fat activists resist the fatpocalypse. She has called for a new fat ethics, acknowledging the role science has played in the oppression of fat people and ensuring that research around fatness centers fat epistemology. Her work appears in scholarly journals including *Fat Studies, Journal of Law, Medicine, and Ethics, Feminist Review*, and *Narrative Inquiries in Bioethics*, as well as online in the *Huffington Post, NPR, The Conversation*, and her blog. Her fat positive radio show, *Friend of Marilyn*, has been showcasing Fat Studies scholarship and fat activism since 2011.

Sonya Renee Taylor is a world-renowned activist, author, artist, spiritual and transformational leader, and the founder of The Body Is Not an Apology, a movement and digital media and education company exploring the intersections of identity, healing, and social justice using the framework of radical self-love. The Body Is Not An Apology's content and message have changed the lives of millions of people across the globe, shifting how we live in and relate to our bodies and the bodies of others, shifting from a relationship of shame and injustice to a relationship bound by love. She is the author of six books, including the best-selling *The body is not an apology* (2nd ed. February 2021), *Celebrate your body (and its changes, too!): The ultimate puberty book for girls* (Rockridge Press, 2018), *The book of radical answers (that I know you already know)* (Dial Press, 2022) and coeditor of *The international handbook of Fat Studies* (Routledge, 2021). Her writing also appears in numerous anthologies and magazines. Sonya is an international-award-winning performance poet and speaker who has appeared across the United States, New Zealand, Australia, England, Scotland, Sweden, Germany, Brazil, Canada, the Netherlands, Bosnia, and more. Sonya and her work have appeared on CBS, CNN, NPR, HBO, BET, MTV, TV One, PBS, MSNBC.com, Today.com, Shape.com, and in the *New York Times, New York* magazine, *Huffington Post, Vogue Australia, Playboy, Self, Ms.* magazine, and many more publications. Sonya was a 2016 invitee to the Obama White House to speak on the intersection of LGBTQIAA+

and disability issues. In 2017, she was selected as an inaugural fellow of the Edmund Hillary Fellowship for global impact change makers in New Zealand. Sonya has shared the stage with such luminaries as Angela Davis, Sonia Sanchez, Amy Goodman, Carrie Mae Weems, Theaster Gates, Harry Belafonte, Dr. Cornel West, Hillary Rodham Clinton, the late Amiri Baraka, and numerous others. She continues to speak, teach, write, create, and transform lives globally. Visit her at www.sonyareneetaylor.com.

Contributors

Sofia Apostolidou is a PhD fellow with the Research Training Group "Minor Cosmopolitanisms" at the University of Potsdam. They studied Philology at the Aristotle University of Thessaloniki and Cultural Analysis at the University of Amsterdam. Together with the activist group The Political Fatties, they have been active in community organising in Greece, the Netherlands and Germany, and have published the collection "Fatties: Aspects of Fatness as a Political Identity". Their academic and activist work come together in their artistic practice, where they employ writing and performance art in order to explore the fat body as a vulnerable, powerful, counter-productive cyborg embodiment.

Amena Azeez is one of India's first plus size fashion bloggers and a body positive activist and influencer. She is also a poet, stylist, fashion consultant and content creator. She covers fashion, beauty, women's lifestyle, body positivity, pop culture, and intersectional feminism on her blog, Fashionpolis. With the aim to create space, visibility and representation for plus size and fat bodies, Amena hopes to dispel the hegemonic cultural standards of beauty and worth and create a size inclusive mainstream beauty, fashion and pop culture narrative. Amena's bylines have appeared in *Femina, Feminism in India, Hauterfly, Live More Zone,* and *Mumbai Mag,* among others. She has been featured on *Miss Malini, BuzzFeed India, Bustle, Grazia, Femina, HT Brunch, Times of India, She The People* and *The Hindu.*

Patricia Cain, PhD, is a weight stigma researcher from Murdoch University in Perth, Western Australia. Her research is informed by both qualitative and quantitative methodology with a focus on critical health psychology, specifically weight stigma and the quantification of discourses around "obesity" and fatness.

Erin Cameron is an Assistant Professor in the Northern Ontario School of Medicine, Lakehead University, Thunder Bay, Canada, co-editor of the award-winning *The fat pedagogy reader: Challenging weight-based oppression through critical education* (Peter Lang, 2016), and co-editor of a special issue of *Fat Studies* devoted to fat pedagogy.

Bertha Chan Hiu Yau is a fat acceptance activist in Hong Kong. She founded Curvasian, a platform for the plus size fashion industry in Asia. Through Curvasian, Bertha promotes fat acceptance and body positivity throughout Asia.

Athia N. Choudhury is a doctoral candidate and Annenberg Endowed Fellow in American Studies and Ethnicity at USC. Her dissertation, *Gut cultures: Decolonial bodies and other unruly matters,* unearths a critical genealogy for the emergence of "health" as a vital dimension to U.S. and Third World nation-building. *Gut cultures* examines the obscured relationship between modern conceptions of health in the U.S. and legacies of empire and militarism through the study of fat, emphasizing representations of women's eating. Her research examines colonial archives, governmental documents, and visual representations of the gut and eating across North

America, Asia, and North Africa – revealing that fat bodies and matter surface through these cultural artifacts as a means to chart how racialization and gender become differently coded throughout the twentieth century. Athia is a dedicated plant mom, unapologetic Gemini, and Boba tea enthusiast.

Laura Contrera is a fat feminist activist, lawyer, and PhD candidate in Gender Studies at Buenos Aires University. Her doctoral investigation focuses on stigmatization and discrimination against fat people as a human rights issue and examines struggles in depathologization in Argentina. She has collaborated in various collective works and, in 2016, co-edited *Cuerpos sin patrones. Resistencias desde las geografías desmesuradas de la carne*. Currently, she teaches Labour Law at the National University of La Matanza, Buenos Aires, and works at the High Court of Justice of the City of Buenos Aires.

Kimberly Dark is a writer, professor and raconteur, working to reveal the hidden architecture of everyday life so that we can reclaim our power as social creators. She's the author of *Fat, pretty and soon to be old*, *The daddies* and *Love and errors*, and her essays, stories and poetry are widely published in academic and popular online publications alike. Her ability to make the personal political is grounded in her training as a sociologist, and you can find her course offerings in Sociology at Cal State San Marcos and Writing/Arts at Cal State Summer Arts.

Graeme Ditchburn, PhD, is Academic Chair of Organisational Psychology at Murdoch University in Perth, Western Australia. His research focuses on individual differences, attitudes, wellbeing, and psychometrics.

Tiana A. Dodson is a fat, Body Liberation Coach who's out to destroy the belief that you have to be skinny to be happy and healthy, loveable, or worthy. Through her work with the Fat Freedom Foundation program, she guides people feminine-of-center to reconnect with their bodies, destigmatize fatness, and learn about the harms of health being a measure of worth all while finding how they can live their best fat lives.

Ngaire Donaghue, PhD, is an Adjunct Associate Professor in the School of Humanities at the University of Tasmania. Her research centres around ideological aspects of gender and subjectivity, with a particular focus on critical feminist understandings of embodiment.

Amy Erdman Farrell is the Curley Chair of Liberal Arts and Professor of American Studies and Women's, Gender and Sexuality Studies at Dickinson College in Pennsylvania, USA. She is the author of two books, *Fat shame: Stigma and the fat body in American culture* (New York University Press, 2011) and *Yours in sisterhood: Ms. magazine and the promise of popular feminism* (University of North Carolina Press, 1998). She is also the author of many articles focusing on fat stigma and motherblaming, Fat Studies pedagogy, and fat stigma in the contemporary food activist movements.

May Friedman's research looks at unstable identities, including bodies that do not conform to traditional racial and national or aesthetic lines. Most recently much of May's research has focused on intersectional approaches to Fat Studies considering the multiple and fluid experiences of both fat oppression and fat activism. May works at Ryerson University as a faculty member in the School of Social Work and in the Ryerson/York graduate program in Communication and Culture.

Hannele Harjunen, PhD, is a Senior Lecturer in Gender Studies at the department of Social Sciences and Philosophy at the University of Jyväskylä, Finland. She has written extensively on gender, body norms, and fatness in Finnish and English. Her work has been published in journals such as *Feminist Theory*, *Feminism and Psychology* and *The Fat Studies Journal*. In addition, she has written numerous book chapters and a monograph *Neoliberal bodies and the gendered fat body* (Routledge, 2017). She is currently working on a book on weight discrimination in Finland.

April Herndon, PhD, is a Professor of English at Winona State University in Winona, MN. April's work, including her book *Fat blame*, examines the disjuncture between conversations about fatness as a social issue and interventions aimed at individual bodies, interventions that pay little attention to social factors. Her work interrogates ideas of "health" as a neutral concept, arguing that size, race, gender, and class often collide in ideas of who is and is not "healthy" in American society. When she's not writing and teaching, April enjoys swimming, biking, yoga, gardening, playing her ukulele, and sitting with her cats.

Natalie Ingraham, PhD, MPH is an Assistant Professor of Sociology at California State University, East Bay. She earned her PhD in Sociology from UC San Francisco. Her research examines the intersections of body size, gender, sexuality and health. She has conducted qualitative research on gender and reproductive health as a staff research associate at Advancing New Standards in Reproduction Health (ANSIRH) at UCSF and in the Dept. of Social Welfare at UC Berkeley. She completed a BS in Psychology from University of Science and Arts of Oklahoma and a Master of Public Health degree from Indiana University, Bloomington.

Dr. Katariina Kyrölä is a Kone Foundation Senior Research Fellow and a Lecturer in Gender Studies at Åbo Akademi University, Finland. Kyrölä is the co-editor of *The power of vulnerability: Mobilising affect in feminist, queer and anti-racist media cultures* (Manchester University Press, 2018) and the author of *The weight of images: Affect, body image and fat in the media* (Routledge, 2014) as well as articles in, for example, *Feminist Theory*, *Sexualities*, *Subjectivity*, and *Social Media + Society*.

Jenny Lee, PhD, was a Senior Lecturer in Creative Writing and Literary Studies, and a research fellow in The Institute for Health and Sport at Victoria University, Australia. In addition to publishing scholarly and autoethnographic papers, she publishes memoir, short stories and narrative non-fiction. Her autoethnographic publications include "You will face discrimination: Fatness, motherhood and the medical profession" in *Fat Studies Journal* (2020), and "Stigma in practice: Barriers to health for fat women" with Dr Cat Pausé in *Frontiers of Psychology* (2016).

Emily McAvan is an Australian writer whose work examines the meeting point between bodies, texts and culture. She is the author of *Jeanette Winterson and religion* (Bloomsbury, 2020) and *The postmodern sacred* (McFarland, 2012). Her work has appeared in *Journal of Postcolonial Writing*, *Literature and Theology*, *Critique: Studies in Contemporary Fiction* and numerous other journals.

Nomonde Mxhalisa is a fat, Black feminist in love with stories. She is fascinated by the ways people's lived realities shape their joys and pains and believes that there is healing to be found in the stories we choose to tell and salvation – perhaps – in who we choose to tell them to. Radical softness is her weapon of choice in a world that often casts her as a hard, fat, Black obstacle. Food, hunger, sex, access, and desirability are her favourite topics and she is currently pursuing a Master of Social Science in Gender and Urban Food Security. Her background is in journalism, documentary film making, communications and marketing. She has collaborated with Love Intersections, a Canada-based media arts collective made up of queer artists of colour, who use multimedia to share the stories of queer, trans, non-binary and intersex people. Nomonde currently works for a conservation non-profit in South Africa that focuses on harmoniously bringing people and nature together for the benefit of all.

Sam Orchard is committed to building a world where our many differences and complexities are celebrated. He writes comics, essays and children's books, creates animated videos, podcasts, and resources with this aim. Sam's recent activism projects include "We Are Beneficiaries" and "Out Loud Aotearoa". As part of these he organized and engaged other artists and writers to drive social change in New Zealand. These projects gained international attention across social media and news sites, amplifying viewpoints which are often missing from public discourse. Sam's comics and resources about sexuality, sex and gender have been used internationally by SOGI advocates. Sam is currently working on his first full length graphic novel.

Sonalee Rashatwar (she/they) grew up as a fat kid and is now a superfat queer non-binary South Asian clinical social worker in Philadelphia, US, popularly known as TheFatSexTherapist on Instagram. She specializes in treating sexual trauma, body image, and racial or immigrant identity issues, while offering fat positive sexual healthcare. They co-own a private practice in West Philadelphia called the Radical Therapy Center.

Kath Read is originally from Brisbane, Australia, and in 2019 migrated to Wellington, New Zealand. After spending 20 happy years as a public librarian in Brisbane, she decided to follow her dream to move to Aotearoa, New Zealand and now works in the private sector. She had an epiphany at age 35 that saw her realising that if she did not give up trying to be thin, she would be giving up her life, both figuratively and literally, so she trotted out the rainbow tights, cute frock and sparkly Doc Martens and marched out into the world to change how people with fat bodies are perceived and treated. After more than a decade of fat activism she has been involved with academia, business and grassroots activities alike.

Esther D. Rothblum, PhD, is Professor of Women's Studies at Diego State University and editor of *Fat Studies: An Interdisciplinary Journal of Body Weight and Society*. She has edited over 20 books, including *Overcoming fear of fat* (with Laura Brown in 1989) and *The Fat Studies reader* (with Sondra Solovay in 2009). She is a member of the advisory board of the National Association to Advance Fat Acceptance and a founding co-chair of the Size Acceptance Caucus of the Association for Women in Psychology.

Constance Russell is a Professor in the Faculty of Education at Lakehead University, Thunder Bay, Canada where she teaches courses in social justice education, critical food education, environmental education, and animal-focused education. She was the co-editor of the award-winning *The Fat pedagogy reader: Challenging weight-based oppression through critical education* (Peter Lang, 2016). She also was given the 2017 North American Association for Environmental Education's Outstanding Contributions to Research in Environmental Education Award.

Hunter Ashleigh Shackelford is a Black fat storyteller, visual artist, data futurist, and shapeshifter. Hailing from the South, Hunter creates cultural art and uplifts stories centering Black fat folks, gender fugitivity, and care work. When they're not performing wellness, they're thriving in authenticity. They're the baddest to ever do it. Find more of their work at: HunterAshleigh.com.

Allison Taylor is a PhD candidate in the department of Gender, Feminist and Women's Studies at York University. Taylor's SSHRC-funded, doctoral research explores queer fat femme identities, embodiments, and negotiations of femmephobia, fatphobia, and other intersecting oppressions in queer communities in Canada. Her research interests include Fat Studies, critical femininity studies, queer theory, and critical disability studies. Her work has appeared in publications such as *Fat Studies: An Interdisciplinary Journal of Body Weight and Society*, *Psychology & Sexuality*, and the *Journal of Lesbian Studies*.

Dr. Darci L. Thoune is Professor of English and First-Year Writing Program Coordinator at the University of Wisconsin-La Crosse where she teaches first-year writing and upper-level writing courses. Her research focuses on first-year writing, writing program administration, and fat activism. She has published in *WPA Journal*, *JoSoTL*, *Composition Studies*, *Fat Studies*, and in several edited collections.

Tara Margrét Vilhjálmsdóttir is a 33-year-old social worker and an intersectional fat acceptance activist. She identifies as a white, hetero, cis-gender, middle-class, disabled superfat woman. She is a founding member and current president of the Icelandic Association for Body Respect. She lives in Reykjavík with her husband.

Stephanie von Liebenstein MA, born 1977, is founder, long time president and now vice president of the German Association against Weight Discrimination (Gesellschaft gegen Gewichtsdiskriminierung e.V.), the largest German fat acceptance organisation. She was the first to publicly use the German translation of "weight discrimination" ("Gewichtsdiskriminierung") in Germany. Besides numerous appearances on TV and in the press, Stephanie has published and presented extensively on weight discrimination, especially its legal implications. In 2016, she was on the expert podium of the German Federal Anti-Discrimination Agency advocating the inclusion of weight into German antidiscrimination legislation. From 2011 to 2014, she was member of the *Fat Studies* (ed. Esther Rothblum) Editorial Board.

Francis Ray White is a senior lecturer in Sociology at the University of Westminster, London, UK. Their research draws on fat, queer and (trans)gender theory and they have written variously about the construction of fat bodies as anti-social and deathly in the discourses of the 'obesity epidemic', medical constructions of fat sexuality, and trans/non-binary fat embodiment. Francis's work has been published in the journals *Somatechnics* (2012), *Fat Studies* (2014) and *Sexualities* (2016) and in edited collections including *Thickening fat* (Routledge, 2019) and *Non-binary lives* (JKP, 2020).

Dr. Jason Whitesel writes, teaches, and gives talks on queer studies, stigmatized groups' embodied resistance to injustice, and the intersectionalities of race/ethnicity, class, gender, sexuality, body weight, appearance, age, dis/ability, and nationality, and how interlocking identities define some lives as less/more valuable than others. He has authored *Fat gay men: Girth, mirth, and the politics of stigma*, and coedited a special double issue on "Fat Activism" for *Fat Studies*, in addition to publishing in peer-reviewed journals and collections. He is jointly employed in Sociology and Gender Studies at Illinois State University.

ACKNOWLEDGEMENTS

This Handbook has taken several years to pull together and has involved a huge amount of work from the editors, the contributors, and the administrative and publishing team at Routledge. The Editors are greatly indebted to the authors who have contributed chapters from around the world; this Handbook would not exist without your generosity and commitment to building our field. We also wish to thank Professors Esther Rothblum and Kathleen LeBesco for their guidance and support throughout the process. And Sarah (Shoog) McDaniel for the gorgeous art on the cover of the Handbook.

We'd like to thank the bounty of fat scholars and activists who have informed the trajectory of our work over our careers. The wisdom, wit, and fortitude of fat liberationists around the globe brought us into each other's lives and those same people have poured richly into the well from which the resilience to see this work to completion was drawn. You are too many to name but we hold you dearly in our hearts.

We are appreciative of each other as well, knowing that we have been working to pull this together on top of multitudes of other projects, international relocations, deaths, celebrations, and more. We are grateful for our colleagues, our friends, our families, our furry friends; all who helped support us along the way. We have worked together across oceans, committed to this project and to each other, and we are very proud of this finished collection.

1

FATTENING UP SCHOLARSHIP

Cat Pausé and Sonya Renee Taylor

Fat Studies is a post-disciplinary field of study that centres the fat body and lived experiences of fat people. "The field of fat studies can offer a revelatory new lens on the central human question of embodiment, a theoretical approach that will have direct political and social effects" (Wann, 2009, p. xxi). Fat Studies scholars identify and discuss mainstream and alternative discourses on fatness, analyse size as a social justice issue at the intersection of oppression, and critically appraise size oppression as it is manifested in various societal institutions (medicine, media, education, etc). In the inaugural issue of the *Fat Studies* journal, Editor-at-Large Esther Rothblum (2012) defines Fat Studies as "a field of scholarship that critically examines societal attitudes about body weight and appearance, and that advocated equality for all people with respect to body size … Fat studies scholars ask why we oppress people who are fat and who benefits from their oppression" (p. 3). In many calls for papers, this definition of the discipline can be found,

> Fat Studies is an interdisciplinary, cross-disciplinary field of study that confronts and critiques cultural constraints against notions of "fatness" and "the fat body"; explores fat bodies as they live in, are shaped by, and remake the world; and creates paradigms for the development of fat acceptance or celebration within mass culture. Fat Studies uses body size as the starting point for a wide-ranging theorization and explication of how societies and cultures, past and present, have conceptualized all bodies and the political/cultural meanings ascribed to every body. Fat Studies reminds us that all bodies are inscribed with the fears and hopes of the particular culture they reside in, and these emotions often are mislabeled as objective "facts" of health and biology. More importantly, perhaps, Fat Studies insists on the recognition that fat identity can be as fundamental and world-shaping as other identity constructs analyzed within the academy and represented in media.[1]

We are very proud to present this *International Handbook of Fat Studies*. Following the model of existing Handbooks, this collection is not intended as a textbook, but as a single-volume reference work aimed at academics and students working in Fat Studies as well as various fields of social science, health science, public health, popular culture, and current socio-political debates and trends. It is intended to be international in scope, both by addressing global and national issues, and in terms of scholars and activists enlisted as contributors.

Contributors to this Handbook hail from fifteen countries around the world. Many of the contributors responded to the call for papers (*CFP*) for this collection, while some were belly bumped to join. We expect this Handbook to challenge traditional ideas about fatness, review existing discourses about fatness, and produce new debates about fatness, in the context of the shifting and developing field of Fat Studies. We recognize, though, that there are gaps. Some of these gaps exist due to contributions that failed to materialize; some exist because of the paucity of scholarship on a singular topic. We have done our best to ensure that this Handbook represents a wide range of Fat Studies scholarship and activism.

In the Introduction to the *Fat studies reader* (2009), Solovay and Rothblum highlight important academic points in early Fat Studies as well as early activism points. In including key early U.S. activism in the chapter, they acknowledge the importance of fat activism to the field of Fat Studies and the production of fat knowledge, practices, and ethics. Wann (2009) argues that the field of Fat Studies "offers a crucial corollary to fat pride community and fat civil rights activism" (p. x). The inclusion and recognition of both academic and activist work in the space of Fat Studies is one of the greatest strengths of the discipline.

Long before there was a field of Fat Studies, fat activists were writing books about the fat experience and the need for fat liberation (Bovey, 1994; Erdman, 1996; Fraser, 1997; Garrison & Levitsky, 1993; Goodman, 1995; Louderback, 1970; Millman, 1980; Schoenfielder & Wieser, 1983; Thone, 1997; Wiley, 1994). The earliest of these is Lew Louderback's *Fat power*; Louderback's publication of the article, "More people should be FAT" in the *Saturday Evening Post* in 1967 was one of the precursors to the creation of the National Association to Advance Fat Americans (now known as the National Association to Advance Fat Acceptance). Most well-known is probably Marilyn Wann's *Fat!So?* published in 1998 by Ten Speed Press. Ten Speed Press is one of the publishing houses that has proven itself to be relatively fat friendly; other friendly presses include Pearlsong Press and Demeter Press.

In addition, scholars were exploring fat stigma (Brown & Rothblum, 1989[2]; DeJong, 1980; Harris et al., 1982; Larkin & Pines, 1979; Rothblum et al., 1988; Tiggemann & Rothblum, 1998), social constructions of fatness and health (Sobal & Maurer, 1999a, 1999b), the legal oppression of fat people (Solovay, 2000), fat history (Schwartz, 1986; Stearns, 1997), and fat identity (Braziel & LeBesco, 2001[3]; Cooper, 1998). Many more were doing work that was critical of the obesity epidemic paradigm and disrupting common sense assumptions about fatness and fat people. Cooper (2010) attempts to "map the field" of Fat Studies as it emerged in her piece, "Fat Studies: Mapping the field". We do not attempt to recreate her work here but would like to acknowledge many of the texts[4] that have contributed to Fat Studies scholarship.

Important theoretical and empirical work has been done by LeBesco (2004), Kirkland (2008), Farrell (2011), Boero (2012), Kwan and Graves (2013), Gailey (2014), Whitesel (2014), Harjunen (2016), Kyrölä (2016), Murray (2008), Saguy (2014), and Cooper (2016). Ley-Navarro (2010) and Strings (2019) have published books that expand the scholarship beyond the traditionally white western framework in the field (see also the forthcoming Luna et al., 2020).

Edited texts have provided opportunities for scholars within the field to organize material around specific topics, such as education and pedagogy (Cameron & Russell, 2016), sex (Hester & Walters, 2015), motherhood (Verseghy & Abel, 2018), and queering fat embodiment (Pausé et al., 2014). Tomrley and Naylor's (2009) *Fat studies in the UK* was an output of a one-day seminar in York hosted by the editors; in a similar fashion, Friedman, Rice, and Rinaldi (2019) brought together the contributors to *Thickening fat* for a two-day symposium at Ryerson University in 2018. *The fat studies reader*, published in 2009 by Rothblum and Solovay, has long been considered one of the formative texts in the discipline.

And many Fat Studies scholars and fat activists have material on hand from scholars whose work falls outside of our field, but aides us in making arguments relevant to fat liberation (for example, see Bacon, 2008; Campos, 2004; Gaesser, 2013; Gard, 2010; Gard & Wright, 2005; Oliver, 2006).

But the material that Fat Studies draws from has always included work from outside of the academy. Contributions to Fat Studies scholarship can be found in blogs, podcasts, documentaries, and more. For the purposes of this introduction, we thought we would present key published material that sits outside of the academy but is very much important to the field of Fat Studies.

Essays have long been used to explore fatness, fat bodies, and the lives of fat people (Chastain, 2014; Schoenfielder & Wieser, 1983; Wiley, 1994). Schoenfielder and Wieser's (1983) *Shadows on a tightrope: Writings by women on fat oppression* is one of the earliest collections of writings by fat women; it includes articles, narratives, and poems. It also includes material that had been distributed by Fat Liberation Publications in the 1970s. Poetry (Donald, 1986; Nicols, 1984; Zellman, 2009) and fiction, including short stories (Holt & Leib, 2012; Jarrell & Sukrungruang, 2003; Koppelman, 2003; Thompson, 2019), have been another vehicle for material that questions the social construction of fatness and imagines a range of fat embodiments. Thompson (2019), for example, imagines a future world where fat people continue to be oppressed through new technologies and regulations; the stories end on a hopeful note, though, as we meet a character who rescues fat people from this future world and takes them somewhere else, someplace where they are liberated. Julie Murphy (2017, 2019) has published several young adult books featuring a fat protagonist and recently penned an origin story for the fat superheroine, Faith (2020).[5] And Sarai Walker's (2015) novel *Dietland* was made into a television series. Other fat positive television includes an adaptation of Murphy's *Dumplin'* for a Netflix film and an adaptation of Lindy West's *Shrill* as a TV series on Hulu.

Non-fiction empowerment and self-help books have often sought to help individuals mitigate the personal impacts of fat oppression while offering critique and commentary regarding the social and systemic manifestations of fatphobia. Self-help books from fat activists range from personal stories with lessons (Baker, 2015, 2018; Hagen, 2019; Shanker, 2004; West, 2017) to more instructive texts (Blank 2011, 2012; Frater, 2005; Harding & Kirby, 2009; Kinzel, 2012; Lyons & Burgard, 1990; Taylor, 2018; Wann, 1998), although to be fair it is a difficult needle to thread. And memoir has long been a powerful vehicle for fat stories; from Cameron Manheim's (2000) *Wake up, I'm fat!* to Pattie's Thomas's (2005) *Taking up space*; fat memoir seems to be having a particular resurgence at present, with several titles being released recently (Byer, 2020; Cottom, 2019; Dark, 2019; Gay 2018; Laymon, 2019) or slated for release (Cox, 2020; Yeboah, 2020).

For decades fat activists and scholars have sought to make visible the experiences and barriers of fat life. This Handbook sits alongside these contributions and attempts to bring together the decades of work done in the service of understanding the fat condition and achieving fat liberation.

Fat activism

If the work of Fat Studies is to confront and critique cultural constraints against notions of "fatness" and "the fat body" and explore fat bodies as they live in, are shaped by, and remake the world; and theorize how society conceptualizes and pathologizes fat bodies; then the fat activist has been charged and continues to answer the question of "what then?" As Amy Farrell posits in her chapter "Feminism and fat":

Feminists across the spectrum (radical, liberal, cultural, socialist, African American, lesbian) and in various formats (*Ms.* magazine, Combahee River Collective, Redstockings, the protests against the Miss America Pageant) argued that the beauty industries exploited women financially, sapped their energy, turned them into objects for male pleasure, and hurt their bodies and souls.

(p. 54)

To this end, activists, armed with this information, have led in the work of boycott initiatives and retail disruption. Activists have shouted down actions of an oppressive and exploitative beauty industry and specifically fat activists have translated and amplified the knowledge of academia so that it might operate in the realm of social change.

In the conclusion of the chapter "Fat and trans", Francis Ray White proposes, "As a necessarily unfixed location, then, fat/trans can perhaps operate as the juncture that reveals the unsustainability of separating gender and fat for anyone"(p. 86). If indeed fat/trans academic theory illuminates the unsustainable nature of positioning the two as unrelated, it is the fat trans activist who has been charged with creating the conditions that shift the fixed understanding and interpretations of gender and weight through challenging the social, political and economic artifices of our society.

Current fat activist groups can be located around the world, including the Political Fatties in Greece, Taller Hacer La Vista Gorda in Argentina, Dik Gelukkig and Fat Positivity Belgium in Belgium, and NOLOSE in the United States. Orgullo Gordo in Spain, Fetter Widerstand in Germany, Yes2Bodies in Switzerland, and Allegro Fortissimo in France. The Gesellschaft gegen Gewichtsdiskriminierung in Germany, Edinburgh Fat Club in Scotland, the Icelandic Association of Body Respect in Iceland, and Malmö Fat Front in Sweden.

In trying to present an overview of fat activism, we are mindful of the criticism that visible fat activism, especially within the Global North, has been the purview of white fat activists. Excellent critiques of white supremacy within fat activist spaces have been produced by Tara Shuai (2008) and others; as a part of NOLOSE, Shuai et al. (2012) published a letter to white fat activists, holding them to account for reproducing white supremacy in their activism. The group writes,

> The time has been long in the coming to again address the prevalent attitudes of socio-economic privilege and white-centric thought in fat activism. When open and authentic conversations about race and class fail to happen, we see these attitudes in the ways that people are left out of conversations. We see people who live with great privilege speaking as authorities on the impact of racism and classism, without basing their approach in the ally model ... We see white allies responding defensively and closing down conversations when presented with clear questions about taking steps to do their own work of finding ally mentors, addressing the ways their own acknowledged and unacknowledged privilege directly affects members of their community, and engaging in thoughtful dialogue about the interconnectedness of oppressions and the diverse ways those oppressions affect different members of our communities . . . We are looking forward to a stronger, more representational expression of fat community in which POC and poor people's voices are heard, their experiences are respected, and their work to strengthen their individual communities is supported just as they work to support others.

(2012, para 8, 15)

It Gets Fatter member, Ahmad, argues that white fat activists need to amplify the voices of fat people of colour, especially when offered media attention. Ahmad (2015) encourages white fat activists to consider the attention they receive and reflect on the role that white supremacy plays in those opportunities.

Farrell (2019) notes that we often resort to telling the same history of fat activism; the history of white fat activism within the United States, which suggests this is the only history – or the only history that matters. She warns, "[the] repetition flattens fat, erasing complexity and contradiction, ignoring other voices" (p. 12). In our first attempt at writing about fat activism, we had over 4,000 words that largely told these same stories again. We decided to turn away from doing that work and to highlight fat activism around the world that are important parts of our community but have not received the same attention. In our commitment to meeting these challenges, we are presenting important snapshots of fat activism from non-white activists; specifically, fat people of colour from the Global South.

Latasha Ngwube is the founder of a plus size lifestyle online magazine in Nigeria, *#AboutThatCurvyLife* and the owner of fashion line, *The Curvy Monroe*. Her online magazine is "Africa's largest platform embracing the plus-size community" (Ngwube, n.d.). And her fashion line provides "stylish, comfortable, modern, feminine, and functional clothes to curvy women" (Bellanaijastyle.com, 2019). Ngwube is also an Assistant Editor of Vanguard's *Allure* magazine. As she shared in her cover story with *Accelerate* magazine, "I'm allowed to call myself beautiful … I'm allowed to wear nice clothes, I'm allowed to want for myself what any other person of any other size wants" (Vincent-Otiono, 2020, para. 14). Ngwube has been working to ensure that fat people in Nigeria have equal access to fashion and influencer culture (BBC News Africa, 2016). In 2016, she persuaded the biggest fashion event in Africa, Lagos Fashion Week, to include plus size models on the runways (CNN, 2016).

Malu Jimenez is an academic and activist in Brazil. Her PhD explores fatphobia, resistance, and activism. Jimenez maintains a blog, Lute como uma gorda (*Fight like a fat*; Jimenez, n.d.), founded the network Estudos do Corpo Gordo Feminino (Female Body Fat Studies), writes pieces for popular media online (Jimenez, 2020), and offers online courses in Fat Studies and fat politics. She represented Brazil at the first fat activist meeting of Latin America in Bogota, Columbia, in 2019 (Jimenez, n.d.; Queiroz, 2020). Jimenez shared with Peita,

> Fighting like a fat woman for me has been facing fatophobia every day of my life, in places that I believed to be safe, with people who loved me and for that reason have not stopped being fatphobic. It means facing disgust and disapproval, it means being intellectually devalued for being fat. It is having socially denied happiness, humanity and transforming all of that into activism.
>
> *(2020, para 2)*

Jimenez is one of the organizers of the online fat festival, Gordosfera, and part of the feminist collective, Gordas xômanas. The collective holds lectures, events, book clubs, and activism events (Marimon, 2020).

Ameya Nagarajan and Pallavi Nath are a Delhi-based duo who host the podcast, *Fat. So?* In their podcast, their intimate conversations range from using the word fat in casual chatting, exercising as a fat person, fat sexuality, and everyday things that fat people may experience (like concern about fitting into/breaking chairs). Nagarajan shared with Asian Age, "Our main intent is to fight the fat-phobia that is deeply ingrained in society. We talk about all the facets of our experiences as fat women, and other people's as well" (Charkravorty, 2019, para 5). They produce a podcast, blog, and host Instagram lives, often with guests to chat about fat-related issues. And they bring to the fore the privileges they have and how they shape their experiences of their fatness. Nath notes, "We are both very aware of our privilege as educated, exposed-to-the-world, reasonable well-to-do women and we cannot even begin to imagine how things would have been if we did not have this background of the parents we had" (Spark Magazine, 2020, para 9).

For those interested in learning more about the scholarship of fat activism, we would point to the work available from around the world. Casadó-Marín and Gracia-Arnaiz (2020) have examined fat activism in Spain; von Liebenstein (2012) has explored fat activism in Germany and the founding of Gesellschaft gegen Gewichtsdiskriminierung. Ellison (2013) examines fat activism in Canada; Maor (2013) has done work on the fat acceptance community in Israel. And a handful of scholars have tried to present histories of fat activism (Farrell 2011, 2019; Levy-Navarro, 2010; Simic, 2015; Stimson, 2003), most notably Charlotte Cooper. On her blog, *Obesity Timebomb*, Cooper reminds fat activists to document their work, and suggests a range of formats to do so, such as zines, online publications, print publications; "create a paper trail for your activism, create evidence that it happened" urges Cooper (2008).

Cooper has compiled fat activist events in her blog, *Obesity Timebomb* (especially the "Roots of Fat Activism Series" in 2016), and her zine, *A queer and trans fat activist timeline* (Cooper, 2011, 2012). In Cooper's (2016) *Fat activism: A radical social movement*, she brings it together and suggests that fat activist work can be classified into five categories. And she argues that fat activism needs to recapture the radical energy of earlier feminist groups, embracing anti-assimilationist activism and ambiguity. Cooper worries that fat activism has become stagnant; she points to the rise in body positivity as one example of this. Cooper also suggests that fat activism is under threat by those who would achieve liberation for some (the "healthy", good fatties) at the expense of the rest.

Levy-Navarro (2010) urges that "fat histories must also work to explore alternative realities, which they can do in part by exploring the very different way that the fat body can be understood by nondominant cultures in the West as well as by non-Western cultures worldwide" (p. 16); she is speaking of fat histories more generally, we would agree it is equally important for histories of fat activism and Fat Studies scholarship. Cooper (2016) acknowledged this in her book as well; she tells a story of fat activism history, but there are many other stories to share. We hope that as Fat Studies continues to grow, especially outside of the English language, more of these histories will be documented and shared across the world.

Fat Studies

The domain of the fat activist has often been to usher in fat liberation at the site of the individual body. Fat Studies scholars engage in a similar quest for liberation, focusing more on sites and domains of the academy, such as conferences. Wann (2009) locates the beginnings of Fat Studies as a field at a 2004 conference and event at Columbia University. The conference, "Fat Attitudes: An Examination of an American Subculture and the Representation of the Female Body", was hosted by Columbia University Teachers College. An accompanying art show, *Fat attitudes: A celebration of large women*, tied fat activism directly to Fat Studies scholarship. A few years later Smith College hosted the conference, "Fat and The Academy". Rothblum and Solovay (2009) suggest 2006 as a tipping point for the emerging discipline, as three national events brought scholars and activists together to advance the scholarship of fatness. First, the Smith College conference. Then, a dedicated Fat Studies stream at the American Culture Association/Popular Culture Association conference (which continues today). And finally, a conference held by the Association for Size Diversity and Health.

The University of Cambridge's Centre for Research in the Arts, Social Sciences, and Humanities (CRASSH) hosted "Bodies of Evidence: Fat Across Disciplines in 2007". Not a Fat Studies conference as evidenced in the description, many in attendance held the common anti-fat views that being fat was unhealthy (Söderqvist, 2007; Tomrley, 2009). And the conference was supported by Big Pharma (specifically, GlaxoSmithKline) (Cooper, 2009b). But many of the papers presented were critical of the pathologization of fatness, such as Dr. Petra Jonvallen's work, *Obesity in the belly of Big Pharma: One example of how body fat is turned into a medical problem*. And the conference closed with a presentation from Katie LeBesco; LeBesco gave a powerful talk in which she linked activism, politics, and power (Tomrley, 2009).

"Fat Studies UK" was hosted by Corinna Tomrley and Ann Naylor at the University of York in 2008. This one-day seminar brought together key thinkers in Fat Studies in the UK, including Charlotte Cooper, Lee Monaghan, and Lucy Aphramor. According to the programme,

> the objectives of the day [were] to discuss the discipline of Fat Studies in a UK context; acknowledge the importance of fat activism and politics to explore the links between activism and research; and to bring together like-minded researchers, activists, and supporters of size acceptance in the UK" (Tomrley & Naylor, 2009, p. 117). Work presented at the seminar was subsequently published in an edited collection, *Fat Studies UK*.
>
> *(Tomrley & Naylor, 2009)*

In 2010, Samantha Murray hosted "Fat Studies: A Critical Dialogue at Macquarie University" in Sydney, Australia. As noted in the CFP, "This two-day event will put Australasian Fat Studies into conversation with critical fat scholarship from around the globe by gathering together scholars from across a spectrum of disciplinary backgrounds, as well as activists, health care professionals, performers and artists" (as cited in Read, 2010, para 7). The keynotes were Charlotte Cooper and Karen Throsby, and the attendees included activists and scholars alike, including critical obesity researcher, Michael Gard.[6] Work presented at the conference contributed to a special issue of *Somatechnics* on fat bodily being (Murray, 2012a) and a special issue of *Feminism & Psychology* on fatness (Murray, 2012b).

Between 2010 and 2012, Universities across the UK hosted an Economic and Social Research Council (*ESRC*) seminar series on Fatness and Health (Cooper, 2009b). The first seminar focused on Embodiment, and included presentations from Corinna Tomrley, Lee Monaghan, and a keynote from Charlotte Cooper. The second focused on Health at Every Size and included a keynote from Lucy Aphramor. The third focused on Fat Activism and included presentations from Hannele Harjunen, Caroline Walters, and Samantha Murray. The fourth focused on the methodologies and politics of fat scholarship and included a keynote from Jacqui Gringras. Having ESRC funding allowed the events to provide student bursaries, free admission, and host materials such as narrated slides and audio files of the talks online (Cooper et al., 2010). The availability of on-demand access to the seminar materials allowed individuals unable to attend the opportunity to engage with the materials presented, albeit in a limited way. This is an important part of building Fat Studies as an international discipline; when such events occur, planning should include how to promote engagement with those interested in fat scholarship around the world.

Almost a decade after the Columbia University conference, Massey University hosted "Fat Studies: Reflective Intersections (FSNZ)" in Wellington, New Zealand. FSNZ12 provided a space for Fat Studies scholars and fat activists to come together and share pedagogy, scholarship, activism, and art. It received a great deal of attention in the New Zealand media, and while most attendees were engaged in Fat Studies scholarship and activism, only one of the invited speakers (Samantha Murray) was a recognized scholar in the field. Work presented at the conference contributed to a special issue of *Fat Studies* on reflective intersections (Pausé, 2014).

Four years later, Massey hosted "Fat Studies: Identity, Agency, Embodiment" in Palmerston North, New Zealand. FSNZ16 was live-streamed and had a handful of remote speakers; this allowed for presentations from individuals from seven countries (Burford et al., 2018). FSNZ16 was bookended by community events: "Fat Out Loud", a spoken word event at the local library the night before the conference, and the opening of an exhibit of The Adipositivity Project (the photo-activism of Substantia Jones, a FSNZ16 keynote) at Te Manawa on the closing night. FSNZ16 marked the first time the conference had one academic keynote and one activist keynote; the commitment to continuing this equity is noted on the conference website for FSNZ. FSNZ is notable for being the only dedicated Fat Studies conference in the world, but its location in New Zealand makes attending inaccessible for many involved in the field.

On 30 May 2017, Women's and Gender Studies et Recherches Feministes hosted a "Feminist Fat Studies" mini-conference in conjunction with the annual Women's and Gender Studies et Recherches Feministes conference. The mini-conference offered four sessions on Fat Studies, with papers exploring temporality, health, identity, fatshion, and more; the overarching theme was fat in the Canadian context. The mini-conference keynote plenary focused on intersectionality, with Idil Abdillahi, Jill Andrew, Carla Rice, and Jake Pyne contributing (Ryerson University, 2017).

Later that year, Ludwig Maximilians University in Munich, Germany, hosted "Doing Fat: Performance and Representation of Fat Bodies". This symposium was organized by Friedrich Schorb and Anja Hermann, and included presentations from scholars and fat activists. Keynotes were given by the Chairwoman of Gesellschaft gegen Gewichtsdiskriminierung (Germany Society against Weight Discrimination), Natalie Rosenke, as well as the founder of the group, legal scholar Stephanie von Liebenstein. Additionally, Cat gave a keynote on the future of Fat Studies scholarship (Ludwig Maximilians University, 2017).

In January 2018, the Political Fatties (supported by the Netherlands Institute of Cultural Analysis and the Amsterdam School of Cultural Analysis) hosted "Politics of Volume". This one-day symposium brought together scholars, activists, and artists to share their work and talk about the politics of fatness. Comedienne Sofie Hagan read a selection from her new book, *Happy fat*. Dina Amlund, Laurara Contrera, Sofia Apostolidou and Corina Coolen presented papers that disrupted fat politics outside of the Global North. And Cat gave a keynote on fat politics and bad fatties in cyberspace (Political Fatties, 2017). A month later, Ryerson University hosted "Thickening Fat: Dialogues on Intersectionality, Social Justice and Fatness". This two-day symposium brought together scholars, activists, and artists from around the world to share their work and workshop their chapters for the edited text of the same name (Bodies in Translation, 2018).

In early 2019, scholars at Leeds University hosted a symposium called "Artful Fat" as part of the Sociological Review Foundation Seminar Series. The one-day event brought together individuals who bridge the arts and social sciences to produce knowledge on fatness; speakers included Bethan Evan, Stacy Bias, and Cath Lambert (Barker, 2019). And in mid-2020, "Fat Studies: Past, Present, Futures" was set to run in Auckland, New Zealand (more on this below).

We do not suggest that this has been a full review of all Fat Studies conferences, symposia and events that have occurred but have attempted to track the organization of these events as best we could. Burford, Henderson, and Pausé (2018) argue that conferences are spaces of public pedagogies, where teaching and learning occurs. Fat Studies conferences allow for those interested in the field to come together and share, create, and co-construct knowledge. Equally important, these spaces allow for like-minded people to come together with a shared vocabulary and shared sense of purpose (Read, 2016). Fat Studies streams exist at the American Culture Association/ Popular Culture Association conference, the National Women's Studies Association conference, and the Allied Media conference. These are yearly opportunities for scholars to come together and share ideas and build communities. For academic disciplines on the margins, this fostering of community cannot be overvalued.

Charlotte Cooper (2009a), though, has questioned the efficacy of using conferences to develop the discipline of Fat Studies. She astutely notes that conferences are exclusive spaces,

> available only to those who know how they work, who are already in the loop. They are also expensive and make regular attendance for outsiders untenable, especially for those who live far away or have a small income or must manage other commitments.
>
> *(p. 332)*

It is worth noting that the yearly streams identified above are all within the United States.

Cooper argues that those who organize such events should work to ensure that there is a way for those not physically in the room to engage with the material and with those in the room; she suggests a bare minimum of offering presentation materials online. Many of the conferences and symposia reviewed here have made strides to provide materials to those unable to attend in person.[7] Perhaps most advanced is the online streaming availability of FSNZ conferences; individuals can watch the presentations in real time and ask questions using social media (Burford et al., 2018). And for FSNZ20, the emergence of COVID-19 forced the planned in-person conference online in its entirety. Moving online opened new opportunities, especially for those interested in attending; while FSNZ16 had approximately 100 people in attendance (40 in the room and 50 joining online), FSNZ20 had almost 400 individuals participate. FSNZ22 is being planned as a dedicated online Fat Studies conference.

Over the last sixteen years, the field of Fat Studies has emerged as a crucial locus of research and scholarship addressing the lives of fat people and society. Inherent in such emergent spaces are threats and challenges that must be explored if the field is to withstand the scrutiny of time.

Threats to Fat Studies

We assess threats both external and internal to Fat Studies scholarship. Externally, we argue that the decreasing support of liberal arts subjects in tertiary institutions around the world poses a threat to Fat Studies. We point to increasing attacks from conservatives against liberal arts subjects. Internally, we suggest that the reproduction of white supremacy poses a threat to Fat Studies. We also point to the blurring of lines between those who study fatness from a Fat Studies perspective, and those who study fatness not from a Fat Studies perspective. We close with our concerns with non-fat individuals engaging in Fat Studies scholarship.

Academic disciplines outside of science and technology are under increasing scrutiny, as governmental underfunding of the tertiary sector squeezes these institutions to find cost saving measures (Dutt-Ballerstadt, 2019; Long, 2018). Humanities, Education, and Social Sciences are the backbone of a liberal arts education, and also the most at risk (Ferrall, 2011). The most vulnerable of these are often disciplines that are perceived as being based in ideology, rather than scientific endeavour, such as Gender Studies, Queer Studies, and Fat Studies. In New Zealand, Victoria University closed its Gender Studies course in 2010 (Fisher, 2010). Then Tertiary Education Union President Tom Ryan pointed to this as an example of "the pressure that's being put on liberal arts areas [which are] seen as less deserving of support than science and technology" (Fisher, 2010, para 18). In Hungary, Prime Minister Orban banned courses in Gender Studies; conservative forces across Europe are working towards similar banning and the eradication of scholarship that is perceived to threaten white supremacy, patriarchy, and capitalism (Apperly, 2019).

Fat Studies scholarship has received a great deal of scrutiny and mocking from conservative pundits, especially in the United States. The Clare Boothe Luce Center for Conservative Women decried the offering of a Fat Studies course at Oberlin College, claiming that instead of highlighting fat stigma and oppression, students should be educated about the dangers of the growing obesity epidemic (Laoutaris, 2018). The National Review suggested that Fat Studies was less an academic discipline and more an exercise in group therapy (Bawer, 2017); Bawer argues that Fat Studies is not about facts or knowledge, but victimhood. Abigail Alger wrote in the conservative Campus Reform that Fat Studies is "part of a dangerous dumbing down of liberation education in which the pursuit of knowledge is replaced by frantic social programming and promotion of state programs" (Alger, 2009, para 6). Alger decried Fat Studies as yet another Identity Study that is harming higher education. Alger suggests that Identity Studies do not produce knowledge, encourage growing government intervention, and label anyone with opposing views a bigot. That same publication, *Campus Reform*, celebrated in early 2018 when the offerings of Fat Studies courses at Universities began to decline (Airaksinen, 2018).

Fat Studies[8] is also under threat from within by white supremacy. As noted in Charlotte Cooper's (2009a) chapter in the *Fat studies reader*, the majority of the scholarship being published in the field of Fat Studies is from the United States; most of it from white scholars about white fatness. When Cat guest edited a special edition of the Fat Studies journal on intersectionality in 2014, she failed to secure any articles addressing issues of race or ethnicity. For this Handbook, Cat and Sonya were unsuccessful in including a scholarly chapter about race. We did include two chapters on the topic from activists, and we are proud of those chapters; they add a great deal to the Handbook and to the larger study of fatness. But the academic offerings in the field are still greatly limited to white people, mainly in the West and Global North. As a field, we need to ensure that we are not simply reproducing white supremacy by elevating the experiences of white fat people. We need to ensure that non-white fat people are centred in our work and amplify the voices of fat people of colour; this must be a priority in both activism and scholarship.

Many scholars are interested in fatness and the fat body; this is not a field of study left only to Fat Studies scholars. Perhaps on the opposite end of the field from Fat Studies are Obesity Studies. Obesity Studies scholars pathologize fatness and seek to eradicate fat bodies. No potential blurring exists between Obesity Studies and Fat Studies. The other two predominant disciplines in this field are Weight Science and Critical Obesity Studies. Critical Obesity Studies has built a literature that disrupts the epistemological, ontological, and methodological assumptions made by those in Obesity Studies. Critical Obesity Scholars (such as Jan Wright, Michael Gard, and Deborah Lupton) highlight the flaws, errors, and erroneous assumptions that underpin the work of Obesity Studies. Weight Science encompasses those who are interested in understanding fatness, often for the purpose of preventing or reducing the occurrence in a population. Almost paradoxically, many of these same scholars have also turned their attention to eliminating fat stigma (seeming to fail to understand that they cannot prevent the stigma of fatness while working to eliminate fatness). There are many overlaps and crossovers among Critical Obesity Studies, Weight Science, and Fat Studies (for more on the similarities and differences between the three, see Pausé, forthcoming). And Fat Studies does itself a service by engaging in collaborative efforts when appropriate with scholars from these fields, and drawing from their literature when appropriate. But Fat Studies is discrete from Critical Obesity Studies and Weight Science, and it is a disservice to all of the fields for scholars to conflate them or dismiss the distance between them as inconsequential. Fat Studies, as a field, focuses the fat body and fat person within the centre of their scholarship. They are the only field to do this. And they are the only field in which fat liberation underpins the scholarship. This commitment to liberation can be seen throughout this Handbook, as half of our contributing authors are from the fat activist community.

The final internal threat to Fat Studies is one which we present with caution. Charlotte Cooper (2016) and Cat (2012, 2019) have both argued for the importance of a fat epistemology. A fat epistemology recognizes that fat people know the most about being fat people. A fat epistemology acknowledges that fat people can be producers of knowledge about fatness and being fat. The chapter from Kath Read provides a powerful illustration of fat epistemology. In her online piece, "Everything that we know about obesity is an indictment of white supremacy", Hess Love (2019) argues,

> Everything we know about obesity is wrong, and everything about who we listen to on the subject of fatness and fatphobia is bullshit. We need to listen to the people that live this day in and day out and do not intend to ride on the boundaries of it or escape it, but to be liberated within it.
>
> *(para 6)*

But we believe that centring the voices and lived experiences of fat people is not enough. We believe that non-fat people engaging in Fat Studies scholarship are a threat to Fat Studies. We do not make this argument lightly and appreciate that this view may alienate us from non-fat scholars who have contributed important work to the field.

We appreciate that many allies have acknowledged their thin privilege and the role it plays in their work; most well-known perhaps is the keynote address Professor Lindo Bacon gave at the National Association to Advance Fat Acceptance conference in 2009. In the keynote, Professor Bacon (2009) spoke of how their thin privilege has shaped their life, scholarship, and how said scholarship is perceived by others. But acknowledging the privilege that one individual has does not afford them the position and entitlement to engage in scholarship which may, by lack of group membership, result in the othering of a vulnerable peoples. Sociologist Robert Merton (1972) coined this idea *extreme insiderism*; the belief that only members of a group should research the group. We believe that it is necessary to complicate this idea with greater nuance. The appropriateness of whether an "outsider" of a group should study said group demands an analysis of power dynamics inherent in identity construction in the western context. White people study Blackness just as thin people study fatness and able-bodied people study disability. The complexity in such study lies in the interplay between identity and social validation. When those with identities of less positional power study the dominant group, it serves to better understand and disrupt structures of dominance. However, when those who hold socially dominant identities study groups that have been marginalized, they reify the positional power of their identity. They are rendered the "experts" by virtue of already being perceived as more credible, valuable, and knowledgeable than those from within the marginalized group. Additionally, within this dynamic is the studying of the "other". This othering perspective positions the scholar as objective; a vantage point that is impossible. The scholar will inevitably bring to their study the biases born of dominant identity which include rendering those not of dominant identity as the "object" of study, again reinforcing the structures of positional power. Cat recognizes the problematics present if she were to decide to study and publish about blackness, or queerness, or being trans. Sonya, as a cis black queer neurodivergent woman, recognizes the choice to study and publish about trans identity as a 'scholar' would reinforce the dynamics of power that limit actual scholarship from trans people. This does not preclude us from studying race/ethnicity, ability, gender, sexual orientation. Just as it does not preclude a non-fat person in studying bodies and body size. It does however invite us to consider where we are recreating structural oppression. We would argue that no matter the good intent, non-fat scholars engaging in Fat Studies scholarship cannot help but reinforce the structural and systemic dynamics of fatphobia and fat bias.

The future

In acknowledging the threats to Fat Studies scholarship, we do not wish to suggest we believe the future for the field is bleak. If anything, we believe that the future of Fat Studies is very fat. There are many opportunities arising for Fat Studies scholarship, including increased interest from postgraduate and undergraduate students, the use of technology to connect scholars around the world, and the continued commitment of the field to engage with fat activism.

We are excited about the increasing amount of Fat Studies scholarship produced around the world, especially the work being conducted in languages outside of English. Within the last few years, several texts have been published that explore the work being done in Germany and Argentina, for example. *Fat studies in Deutschland: Hohes körpergewicht zwischen diskriminierung und anerkennung*, edited by Rose and Schorb (2017), presents a range of academic and activists work within Germany. And *Cuerpos sin patrones* by Contrera and Cuello (2016) brings together a range of writings from scholars and activists on the topic, woven together in an analysis by Contrera and Cuello to demonstrate the social construction of fatness as a tool for political oppression. We are confident these are not the only two examples of Fat Studies scholarship outside of the English language; we hope to discover them all and share them widely.

There is also growing interest in Fat Studies as an academic field from both postgraduate and undergraduate students around the world. During her European sabbatical, Cat was thrilled to spend time with postgraduate students across the continent who were keen to engage in Fat Studies scholarship. These students were from a range of disciplines, but all had a similar commitment to centralizing fatness in their work. They were well read in Fat Studies texts, somewhat connected to one another through social media, and eager for opportunities to learn and engage with scholarship. An example of this was the "Politics of Volume". As noted earlier, *Politics of volume* was organized by a group of postgraduate students, the Political Fatties. Supported by the Netherlands Institute of Cultural Analysis and the Amsterdam School of Cultural Analysis, the one day event of fat politics showcased a diverse range of presentations, workshops, and provided space for "researchers, activists, and artists [to] problematize, analyse, and reflect on the ways fatness is experienced, marginalized, and represented both within mainstream media and institutions as well as within body positive/fat acceptance spaces" (Political Fatties, 2017, para 3).

Outside of Europe, there are growing numbers of postgraduate students engaging in Fat Studies scholarship as well. In New Zealand, for example, there are several postgraduate students doing this work across the country. One such scholar, George Parker, is completing their PhD through publication; their contributions to the literature on anti-fat attitudes in maternity care have been invaluable additions, especially given the diversity of their participants (Parker, 2014, 2017). At the 2019 meeting of the Sociological Association of Aotearoa New Zealand, there was a dedicated Fat Studies stream where several postgraduate students, including George Parker, presented their scholarship.

The interest in Fat Studies is not only located in postgraduate students. Undergraduate students across the world are also signalling their interest in learning more about fatness through a Fat Studies lens. Courses in Fat Studies have been taught across the United States, in New Zealand, and in Australia (Watkins et al., 2012). In 2016 Fat Studies courses were being offered at five tertiary institutions in the United States: Dickinson College, Oregon State University, Tufts University, University of Maryland College Park, and Willamette University (Hasson, 2016).

In addition to completing Fat Studies work in tertiary institutions, other opportunities have arisen. One such opportunity is the Fat Studies MOOO, a massive online open offering hosted by Cat. Each MOOO is a discrete engagement, focusing on a single topic and guest scholar. Guest scholars provide materials for participants to engage with before the session. The MOOOs take place using Zoom, making them accessible to anyone anywhere in the world with internet access. Since 2018, fifteen MOOOs have seen participants study weight and the law, fatness and neoliberalism, anti-racism and fatness, fatness and disability, fat pedagogy, fat in art history, and fat reproductive justice; more are planned for 2021. This is just one example of using technology to further the field of Fat Studies. Another is #FatStudyGroup. This hashtag was created by fat activist Kivan Bay (@KivaBay) on Twitter, as a resource for individuals who are interested in Fat Studies to engage with one another. There are many active producers on this tag, including Kivan Bay, Da'Shaun Harrison (@DaShaunLH), and Cat (@FOMNZ). The tag is used to share readings, presentations, and to co-construct knowledge. Kivan has noted that the use of the tag makes the scholarship of Fat Studies more accessible; they note, "I have heard from people who participate in the #FatStudyGroup threads who have cognitive dysfunction that otherwise hinders their ability to read long essays that threads, are, miraculously, easier for them to engage with" (Bay, 2018, para 6).

The use of #FatStudyGroup allows for academics and activists alike to build the field of Fat Studies together, which is another key opportunity for the discipline. As noted by Cooper in 2010, "one of the strengths of Fat Studies is that it supports the work of people who have direct experience of fat embodiment, grassroots activists and other autonomous voices, it is not simply the product of remote expert curiosity" (p. 1028). Arguably, fat activism and Fat Studies are siblings whose epistemologies come forth through a shared necessity to understand and traverse a fat pathologizing society and in theory and practice humanize the fat body. Fat activists are making the provocations that paired with academic theory are shifting the material realities of fat bodies in society. This pairing of scholarly and activist work is not a new undertaking and can be seen throughout history in the works of scholar activists such as Audre Lorde and in the present use of the theory of intersectionality, a term coined by legal scholar Kimberle Crenshaw, to frame modern social justice issues from gender to race to disability. When recruiting for this International Handbook, we felt strongly that we needed to include a wide range of fat activists as contributing authors. Fat activists in this Handbook serve as the connective tissue giving scholarly chapters range of motion, operational vitality and real-world application. It is the voice of the fat activist who reminds us that theory must be married to praxis: epistemologies exist in our bodies, and it is with these fat bodies that we might hope to create a world expansive enough for each of our unique and celebrated existences.

To close

This *International Handbook of Fat Studies* meets the world at a time of great upheaval. A moment in history where those navigating lives at the intersections of various oppressions are demanding change and one where those who have been historically nescient to these experiences are being ushered into greater awareness. Fat Studies and fat activism sit at the precipice of an emerging world, one where fat bodies and their liberations cannot be disaggregated from the liberation of all oppressions. We believe the work in this book invites you, the reader, into a more nuanced and yet expansive landscape of fat scholarship. We believe there is also a necessary summons into the queries, harms, and hopes of fat lives beyond the too often foregrounded western narratives. Most importantly, within these pages is an offering for Fat Studies and all who are impacted by the field to live juicier, more abundant, more robust existences. We hope we fatten up your world.

Notes

1 We were unable to source the original credit for this; we believe it was first used in a CFP for the Fat Studies stream at the PCA/ACA, and we do know that Julia McCrossin, Lesleigh Owen, and Stefanie Snider all contributed/revised it along the way.
2 This was comprised of articles from a special issue of the journal *Women & Therapy* that focused on fat oppression and psychotherapy.
3 It could be argued that this edited collection was the first Fat Studies collection.
4 We have worked to include as much of the scholarship in this area in English as possible; forgive us for any omissions. We want to highlight Rose and Schorb (2017) and Contrera and Cuello (2016) as non-English Fat Studies texts.
5 Check out Herbie Popnecker, a fat superhero from 1958–1967 with the American Comics Group ("Herbie Popnecker"; Murphy, 2012).
6 Gard was a keynote earlier that year the University of Otago's "The Big Fat Truth Symposium" (University of Otago, 2010). The three-day event aimed to "foster critical debate about obesity and physical activity", with six invited keynotes. Three of these keynotes, Steven Blair, Paul Campos, and Michael Gard, took critical approaches to obesity; the other three did not.
7 A fully online event, the Fat Studies MOOO, is discussed later in the chapter.
8 And fat activism.

References

Ahmad, A. (2015, January 23). Dear white fatties (and other socially visible fat activists). Fat!So? http://www.fatso.com/stories/dear-white-fatties-and-other-socially-visible-fat-activists
Airaksinen, T. (2018, Jan 17). Colleges dropping "fat studies" courses in 2018. *Campus Reform*. https://www.campusreform.org/?ID=10393
Alger, A. (2009, Oct 23). Why Fat Studies (and all identity studies) hurt higher education. *Campus Reform*. https://web.archive.org/web/20091125184954/https://www.campusreform.org/blog/fat-studies
Apperly, E. (2019, Jun 15). Why Europe's far right is targeting gender studies. *The Atlantic*. https://www.theatlantic.com/international/archive/2019/06/europe-far-right-target-gender-studies/591208/
Bacon, L. (2008). *Health at every size*. Dallas, TX: BenBella Books.
Bacon, L. (2009). *Reflections on fat acceptance: Lessons learned from privilege*. [Keynote presentation]. National Association to Advance Fat Acceptance conference. https://lindabacon.org/wp-content/uploads/Bacon_ReflectionsOnThinPrivilege_NAAFA.pdf
Baker, J. (2015). *Things no one will tell fat girls: A handbook for unapologetic living*. New York: Basic Books.
Baker, J. (2018). *Landwhale: On turning insults into nicknames, why body image is hard, and how diets can kiss my ass*. Berkeley: Seal Press.
Barker, D. (2019, Oct 23). Artful fat: Lessons from Leeds. *The Sociological Review*. https://www.thesociologicalreview.com/artful-fat-lessons-from-leeds/
Bawer, B. (2017, Aug 21). The fatuity of Fat Studies. *National Review*. https://www.nationalreview.com/2017/08/fat-studies-academic-nonsense-disguised-scholarship/
Bay, K. (2018, Feb 23). Threader. https://threader.app/thread/967019062466289664
BBC News Africa. (2016, November 25). Latasha Ngwube – African women you need to know. YouTube. https://youtu.be/9tOg-Osi8xs
Bellanaijastyle.com (2019, August 27). Every curvy girl will fall in love with the first drop of Latasha Ngwube's 'The Curvy Monroe' collection. Editor: *Bella Stylista*. https://www.bellanaijastyle.com/latasha-ngwubes-curvy-monroe-about-that-curvy-life-grey-velvet/
Blank, H. (2011). *Big, big love: A sex and relationships guide for people of size (and those who love them)*. Berkeley: Ten Speed Press.
Blank, H. (2012). *The unapologetic fat girl's guide to exercise and other incendiary acts*. Berkeley: Ten Speed Press.
Bodies in Translation. (2018). Thickening fat: Dialogues on intersectionality, social justice & fatness. Re-Vision: The Centre for Art & Social Justice. *Vimeo* [Online]. https://vimeo.com/292392249
Boero, N. (2012). *Killer fat: Media, medicine, and morals in the American "obesity epidemic"*. New Brunswick, NJ: Rutgers University Press.
Bovey, S. (1994). *The forbidden body: Why being fat is not a sin*. Telford, PA: Pandora.
Braziel, J. E., & LeBesco, K. (2001). *Bodies out of bounds: Fatness and transgression*. Berkeley: University of California Press.

Brown, L. S., & Rothblum, E. D. (1989). *Overcoming fear of fat*. New York: Harrington Park Press.

Burford, J., Henderson, E. F., & Pausé, C. J. (2018). Enlarging conference learning: At the crossroads of Fat Studies and conference pedagogies. *Fat Studies*, 7(1): 69–80.

Byer, N. (2020). *#VERYFAT #VERYBRAVE: The fat girl's guide to being #brave and not a dejected, melancholy, down-in-the-dumps weeping fat girl in a bikini*. Kansas City, MO: Andrews McMeel Publishing.

Cameron, E., & Russell, C. (2016). *The fat pedagogy reader: Challenging weight-based oppression through critical education*. New York: Peter Lang.

Campos, P. (2004). *The obesity myth: Why America's obsession with weight is hazardous to your health*. New York: Gotham Books.

Casadó-Marín, L., & Gracia-Arnaiz, M. (2020). "I'm fat and proud of it": Body size diversity and fat acceptance activism in Spain. Fat Studies, 9(1): 51–70.

Chakravorty, R. (2019, November 17). Sharing the big fat truth. Asian Age. https://www.asianage.com/life/more-features/171119/sharing-the-big-fat-truth.html

Chastain, R. (2014). *The politics of size: Perspectives from the fat acceptance movement* [2 volumes]. Santa Barbara, CA: ABC-CLIO.

CNN (Staff writer). (2016 November 12). Curves steal the spotlight during LFDW. CNN. https://edition.cnn.com/style/gallery/about-that-curvy-life/index.html

Contrera, L., & Cuello, N. (2016). *Cuerpos sin patrones*. Buenos Aires: Madreselva Editorial.

Cooper, C. (1998). *Fat and proud: The politics of size*. London: Women's Press.

Cooper, C. (2008, October 13). How to document fat activist histories. Obesity Timebomb. http://obesitytimebomb.blogspot.com/2008/10/making-history.html?m=1 Cooper, C. (2009a). Maybe it should be called Fat American Studies. In E. Rothblum & S. Solovay (Eds.), *The Fat Studies reader* (pp. 327–333). New York: New York University Press.

Cooper, C. (2009b, May 27). Government support for Fat Studies and HAES in the UK. *Obesity Timebomb*. http://obesitytimebomb.blogspot.com/2009/05/government-support-for-fat-studies-and.html

Cooper, C. (2010). Fat Studies: Mapping the field. *Sociology Compass*, 4(12), 1020–1034.

Cooper, C. (2011). A queer and trans fat activist timeline. Charlotte Cooper. http://charlottecooper.net/fat/fat-research/a-queer-and-trans-fat-activist-timeline/

Cooper, C. (2012). A queer and trans fat activist timeline: Queering fat activist nationality and cultural imperialism. *Fat Studies*, 1(1), 61–74.

Cooper, C. (2016). *Fat activism: A radical social movement*. Bristol: Hammerhead Press.

Cooper, C., Evans, B., Colls, R. et al. (2010) Seminar 1: Abject embodiment: Uneven targets of fat discrimination. *Fat Studies and health at every size*. Seminar series, Durham University. https://www.dur.ac.uk/geography/research/researchprojects/fat_studies_and_health_at_every_size/seminars/seminar_one/

Cottom, T. M. (2019). *Thick: And other essays*. New York: The New Press.

Cox, J. (2020). *Fat girls in black bodies: Creating communities of our own*. Berkeley: North Atlantic Books.

Dark, K. (2019). *Fat, pretty, and soon to be old. A makeover for self and society*. Chico, CA: AK Press.

DeJong, W. (1980). The stigma of obesity: The consequences of naïve assumptions concerning the cause of physical deviance. *Journal of Health and Social Behavior*, 21(1), 75–87.

Donald, C. M. (1986). *The fat woman measures up*. Charlottetown, P.E.I.: Ragweed.

Dutt-Ballerstadt, R. (2019, Mar 1). Academic prioritisation or killing the liberal arts? *Inside Higher Education*. https://www.insidehighered.com/advice/2019/03/01/shrinking-liberal-arts-programs-raise-alarm-bells-among-faculty

Ellison, J. (2013). Weighing in: The "evidence of experience" and Canadian fat women's activism. *Canadian Bulletin of Medical History*, 30(1), 55–75.

Erdman, C. K. (1996). *Nothing to lose: A guide to sane living in a larger body*. San Francisco: Harper.

Farrell, A. (2011). *Fat shame*. New York: New York University Press.

Farrell, A. (2019). Origin stories: Thickening fat and the problem of historiography. In M. Friedman, C. Rice, & J. Rinaldi (Eds.). *Thickening fat: Fat bodies, intersectionality, and social justice* (pp. 29–39). New York: Routledge.

Ferall, V. E. (2011). *Liberal arts at the brink*. Cambridge: Harvard University Press.

Fisher, A. (2010, Dec 1). Axing gender studies "setback to rights". *Stuff*. http://www.stuff.co.nz/national/education/4407891/Axing-gender-studies-setback-to-rights

Fraser, L. (1997). *Losing it: America's obsession with weight and the industry that feeds on it*. New York: Dutton.

Frater, L. (2005). *Fat chicks rule! How to survive in a thin-centric world*. Brooklyn, NY: IG Publishing.

Friedman, M., Rice, C., & Rinaldi, J. (2019). *Thickening fat: Fat bodies, intersectionality, and social justice*. New York: Routledge.

Gaesser, G. A. (2013). *Big fat lies: The truth about your weight and your health.* Carslbad, CA: Gurze Books.

Gailey, J. (2014). *The hyper(in)visible fat women: Weight and gender discourse in contemporary society.* New York: Springer.

Gard, M. (2010). *The end of the obesity epidemic.* London: Routledge.

Gard, M., & Wright, J. (2005). *The obesity epidemic: Science, morality, and ideology.* London: Routledge.

Garrison, T. N., & Levitsky, D. (1993). *Fed up! A woman's guide to freedom from the diet/weight prison.* New York: Carol & Graf Publishers.

Gay, R. (2018). *Hunger: A memoir of (my) body.* New York: Harper Perennial.

Goodman, W. C. (1995). *The invisible woman: Confronting weight prejudice in America.* Carlsbad, CA: Gurze Books.

Hagen, S. (2019). *Happy fat: Taking up space in a world that wants to shrink you.* London: 4th Estate.

Harding, K., & Kirby, M. (2009). *Lessons from the Fat-o-sphere: Quit dieting and declare a truth with your body.* New York: Penguin.

Harjunen, H. (2016). *Neoliberal bodies and the gendered fat body: The fat body in focus.* London: Routledge.

Harris, M. B., Harris, R. J., & Bochner, S. (1982). Fat, four-eyed and female: Stereotypes of obesity, glasses, and gender. *Journal of Applied Social Psychology, 12,* 503–516.

Hasson, P. (2016, Jan 11). The next big thing? "Fat Studies" courses, fat awareness groups spread across universities. *Daily Caller.* https://dailycaller.com/2016/01/11/fat-studies-courses-fat-awareness-groups-spread-across-universities/

"Herbie Popnecker". *Wikipedia.* https://en.wikipedia.org/wiki/Herbie_Popnecker

Hester, H., & Walters, C. (2015). *Fat sex: New directions in theory and activism.* New York: Routledge.

Holt, K. T., & Leib, B. R. (2012). *Fat girl in a strange land.* Somerville, MA: Crossed Genres Publications.

Jarrell, D., & Sukrungruang, I. (2003). *What are you looking at? The first fat fiction anthology.* Austin: Harcourt, Inc.

Jimenez, M. (n.d.) Blog: Lute como uma gorda. https://lutecomoumagorda.home.blog/

Jimenez, M. (2020, June 24). Gordofobia na pandemia mata mais do que a Covid-19. Guru Da Cicade. https://gurudacidade.com.br/2020/06/24/gordofobia-na-pandemia-mata-mais-do-que-a-covid-19-por-malu-jimenez/

Kinzel, L. (2012). *Two whole cakes: How to stop dieting and learn to love your body.* New York: The Feminist Press.

Kirkland, A. (2008). *Fat rights: Dilemmas of difference and personhood.* New York: New York University Press.

Koppelman, S. (2003). *The strange history of Suzanne LaFleshe. And other stories of women and fatness.* New York: The Feminist Press at the City University of New York.

Kwan, S., & Graves, J. (2013). *Framing fat: Competing constructions in contemporary culture.* New Brunswick, NJ: Rutgers University Press.

Kyrölä, K. (2016). *The weight of images.* New York: Routledge.

Laoutaris, R. (2018, Sept 11). Ridiculous campus courses: Oberlin College's "Inquiries in Critical Fat Studies". Clare Boothe Luce Center for Conservative Women. https://cblwomen.org/ridiculous-campus-courses-fat-studies/

Larkin, J. C., & Pines, H. A. (1979). No fat persons need apply. *Sociology of Work and Occupations, 6,* 312–327.

Laymon, K. (2019). *Heavy: An American memoir.* New York: Scribner.

LeBesco, K. (2004). *Revolting bodies? The struggle to redefine fat identity.* Amherst: University of Massachusetts Press.

Levy-Navarro, E. (2010). *Historicizing fat in Anglo American culture.* Ohio State University Press.

Long, J. (2018, Aug 1). "Declining student interest" threatens Victoria University of Wellington's arts faculty. *Stuff.* https://www.stuff.co.nz/national/education/105915797/declining-student-interest-threatens-victoria-university-of-wellingtons-arts-faculty

Louderback, L. (1970). *Fat power: Whatever you weigh is right.* New York: Hawthorn Books.

Love, H. (2019). Everything that we know about obesity is an indictment of white supremacy. *WearYourVoice Mag.* https://wearyourvoicemag.com/obesity-fatphobia-white-supremacy/

Ludwig Maximilians University. (2017). *Symposium "Doing Fat". Performance and Representation of Fat Bodies.* Institute of Sociology. https://www.gender.soziologie.uni-muenchen.de/veranstaltungsarchiv/vergangene_veranst/andere/catpause/index.html

Luna, C., George, S. M., Lee, E. K., & Solovay, S. (2020). *Body sovereignty: Fat politics and the fight for human rights.* Santa Barbara, CA: ABC-CLIO.

Lyons, P., & Burgard, D. (1990). *Great shape: The first fitness guide for large women.* Palo Alto, CA: Bull.

Manheim, C. (2000). *Wake up, I'm fat!* New York: Broadway Books.

Maor, M. (2013). "Do I still belong here?" The body's boundary work in the Israeli fat acceptance movement. *Social Movement Studies, 12*(3), 280–297.

Marimon, M. (2020, April 24). Lute como uma gorda! Ciadadao Cultura. https://www.cidadaocultura.com.br/lute-como-uma-gorda/

Merton, R. K. (1972). Insiders and outsiders: A chapter in the sociology of knowledge. *American Journal of Sociology, 78*(1), 9–47.

Millman, M. (1980). *Such a pretty face: Being fat in America.* New York: W. W. Norton & Company.

Murphy, J. (2017). *Dumplin': Go big or go home.* New York: Balzer + Bray.

Murphy, J. (2019). *Puddin'.* New York: Balzer + Bray.

Murphy, J. (2020). *Faith: Taking flight.* New York: Balzer + Bray.

Murphy, S. (2012, Feb 14). Herbie Popnecker: The little fat nothing that saved the world (regularly). *Obesity Timebomb.* http://obesitytimebomb.blogspot.com/2012/02/herbie-popnecker-little-fat-nothing.html

Murray, S. (2008). *The fat female body.* New York: Palgrave MacMillan.

Murray, S. (2012a). Fat bodily being. *Somatechnics, 2*(1), v–viii.

Murray, S. (2012b). Rethinking fatness – A critical dialogue. *Feminism & Psychology, 22*(3), 287–289.

Ngwube, L. (n.d.). About. AboutthatCurvyLife. https://www.aboutthatcurvylife.com/about/Nicols, G. (1984). *The fat Black women's poems.* London: Virago Press.

Oliver, J. E. (2006). *Fat politics: The real story behind America's obesity epidemic.* Oxford: Oxford University Press.

Parker, G. (2014). Mothers at large: Responsibilizing the pregnant self for the "obesity epidemic". *Fat Studies, 3*(2), 101–118.

Parker, G. (2017). Shamed into health? Fat pregnant women's views on obesity management strategies in maternity care. *Women's Studies Journal, 31*(1), 22–33.

Pausé, C. J. (2012, Apr 5). On the epistemology of fatness. *Friend of Marilyn.* https://friendofmarilyn.com/2012/04/05/the-epistemology-of-fatness/

Pausé, C. J. (2014). X-static process: Intersectionality within the field of fat studies. *Fat Studies, 3*(2), 80–85.

Pausé, C. J. (2019). Ray of light: Standpoint theory, Fat Studies, and a new fat ethics. *Fat Studies, 9*(2), 175–187. doi.org/10.1080/21604851.2019.1630203

Pausé, C. J. (forthcoming). Devil pray: Fat Studies in an obesity research world. In M. Gard, D. Powell, & J. Tenorio (Eds.), *Handbook of critical obesity studies.* London: Routledge.

Pausé, C. J., Wykes, J., & Murray, S. (2014). *Queering fat embodiment.* London: Ashgate.

Political Fatties. (2017). What is "Fatties: The Politics of Volume"? *Politics of Volume.* https://politicsofvolume.wordpress.com/

Queiroz, J. (2020, February 2). Pesquisadora usa experiências próprias para produzir tese sobre gordofobia. RD News. https://www.rdnews.com.br/cidades/pesquisadora-usa-experiencias-proprias-para-produzir-tese-sobre-gordofobia/123447

Read, K. (2010, May 30). "Fat Studies: A Critical Dialogue" Conference – registrations now open. *Fat Heffalump.* https://fatheffalump.wordpress.com/2010/05/30/fat-studies-a-critical-dialogue-conference-registration-now-open/

Read, K. (2016, Aug 1). There's no comfort like community. *Fat Heffalump.* https://fatheffalump.wordpress.com/2016/08/01/theres-no-comfort-like-community/

Rose, L., & Schorb, F. (2017). *Fat studies in Deutschland: Hohes körpergewicht zwischen diskriminierung und anerkennung.* Weinheim, Germany: Belt Juventa Verlag.

Rothblum, E. (2012). Why a journal on Fat Studies? *Fat Studies, 1*(1), 3–5.

Rothblum, E., & Solovay, S. (2009). *The fat studies reader.* New York: New York University Press.

Rothblum, E. D., Miller, C. T., & Garbutt, B. (1988). Stereotypes of obese female job applicants. *International Journal of Eating Disorders, 7*, 277–283.

Ryerson University (2017). Women's and Gender Studies et Recherches Feministes Conference Congress 2017 of the Humanities and Social Sciences. https://www.wgsrf.com/uploads/2/4/8/8/24888219/wgsrf_final_conf_program_2017.pdf

Saguy, A. (2014). *What's wrong with fat.* London: Oxford University Press.

Schoenfielder, L., & Wieser, B. (1983). *Shadow on a tightrope: Writings by women on fat oppression.* San Francisco: Aunt Lute Book Company.

Schwartz, H. (1986). *Never satisfied. A cultural history of diets, fantasies, & fat.* New York: Anchor Books.

Shanker, W. (2004). *The fat girl's guide to life.* New York: Bloomsbury.

Shuai, T. (2008, March 21). A different kind of fat rant: People of color and the fat acceptance movement. Fatshionista. https://web.archive.org/web/20100501202754/http://www.fatshionista.com/cms/index.php?option=com_content&task=view&id=180&Itemid=69

Shuai, T., Mozee, G., Tovar, V., Fontaine, G., Feminista, M., Starkey, J., Ongiri, A., Davis, M. T., & Lowe, N. (2012). A response to fat white activism from people of color in the fat justice movement. NOLOSE. https://nolose.org/about/policy/fat-white-activism-poc/

Simic, Z. (2015). Fat as a feminist issue: A history. In H. Hester, & C. Walters (Eds.), *Fat sex: New directions in theory and activism* (pp. 15–36). Surrey: Ashgate.

Sobal, J., & Maurer, D. (1999a). *Weighty issues: Fatness and thinness as social problems.* New York: Walter de Gruyter, Inc.

Sobal, J., & Maurer, D. (1999b). *Interpreting weight: The social management of fatness and thinness.* Piscataway, NJ: Transaction Publishers.

Söderqvist, T. (2007, Sept 6). Bodies of evidence: Fat across disciplines. Medical Museion, University of Cophenhagen. https://www.museion.ku.dk/2007/09/bodies-of-evidence-fat-across-disciplines/

Solovay, S. (2000). *Tipping the scales of justice: Fighting weight based discrimination.* Buffalo, NY: Prometheus.

Solovay, S., & Rothblum, E. (2009). Introduction. In *The fat studies reader* (pp. 1–10). New York: New York University Press.

Spark Magazine (Editors). (2020, January 5). The greatest power podcasting has is the ability to create a space of intimacy. Spark Magazine. http://www.sparkthemagazine.com/the-greatest-power-podcasting-has-is-the-ability-to-create-a-space-of-intimacy/

Stearns, P. N. (1997). *Fat history. Bodies and beauty in the modern west.* New York: New York University Press.

Stimson, K. W. (2003, June 23). Fat feminist herstory, 1969–1993: A personal memoir. Largesse. https://web.archive.org/web/20030623021536/http://largesse.net/Archives/herstory.html

Strings, S. (2019). *Fearing the black body: The racial origins of fat phobia.* New York: New York University Press.

Taylor, S. R. (2018). *The body is not an apology: The power of radical self-love.* Oakland, CA: Berrett-Koehler Publishers.

Thomas, P. (2005). *Taking up space: How eating well and exercising regularly changed my life.* Nashville, TN: Pearlsong Press.

Thompson, A. (2019). *They don't make plus size spacesuits.* Amazon Digital Services.

Thone, R. R. (1997). *Fat: A fate worse than death? Women, weight and appearance.* New York: The Haworth Press.

Tiggemann, M., & Rothblum, E. (1988). Gender differences in social consequences of perceived overweight in the United States and Australia. *Sex Roles, 18*(1/2), 78–56.

Tomrley, C. (2009). Introduction. In C. Tomrley & A. K. Naylor (Eds.), *Fat studies in the UK* (pp. 9–18). York, England: Raw Nerve Books.

Tomrley, C., & Naylor, A. K. (2009). *Fat studies in the UK.* York: Raw Nerve Books.

University of Otago. (2010). Big Fat Truth Symposium. https://www.otago.ac.nz/thebigfattruth2010/

Verseghy, J., & Abel, S. (2018). *Heavy burdens: Stories of motherhood and fatness.* Bradford, ON: Demeter.

Vincent-Otiono, J. K. (2020, August 19). Step into the life of Latasha Lagos. *Accelerate Magazine.* https://acceleratetv.com/the-cover-august-2020-digital-magazine-latasha-lagos/

von Liebenstein, S. (2012). Confronting weight discrimination in Germany — the foundation of a fat acceptance organization. *Fat Studies, 1*(2), 166–179.

Walker, S. (2015). *Dietland.* Boston: Houghton Mifflin Harcourt.

Wann, M. (1998). *FAT!SO? Because you don't have to apologise for your size.* Berkeley: Ten Speed Press.

Wann, M. (2009). Foreword. Fat Studies: An invitation to revolution. In E. D. Rothblum & S. Solovay (Eds.). *The fat studies reader* (pp. ix–xxv). New York: NYU Press.

Watkins, P., Farrell, A., & Hugmeyer, A. D. (2012). Teaching fat studies: From conception to reception. *Fat Studies, 1*(2), 180–197.

West, L. (2017). *Shrill.* New York: Hachette Books.

Whitesel, J. (2014). *Fat gay men: Girth, mirth, and the politics of stigma.* New York: New York University Press.

Wiley, C. (1994). *Journey to self-acceptance: Fat women speak.* Freedom, CA: The Crossing Press.

Yeboah, S. (2020). *Fattily ever after: The fat, Black girls' guide to living life unapologetically.* Melbourne: Hardie Grant Books.

Zellman, F. (2009). *Fat poets speak: Voices of the Fat Poets' Society.* Nashville, TN: Pearlsong Press.

PART 1

Defining fat

Part 1 focuses on the social construction of fatness, and the language used to discuss fatness. Fatness is a social construction; the understanding of who is fat has shifted across time and continues to shift across cultures. Scholars outside of Fat Studies (along with the biomedical community, the press, and most lay people) use the BMI to designate who is fat and who is not. Many activists make distinctions between small fats (those who wear around a 16–18 in US clothes sizes), fats (those who wear between 20–28), super fats (those who wear over size 30 and are often sized out of clothing markets), and infinity/death fats (those who wear over a size 36 and are often unable to find mass produced clothing) (Nischuk, 2012). Many fat people feel aggrieved when those who they do not deem as fat use the label; understandable as fat stigma and discrimination are common in their lives. This might suggest that an individual is fat when they face some form of structural discrimination and oppression; perhaps a healthcare professional making anti-fat assumptions about them, the inability to find clothes in their size in most of the stores available to them, the sneers or mutters of discontent when sitting next to a stranger on public transportation. Cooper (2010) argues that "fat is a fluid subject position relative to social norms, it relates to shared experience" (p. 1021).

Across the world, there are thousands of words that signify fat/being fat. Within English alone, they are plentiful: fat, rotund, Rubenesque, fluffy, big-boned, BBW, plump, stout, heavy, large, chubby, portly, flabby, paunchy, pot-bellied, Falstaffian, overweight, chunky, thick, big, plus size, tubby, corpulent. While each of these words are a signifier for fat/being fat, they each hold different connotations and associations. To be fluffy or chubby might be endearing; to be corpulent and heavy might be shameful. Within the medical and public health community, the labels of overweight and obese have been adopted and used to signify the diseased state and risk to health associated with fatness. Fat activists have long rejected these "O" words, pointing out that to be overweight means there is a normative weight to be, and that to be obese is to pathologise a body size based on an algorithm created in the 1800s. These activists, and Fat Studies scholars alike, prefer the term fat. They have reclaimed this term, arguing that it is the most apt descriptor of their bodies and enjoying the political power that comes with taking it back from the harmful taunting it had been for so long for so many.

This Part begins with a chapter from Associate Professor Darci Thoune, who reflects on who can be called fat, and why who is able to own the designation matters. Thoune asks,

Am I fat? And what does it mean that I can even ask this question? Perhaps a better way to ask the question would be, am I fat enough? Or, even, am I the right kind of fat? The question of who is fat or the complications that arise in trying to define fat reveals layers of complexity. Fat operates as both construct and lived reality, and this requires some unpacking.

(p. 23)

Thoune locates herself as a queer fat femme, and she considers the nuances of claiming a fat identity and the role that other privileges might impact on who does and does not identity as fat. Thoune, like other contributors in this volume, does not shy away from the word fat to describe her body or define this aspect of her identity.

In their chapter, Patricia Cain, Ngaire Donaghue, and Graeme Ditchburn, explore the language used in common social science measures of fat attitudes. They suggest that the language used often measures and contributes to negative attitudes towards fatness. The current measures are filled with material concerning personal qualities and responsibility for fatness; much of the material presents fatness as undesirable. In addition, they highlight how problematic most of the measures are, as they fail to define fatness at the start or ask the participant whether they identify as fat. They muse, "At this point you start to wonder, what are these measures actually doing? Quantifying antifat attitudes or contributing to them?" (p. 26). The authors conclude by calling for new measures of fat attitudes to be developed alongside the fat community.

A member of the fat community, Kimberly Dark's chapter reflects on how the real world impacts the language we use around fatness. She writes,

When I type or say that I am morbidly obese, something occurs in my body that was not happening just a moment before. My pulse quickens and my head throbs. Sometimes I feel panic and I want to cry. I feel like I need to take a deep breath, clear my lungs. I have been handling the themes and language of embodiment for decades and this is still my experience with the language … I'm affected by this classification and language and I carry the classification in the body.

(p. 37)

Dark suggests that acknowledging the harm that the language around fatness engenders, is one way to move past the oppression and into the liberation; she urges us to use language in agentic ways, illuminating pathways that lead to healing and connection.

In the final chapter of this section, Tiana Dodson considers what it means when having a fat body means you do not look the right way for your chosen profession. Dodson writes,

I do not look like the ideal of "health" because I am a fat, multiracial woman with brown skin when the prevailing thought in our healthist and dieting-obsessed culture states that fat people cannot possibly be healthy because healthy people are not fat.

(p. 40)

People read Dodson's fat body as unhealthy, which is a seeming contradiction to her paid employment as a health coach. Dodson suggests, instead, that being fat makes her a better health coach, because she has a more well-rounded idea of what health means and can provide value to a wide range of individuals with different lived experiences. Fatness, according to Dodson, is a great equalizer – there are no other identities that fatness cannot touch. Class, race, gender, sexuality, education, and more – fat people are among them all.

References

Cooper, C. (2010). Fat studies: Mapping the field. *Sociology Compass, 4*(12), 1020–1034.

Nischuk, A. (2012, Dec 20). Beyond superfat: Rethinking the farthest end of the fat spectrum. *The Fat Lip*. http://thefatlip.com/2016/12/20/beyond-superfat-rethinking-the-farthest-end-of-the-fat-spectrum/.

2

"AM I FAT?"

Darci L. Thoune

No, seriously, am I fat? And what does it mean that I can even ask this question? Perhaps a better way to ask the question would be, am I fat *enough*? Or, even, am I the right kind of fat? The question of who is fat and the complications that arise in trying to define fat reveals layers of complexity. Fat operates as both construct and lived reality, and this requires some unpacking.

While we are now beginning to see more nuanced representations of fat folx in the media, (I see you, *Shrill*), this recent representation does not undo years of the "headless fatty" trope (Cooper, 2007) or the host of other essentializing and reductive representations of fat folx that have served as the dominant narratives for fat experiences. Fortunately, an array of voices in the field have taken on the challenge of negotiating the spaces between concepts like *small fat* (Ospina, 2019) and *superfat* (Ash, 2016) and the challenge of intersectionality (Glass, 2016), but so much work still remains and this is where I'm attempting to enter the conversation.

As an academic, I spend an inordinate amount of time in imposter syndrome hell. As an academic who is also a fat activist, I find that my imposter syndrome also bleeds into the fat activism part of my life as well. Without providing my height, weight, dress size, and BMI, I can say with certainty that I am fat, but I do worry that perhaps I am not the right kind of fat or fat enough to be speaking out about fat issues or for other fat people. But, that's exactly what I have set myself up to do.

On the surface, the word *fat* operates simply as a descriptor without negative or positive connotations. In the same way that I have brown hair, I am also fat. But, obviously, fat is so much more than that as well. According to many folx in the health professions, fat means I am unhealthy and headed for an early death, despite empirical evidence challenging the purported causal links between "obesity" and mortality and morbidity (Stoll, 2019). According to many folx in the fashion industry, fat means I am invisible (Dickman, 2018), or only visible as a foil to bodies that they value and want to clothe. According to the airline industry, I am an inconvenience (Bias, n.d.), but it also means dollar signs when fat people have to pay the fat tax seats to fly, in the form of additional seats. And, according to the sadists who design furniture for university classrooms, I do not have the same rights to a comfortable learning environment that straight sized students have (Brown, 2017).

But it is even more complicated than that. Fat also dances around conversations between girls on playgrounds, hangs thick between mothers and daughters at dinner time, and is a cocked weapon on the tongues of every mean-mouthed bully looking to land a low blow. And, it is SO

MUCH MORE THAN THIS. Fat is food and food scarcity and access to food. Fat is Oprah dragging a Radio Flyer filled with 67 lbs of animal fat across the stage on national television. Fat is trying on bathing suits at Target and feeling like shit.

So, does it really matter who identifies as fat when we are literally soaking in a culture filled with fat hatred? I think it does, but I am going to walk a tightrope in trying to unpack the messiness of the question. Lately, I have been trying to hold two complicated ideas in my head at the same time. As a feminist and a queer, my impulse is to make space at the table for everyone. If a straight-size woman says to me that she identifies as fat, I do not think it is my job to convince her otherwise. Part of me thinks (hopes) that if she really does feel fat, then maybe she will advocate for visibly fat people. But, as a visibly fat person, I am also protective of the term *fat* because it means something. As a queer person, I shudder a little bit every time a straight person uses the metaphor of coming out of the closet. Unless you have actually had to utter the words, "I am dating a woman and her name is Sara" to your mother (as one example of coming out), then you have not had to come out of the closet. Similarly, if you have not experienced the shame of being told that you are fat in your doctor's office or any of a host of other humiliations, then maybe you should not be calling yourself fat.

Now, I also have to confess that I am not the least bit interested in being the fat police or being policed for being fat. But, I do think that we have to agree that words matter. And, in as much as words matter, lived experiences matter too. I am the kind of fat that often passes. By passing, I mean that on lucky days I can still shop in regular clothing stores at the very end of the dress sizes. I am the kind of fat that still fits in most spaces. I am the kind of fat that does not draw much attention in the grocery store. This passing provides me with some thin privilege, even though I am far from thin (for more on this subject, see Bacon, O'Reilly, & Aphramor, 2016. Similarly, the kind of queer I am allows me passing privileges as well. I am femme and appear to be in a heterosexual relationship. I frequently have to out myself as queer and I also have to out myself as fat. These are both privileges. So, with all of this privilege, am I really in a position to be calling out others for not being "fat enough", or to tell anyone how they are allowed to use the word? I am still working this out. What I do know is that in the same way that I feel a prickle of suspicion when I hear non-queers using the term "queer" (do you mean it like I mean it?), I feel physically uncomfortable when I hear straight-size women calling themselves fat, or acting as if they understand what it is like to be fat (although this not one thing).

I worry, though, about gatekeeping. I worry too about infighting among folx in the fat community. I worry about how white, cis, able-bodied, and straight the fat activist movement is. But, the more time I spend among fat folx, the less I worry about being fat and the more comfortable I am saying, "I am fat." If I ever need confirmation that fatphobia exists, all I have to do is say I am fat in front of my students or someone outside of the fat community. People stumble over themselves to tell me that I am not fat. Let's think about that for a minute. Maybe what they mean is that I am not *fat like that* or that they like me too much for me to be fat. But, every time this happens, I am reminded that to be fat is, in the eyes of many, to be a failure (Thoune, 2019), to be inadequate, to be other.

But, fuck it, I am fat.

So, while I might fret about being the right kind of fat and I might be self-conscious that I am not the most qualified person to be talking about fat issues, I also feel empowered by my fat identity and this makes me bold.

References

Ash. (2016, Dec 20). Beyond superfat: Rethinking the farthest end of the fat spectrum [Audio podcast]. *The Fat Lip*. http://thefatlip.com/2016/12/20/beyond-superfat-rethinking-the-farthest-end-of-the-fat-spectrum/

Bacon, L., O'Reilly, C., & Aphramor, L. (2016). Reflections on thin privilege and responsibility. In E. Rothblum & S. Solovay (Eds.), *The fat pedagogy reader* (pp. 41–50). New York: New York University Press.

Bias, S. (n.d.). *Flying while fat* [Animated video]. http://flyingwhilefat.com/

Brown, H. A. (2017). "There's always stomach on the table and then I gotta write!": Physical space and learning in fat college women. *Fat Studies*, 7(1), 11–20. doi:10.1080/21604851.2017.1360665

Cooper, C. (2007). Headless fatties. *Dr Charlotte Cooper*. http://charlottecooper.net/fat/fat-writing/headless-fatties-01-07/

Dickman, L. (2018, Jan 22). Why don't luxury brands want to dress fat people? *Ravishly*. https://ravishly.com/luxury-brands-dress-fat-people

Glass, I. (Producer). (2016, Jun 17). 589: Tell Me I'm Fat [Audio podcast]. *This American Life*. https://www.thisamericanlife.org/589/tell-me-im-fat

Michaels, L., Singer, A., Bryant, A., Banks, E., Handelman, M., West, L., & Rushfield, A. (Producers). (2019, Mar 15). *Shrill* [Television series]. Los Angeles, CA: Hulu.

Ospina, M. S. (2019, May 07). The "small fat" complex in body positivity. *Bustle*. https://www.bustle.com/articles/125803-the-small-fat-complex-in-body-positivity-why-its-not-entirely-justified

Stoll, L. C. (2019, Mar 1). Fat is a social justice issue too. *Two Fat Professors*. https://www.twofatprofessors.com/blog/fat-is-a-social-justice-issue-too

Thoune, D. L. (2019, Feb 1). Two f words: Fat and failure. *Two Fat Professors*. https://www.twofatprofessors.com/blog/two-f-words-fat-and-failure

3

QUANTIFYING OR CONTRIBUTING TO ANTIFAT ATTITUDES?

Patricia Cain, Ngaire Donaghue, and Graeme Ditchburn

Suppose you are a researcher and you want to develop and conduct an intervention designed to reduce negative attitudes toward fat people. Before you start, there will be decisions to make: What type of intervention is best? Who will participate? How many participants do I need? Will I have a control group? How will I demonstrate success? This last decision typically involves selecting a means of measurement. So, as an astute researcher, you turn to a selection of antifat attitude measures recommended and endorsed by other academics (Lee et al., 2014; Morrison et al., 2009; UConn Rudd Centre for Food Policy and Obesity, 2015). When reading through this selection, you are struck by the following items: "Jokes about fat people are funny" (Lewis et al., 1995); "Fat people have bad hygiene" (Latner et al., 2008); "Obese people should not expect to live normal lives" (Allison et al., 1991); "It is disgusting when a fat person wears a bathing suit at the beach" (Morrison & O'Connor, 1999); and "Although some fat people are surely smart, in general, I think they are not quite as bright as normal weight people" (Crandall, 1994). At this point you start to wonder, what are these measures actually doing? Quantifying antifat attitudes or contributing to them?

In this chapter, we review key measures of antifat attitudes and examine the assumptions, meaning, and content evident within. We assess the depth and breadth of item content to establish the overall scope of measures and identify where and how these instruments focus attention on problematic representations of fatness and fat people. In doing this we work to highlight how the current approach almost completely overlooks the work that has been done by fat activists and scholars in the field of Fat Studies, as well as how the growing complexity and nuance with which fatness is beginning to be treated in (some) mainstream social discourse (Cain et al., 2017) is overlooked. We seek to expose the limitations within this field of research and highlight the need for future strategies that not only honor all bodies but also reflect the colorful and complex landscape of fat discourse.

Figuring "the fat person" of antifat attitude measurement

As in all measurement of attitudes towards groups of people, antifat attitude measures assume that respondents have a mental model of the figure of "the fat person" on which they base their responses to specific evaluative statements. Assumptions about this figure guide the content of the items that constitute the attitude measure. Two assumptions stand out in relation to the figure of the fat person: first, that fatness is an embodied manifestation of controllable behaviors (primarily eating and exercise); and, second, that the fat figure is an "other". We discuss each of these in turn below.

Attributions of controllability dominate social understandings of fatness (Crandall & Resser, 2005; Weiner et al., 1988). For several decades in Western societies we have had a simultaneous circulation of two key ideas; the "obesity crisis" has connected fatness or "obesity" with poor health, and at the same time, healthism (Crawford, 2006) has located responsibility for health onto the individual, and positioned fat people as responsible for their weight via the idea that fatness is controllable. Despite being highly contested (Campos et al., 2006), this narrative positions fat people as reneging on a key requirement of citizens in neoliberal societies, to engage in responsible self-management that will prevent them from "overburdening" shared social resources (such as health care; see Murray, 2008) A lean body has become the aesthetic of responsible neoliberal selfhood, with the look and size of the body relied upon as an indicator of health (Donaghue & Allen, 2016; Jutel, 2005). The assumption that a fat body is a corporeal manifestation of "unhealthy choices" is reproduced by lay people and health professionals alike, and serves to foster pervasive stigma, creates barriers to health, and undermines wellness (LeBesco, 2011; Lee & Pausé, 2016). When fat people are considered to be responsible for their fatness the overt expression of negative sentiment can be seen as deserved (Crandall & Biernat, 1990). Indeed practices such as fat shaming are often justified as a method for motivating weight loss (Rogge et al., 2004) – which is uncritically assumed to be the desired goal of/for all fat people.

The majority of adults in most affluent western countries are fat; according to the World Health Organization most adults in these countries fall into either "overweight" or "obese" categories (World Health Organization, 2014). Yet, as we will show, antifat measurement neither acknowledges nor reflects this. Participants respond to items that essentially "other" fat people, yet in all likelihood the respondents themselves will be "fat", and as such will be responding to negative items relating to themselves. While the situation in which members of groups targeted by an attitude measure many find themselves completing that measure is not unique to antifat attitudes, the potential harms that might result from this are brought into stark relief by the fact that the "stigmatized" group is the population majority. The complications of measuring (negative) attitudes towards a majority group is further compounded by the vague and permeable boundaries that exist around the category of fatness. Unlike gender or "race", which are (problematically) socially understood as involving discrete categories, fatness exists on a continuum. Most studies measuring antifat attitudes do not define the criteria for fatness, nor do they ask respondents whether they personally identify as fat. Thus when asked to respond to statements about "fat people", respondents are required to conjure their own image of fatness and to decide for themselves (undisclosed to researchers) whether or not they are "fat".

The figure of the fat person assumed in antifat measurement reflects a common narrative, a "negative cultural knowingness" (Murray, 2008, p. 4) based on the assumption that a fat body is irresponsible, and the result of poor individual choices (LeBesco, 2011; Pausé, 2017). The fat person's identity has come to be largely defined by stigma (Harjunen, 2016) based on the assumption that outward appearance reflects an inner "true" self (Jutel, 2005). The fat individual is thus constructed as a "recalcitrant other", a citizen who is, either wilfully or haplessly, failing in appropriate self-governance (Harjunen, 2016; LeBesco, 2011).

How we currently measure antifat attitudes

Quantifying antifat attitudes, like any attitude, involves investigating and measuring a hypothetical or intangible construct (Mueller, 1986). A construct that, according to the popular three-component model of attitudes, manifests through beliefs, feelings, or behaviors (Katz

& Stotland, 1959). Should a researcher ascribe to this particular model, then measuring an attitude would mean measuring overt manifestations of beliefs, feelings, and actions (behavior) toward the target of interest (Katz & Stotland, 1959; Rosenberg & Hovland, 1960). Identifying these components would be important as they have demonstrated theoretical links with the constructs of prejudice, stereotyping and discrimination. Evaluation/attitudes have been linked to prejudice, beliefs to stereotypes, and actions/behavior to discrimination (Lee et al., 2014). If antifat attitudes are the root of stigma, prejudice, and discrimination, it appears logical that to reduce weight-based stigma and oppression we need methods of measurement, to establish where negative attitudes are most prevalent, and so that we can assess strategies for persuasion and attitude change.

There are currently seven measurement instruments used to quantify attitudes towards fat and "obese" people and of the "conditions" of fatness and "obesity" that are recommended (Morrison et al., 2009; UConn Rudd Centre for Food Policy and Obesity, 2015). These measures, in order of publication are; *The Attitudes Toward Obese Persons Scale* (ATOP) and *Beliefs About Obese Persons Scale* (BAOP; Allison et al., 1991), the *Antifat Attitudes Questionnaire* (AAQ; Crandall, 1994), the *Antifat Attitudes Test* (AFAT; Lewis et al., 1995), the *Antifat Attitudes Scale* (AFAS; Morrison & O'Connor, 1999), the *Fat Phobia Scale – Short Form* (FFS-SF; Bacon et al., 2001) and the *Universal Measure of Bias – Fat Scale* (UMB-FS; Latner et al., 2008). It should be noted that while these measures are the most frequently employed (Lee et al., 2014) they are not the only instruments for assessing attitudes toward fatness (for details on other measures see Lacroix et al., 2017).

The **Attitudes Toward Obese Persons Scale (ATOP)** is a 20-item scale developed in conjunction with the Beliefs About Obese Persons Scale (BAOP; Allison et al., 1991). The development of dual scales was to enable the relationship between evaluations of fat people and beliefs about the causes of "obesity" to be investigated. The ATOP consists of items relating to evaluations of fat people with a focus on personal characteristics and perceived self-evaluations.

The **Beliefs About Obese Persons Scale** (BAOP; Allison et al., 1991) is an eight-item scale examining the extent to which respondents believe that "obesity" is within individual control. As mentioned, the BAOP was developed in conjunction with the ATOP to assess the relationship between beliefs about controllability of weight and negative attitudes.

The **Antifat Attitudes Questionnaire** (AAQ; Crandall, 1994) is a 13-item scale. The measure was developed to investigate whether antifat attitudes were structured in a similar way to other symbolic attitudes, such as symbolic racism. Symbolic attitudes are said to develop in relation to established social values and involve emotional responses concerning the degree to which the target group is perceived to be aligned with important social values (Herek, 1986). The AAQ consists of three subscales: "willpower" assesses the belief that weight is a function of personal control, "dislike" assesses antipathy toward fat people, and "fear of fat" measures personal concerns around weight and weight gain. Prejudice toward fat people is operationalized as involving the belief that fat people fail to meet key western values relating to the Puritan work ethic and self-determination (reflected in the "willpower" scale) and are thus legitimately subject to intolerance (reflected in the "dislike" scale). The inclusion of self-relevant items ("fear of fat" scale), allows for the possibility that respondents' own personal relationship to the thin ideal might colour their attitudes towards fat people in general (The AAQ is the only major antifat attitude measure to include a self-reflection scale).

The **Antifat Attitudes Test** (AFAT; Lewis et al., 1995) is a 47-item measure. In developing the AFAT, Lewis et al. (1995) reviewed previous measures of attitudes toward obesity (including Allison et al., 1991 and Crandall, 1994) and expressed particular concern over the inclusion of both self-relevant items and items relating to social attitudes, considering the two concepts conceptually different. For this reason, the AFAT includes only items relating to social attitudes toward fatness. The AFAT includes three subscales: "social/character disparagement" measures both disregard for fat people and the attribution of undesirable personality traits, "physical/romantic attractiveness" measures the perceptions that fat people make undesirable partners, and "weight control/blame" measures beliefs about the personal controllability of weight.

The **Antifat Attitudes Scale** (AFAS; Morrison & O'Connor, 1999) is a five-item scale, also developed to address perceived limitations in existing measures. Morrison and O'Connor also criticized the inclusion of self-relevant items, such as those expressed in the "fear of fat" subscale of the AFAT (Crandall, 1994). The need for a much shorter measure as an alternative to existing long scales was also motivation for developing the five-item instrument.

The **Fat Phobia Scale – Short Form** (FPS-SF; Bacon et al., 2001) is a 14-item, shortened version of the 50 item Semantic Differential Fat Phobia Scale by Robinson, Bacon, and O'Reilly developed in 1993. Semantic differential scales present opposing adjective-pairs (ranging from negative to positive evaluation, such as "good-bad" or "closed-open"), and the participant rates the object, in this case "fat people" somewhere on that continuum. (Henderson et al., 1987). The original 50-item scale has six factors: undisciplined, inactive, and unappealing; grouchy and unfriendly; poor hygiene; passivity; emotional/psychological problems, and stupid/uncreative. The first subscale (undisciplined, inactive, and unappealing) accounted for most of the variance in the long form of the scale, and so to increase utility of the measure in a range of clinical and research settings, this became the basis of the short form (Bacon et al., 2001). It is interesting to note that this is the only measure to use the term "phobia" in relation to fatness. The term "fat phobia" as it is used here relates to the "pathological fear of fatness" (Robinson et al., 1993, p. 468), a fear that is believed to manifest in negative perception and evaluations of fat people. Thus by assessing one's fear of fat, negative attitudes toward fat people are accessed.

The **Universal Measure of Bias – Fat Scale** (UMB-FS; Latner et al., 2008) is a 20-item measure designed to provide a means of comparing weight bias to other common biases. The measure also provides a "standard" measure for evaluating bias across different groups. The measure was developed with reference to three target populations – "fat", "gay" and "Muslim". These populations were selected because they were considered common targets for overt bias in Western Society, and less likely to be prone to "socially desirable" responses (Latner et al., 2008). Items are based on their ability to capture the underlying drivers of bias across disparate groups so as to allow the relative strength of bias to be compared.

Turning now to item content, it becomes obvious that negative appraisals dominate these measures, and given their explicit antifat intention, this could be expected. What is more revealing is the focus of this negativity. Almost half of the items emphasize personal qualities and attributes (42 items). Following this, content centres on the desire to dissociate from fat and "obese" people (22 items), responses to fatness (21 items), perceived causes of fatness (19 items), and appearance (13 items). Lastly, some items (10 items) seem to take on a critical perspective, that is, they represent ideas beyond a normative or negative approach to fatness. Probing further to consider the themes underlying the items, we reveal assumptions and evaluations that despite being arguably anticipated, say things about fat people that should be cause for concern.

Fat people have impaired character

Overall, content relating to personal qualities dominates. Participants completing these measures are continually responding to statements regarding the overall character or personality features ascribed to fat people (of which they indeed may be one). Participants are specifically required to make ratings on attributed traits such as trustworthiness, moodiness or thoughtlessness, self-esteem, and even personal hygiene, as the following items demonstrate. "Fat people obviously have a character flaw, otherwise they wouldn't become fat" (AFAT; Lewis et al., 1995), "Most obese people feel they are not as good as other people" (ATOP; Allison et al., 1991), and "Fat people have bad hygiene" (UMB-FS; Latner et al., 2008).

As anticipated, items are primarily negative in orientation, presenting a picture of "obese" and fat people as lacking in many socially desirable traits and characteristics. Furthermore, these presumed faults or deficits are not even weight related, with items frequently referring to emotional states, such as "Most fat people are moody and hard to get along with" (AFAT; Lewis et al., 1995), "I tend to think that people who are overweight are a little untrustworthy" (AAQ; Crandall, 1994) and "Most fat people are boring" (AFAT; Lewis et al., 1995). This attention illustrates the importance creators of these measurements have placed on character appraisal as a major contributor to the overall evaluation of fat people. Judgments of (negative) personal qualities are deemed important, indicating that disparagement directed toward fat and people is more than simply about body size, rather it is about the "type" of person they are assumed to be.

In specific instances, fat people are depicted as being impaired in some way, for example, "Most fat people are lazy" and "Fat people have no willpower" (AFAT; Lewis et al., 1995). In some cases, inferences suggest that these impairments are the cause of a person being fat, such as "Obesity often occurs when eating is used as a form of compensation for lack of love or attention" (BAOP; Allison et al., 1991). These items focus on the idea that there is something fundamentally wrong with a fat person, particularly around perceived "energy in–energy out" management; fat people are fat because they eat too much or exercise too little (and they eat too much and exercise too little because their character is impaired).

If fat people are believed to be impaired, we might ask, impaired in relation to whom? Although not explicitly stated in the items above, it appears evident that a comparison should be made to "non-fat" or "normal weight" people. Several items do make such judgment explicit, overtly making a comparison, positioning the fat person as inferior to the "normal" weight person. These evaluations occur across different life domains; "Although some fat people are surely smart, in general, I think they tend not to be quite as bright as normal weight people" (AAQ; Crandall, 1994), "Most obese people have different personalities than non-obese people", "Obese workers cannot be as successful as other workers" (ATOP; Allison et al., 1991), and "On average, fat people are lazier than thin people" (AFAS; Morrison & O'Connor, 1999). While these measures explicitly label themselves "antifat", we must start to question whether responding to items that represent fat people as stupid, different, failed, and lazy is really an acceptable practice, given what we know about the impact of internalized weight stigma (Carels et al., 2013). With items such as these, respondents are afforded no opportunity to reflect positive beliefs about fat people; the best option that is possible is disagreement with negative statements.

Fat people are to be avoided

The next category of items focuses on desire to disassociate with or avoid contact with (other) fat people. It follows that these are negatively oriented and include items such as; "I would not like to have a fat person as a roommate", "I don't enjoy having a conversation with a fat person" (UMB-FS; Latner et al., 2008) and, "I can't stand to look at fat people", "I prefer not to associate with fat people" (AFAT; Lewis et al., 1995). There are two domains that depict specifically the spaces where fat people were to be shunned; in employment situations "If I were an employer looking to hire, I might avoid hiring a fat person" (AAQ; Crandall, 1994) and "If I owned a business I would not hire fat people because of the way they look" (AFAT; Lewis et al., 1991). And in relationships, particularly romantic partnerships; "I can't believe someone of average weight would marry a fat person", "I would not want to continue in a romantic relationship if my partner became fat" (AFAT; Lewis et al., 1991) and "I would never date a fat person" (AFAS; Morrison & O'Connor, 1999). Despite the objectionable nature and wording of these items they unfortunately do reflect key domains where fat people are discriminated against (Brewis et al., 2011; Major et al., 2012; Puhl & Brownell, 2001; Puhl & Heuer, 2009).

Interestingly, within this category the AAQ includes self-relevant items, with aversion toward fatness expressed toward the self, or specifically, the potential for future fat. These include "One of the worst things that could happen to me would be if I gained 25 pounds" and "I worry about becoming fat" (AAQ; Crandall, 1994). These items represent the idea that fat is to be avoided at all costs, whether fat is personally embodied or disconnected, they are also written in such a way that assumes the respondent is not currently fat.

Fat people are disparaged

The sentiment of avoidance is echoed by the items categorized here, items that reflect disapproval, ridicule, disgust, contempt, and shame. Some of these items expose broad disapproval and ridicule such as "I hate it when fat people take up more room than they should in a theatre or on a bus or plane" or "Jokes about fat people are funny" (AFAT; Lewis et al., 1995) as well as "I have a hard time taking fat people too seriously" (AAQ; Crandall, 1994). Other items signal explicit disgust "Fat people are disgusting", "It is disgusting to see fat people eating" (AFAT; Lewis et al., 1995) and "It is disgusting when a fat person wears a bathing suit at the beach" (AFAS; Morrison & O'Connor, 1999). Focusing in on disgust for a moment, as an emotional response disgust has been considered a reaction to moral violations relating to tenets of divinity and purity, as well as "degradation of the self and the natural order of things" (Rozin et al., 1999, p. 576). In this context, assessing the response of disgust may have been an attempt to associate fatness and fat people with the sins of "sloth" and "gluttony". Indeed such negative moral judgments have been found to align with the denigration of fat people (Crandall & Martinez, 1996). Unfortunately, for some, disgust and fatness appear connected. Disgust is even deliberately elicited in relation to fat bodies. It is a response often provoked via public health campaigns, rationalized by the argument that disgust is considered a motivator for change, a tactic that has not gone without critique (Lupton, 2015).

Some items within this grouping focused more on contempt and shame and specifically relate to friends and family members. These include: "I'd lose respect for a friend who started getting fat" and "If someone in my family were fat, I'd be ashamed of him or her" (AFAT; Lewis et al., 1995). Apparent in these items, is the idea that even positive feelings toward people one is supposedly close to, are not enough to protect against derogation, should that person become fat. Seemingly, no one is exempt.

Fat people are out of control

This category of items operationalizes the idea that weight is within individual control, with many items featuring assessments of eating and behavior. "Most obese people cause their problem by not getting enough exercise" and "The majority of obese people have poor eating habits that lead to their obesity" (BAOP; Allison et al., 1991). In support of this is the dismissal of other explanations regarded as not within individual control "The idea that genetics causes people to be fat is just an excuse" (AAT; Crandall, 1994). These items reflect an assumption that the fat body is evidence not only of a lack of restraint, but also of some form of misbehavior that fat people try to cover up with "excuses". Such opinions represent the fat life as one lived with reckless abandon, with the fat body proof of such transgressions. These beliefs and assumptions are reflected in items included in most measures. "Fat people only have themselves to blame for their weight" (AFAS; Morrison & O'Connor, 1999), "If fat people really wanted to lose weight, they could" (AFAT; Lewis et al., 1995), "Fat people tend to be fat pretty much through their own fault" (AAQ; Crandall, 1994) and "Fat people tend toward bad behavior" (UMB-FS; Latner et al., 2008). Central to these beliefs is the idea that if people did not engage in these "bad" behaviors – if they "behaved correctly" – then they would not be fat.

There are some deviations from these very individualized attributions, items relating to the biological or external causes of fatness are represented, although to a much lesser extent. "In many cases, obesity is the result of a biological disorder" and "People can be addicted to food, just as others are addicted to drugs, and these people usually become obese" (BAOP; Allison et al., 1991). Evident in these items is more balance between negative and neutral items. While replacing a "bad character" view of fatness with an "addiction" model does shift the moral status of the fat person, these items still reflect a view that fatness is an undesirable state, which needs to be both "explained" and "cured". Nonetheless, these items do provide opportunities for participants to engage with alternative points of view, albeit briefly. Depending on the measure completed, participants may be witness to a shift from negative to more neutral portrayals of fat people. The more neutral items do tend to focus on external however still individualized accounts of why and how someone would come to be fat. Such items continue to position fatness as a condition that requires an explanation.

Fat people are unattractive/Fat people are attractive

The next topic of interest is appearance. The high proportion of items dedicated to this subject signposts the importance placed on evaluating a fat person's attractiveness as a facet of attitudes toward fat people. Some items here relate to the perceived unattractiveness and offensiveness of the fat body, reflecting the idea that people should manage the public display of their fat body so as not to offend others; "Fat people shouldn't wear revealing clothing in public" (AFAT; Lewis et al., 1995) and "Fat people are a turn off" (UMB-FS; Latner et al., 2008). Not all items, however, reflect negative appraisals, juxtaposed with the above judgments is the notion that fat people are appealing with items such as "I find fat people to be sexy" and "I find fat people attractive" (UMB-FS; Latner et al., 2008). Within this category there are as many positively or neutrally worded items as there are negative, demonstrating a shift in perspective and offering participants the opportunity to engage with less oppressive items. The positively framed items tend to appear in the most recently developed measure, the UMB-FS (Latner et al., 2008) perhaps reflecting a more progressive or inclusive perspective by the developers, or perhaps this is related to the scale's applicability for multiple targets. As mentioned, this is the only scale that is not specifically written to be about fat people. The UMB is designed for multiple targets, with "fat people" interchangeable with the targets "gay" and "Muslim". It may be that the multiple applicability of this scale allows for the possibility that fat people have positive qualities to be entertained. Or perhaps this framing does indeed reflect the beginning of a shift away from antifat rhetoric dominating quantification.

Fat people need special consideration

This grouping of items reflects an awareness that fat people are marginalized within society and as such may require protection from discrimination and negative consequences. While not overtly reflecting positive evaluations of fat people, these items measure endorsement of the

belief that fat people's rights are often infringed. The items include: "The existence of organizations to lobby for the rights of fat people in our society is a good idea" (AFAT; Lewis et al., 1995), "I try to understand the perspectives of fat people" and "Special effort should be taken to make sure that fat people have the same rights and privileges as other people" (UMB-FS; Latner et al., 2008). While some may not consider these items altogether "critical" in regard to a critical fat approach to embodiment, politics or scholarship, in this instance we consider them as representing a more critical approach, given that they focus on and recognize the importance of inclusion and equal rights. These items again offer respondents an opportunity to engage with messages that contrast with the dominating messages that epitomise negativity, disparagement, and derision.

Fat people are (actually) ok

Lastly, we identified a group of items that reflect the idea that fat people are really no different to people who are not fat. Despite comparing fat and non-fat people or "obese" and "non-obese" people, these items do the work once again of challenging negative representations. They include; "Obese people are just as healthy as non-obese people", "Obese people are just as self-confident as other people", "Obese people are just as sexually attractive as non-obese people" (ATOP; Allison et al., 1991) and "People who are fat have as much physical coordination as anyone" (AFAT; Lewis et al., 1995). These evaluations represent the flip side of previously identified items focused on (un)attractiveness or poor character, although in more positive, or at least equalizing terms. The inclusion of these topics is again of note as very few measures have presented any alternative perspective, particularly with regard to health and the fat body. Health-related items have typically been excluded from quantification due to concern that such items may potentially reflect concern for a person's health rather than reflecting explicit attitudes toward fatness (Lewis et al., 1995).

Rethinking measurement

From this close reading of antifat attitudes measures, it becomes apparent that researchers attempting to quantify and reduce negative attitudes and evaluations of fat people have more to consider than the measure they employ. They need to consider the possibility that the measure they choose may inadvertently be contributing to the very experience they are trying to eliminate. With respect to the measures we have reviewed, the majority of instruments were developed during the 1990s, a time when the "obesity epidemic" was gaining attention and the "war on obesity" began to be waged (Lupton, 2013). During this time, weight management became a focus for many western countries (Jutel, 2011) with the ensuing public health policies creating what has been termed an adipophobicogenic environment, epitomized by fat hatred and stigma (O'Hara & Taylor, 2014). Unfortunately little has changed, as the overt expression of antipathy towards fat people shows no sign of decline (Andreyeva et al., 2008; Latner & Stunkard, 2003), When it comes to quantifying evaluations of other people or groups, Stangor's (2009) observation that "If we were to study the really bigoted, then perhaps we would feel more comfortable using direct measures" (p. 5) perhaps depicts the atmosphere of measure development at the time. It may be that the reason antifat measurement has taken this current form, is simply – because it could.

It is also worth noting that not all research and researchers concerned about weight stigma are working from a position that accepts fatness as an ordinary aspect of human diversity. In recent years, many researchers have identified weight stigma as a concern because it may lead to diminished dietary intentions (Seacat & Mickelson, 2009), increased calorie consumption (Schvey et al., 2011), and decreased interest in exercise (Nolan & Eshleman, 2016) for reviews see Puhl and Suh (2015), and Vartanian & Porter (2016). In other words, some of the concern about weight stigma derives from the belief that it is a counterproductive to efforts to encourage fat people to "improve" their health via weight loss. This concern among some researchers reflects a recent tendency for some public discourse about fatness to be characterized as a dilemma in which concerns about the mental health and civil rights of fat people (as a result of weight stigma) are set against the unquestioned assumption that fat people must nonetheless continue to be exhorted to lose weight in order to become "healthy" (Cain et al., 2017; Cain & Donaghue, 2018). With this in mind, it is important that critical fat scholars continue to pay attention not only to the nature of the measures used to assess attitudes towards fat people, but also the ends to which such measures are used.

It is becoming increasingly apparent that a refocus of attention is in order, "Who researches fat people and who creates knowledge about fatness is important" (Cooper, 2016, p. 32). One issue made apparent in this review, is that the instruments presented here reflect more an approach to doing research *about* fat people, than *with* fat people, a tactic that is akin to positioning fat people as "abjected objects" (Cooper, 2016, p. 39). Going forward we need to challenge and change this default, and commit to research practices that foreground ethical practice and harm minimization. In short, we need new ways of measuring evaluations of fat people. We need to move away from quantifying negativity and instead focus on measurement that allows for a range of perspectives to be expressed. We need to embrace and include the work of fat activists and scholars, and we need to represent critical fat discourse in measurement. In doing this, we not only have the opportunity to broaden the scope of measurement and understand more about the endorsement of elements of contemporary discourse, we will be able to assess the important progress of fat voices and fat movements as they work to destabilize anti-"obesity" rhetoric and reconstruct what it means to be fat.

References

Allison, D. B., Bastile, V. C., & Yuker, H. E. (1991). The measurement of attitudes toward and beliefs about obese persons. *International Journal of Eating Disorders, 10*(5), 599–607. doi:10.1002/1098–108X

Andreyeva, T., Puhl, R. M., & Brownell, K. (2008). Changes in perceived weight discrimination among Americans, 1995–1996 through 2004–2006. *Obesity, 16*(5), 1129–1134.

Bacon, J. G., Scheltema, K. E., & Robinson, B. E. (2001). Fat phobia scale revisited: The short form. *International Journal of Obesity, 25*(2), 525–257.

Brewis, A. A., Hruschka, D. J., & Wutich, A. (2011). Vulnerability to fat-stigma in women's everyday relationships. *Social Science & Medicine, 73*(4), 491–497.

Cahnman, W. J. (1968). The stigma of obesity. *The Sociological Quarterly, 9*(3), 283–299.

Cain, P., & Donaghue, N. (2018) Political and health messages are differently palatable: A critical discourse analysis of women's engagement with Health at Every Size and Fat Acceptance messages. *Fat Studies, 7*(3), 264–277.

Cain, P., Donaghue, N., & Ditchburn, G. (2017). Concerns, culprits, counsel, and conflict: A thematic analysis of "obesity" and fat discourse in digital news media. *Fat Studies, 6*(2), 170–188.

Campos, P., Saguy, A., Ernsberger, P., Oliver, E., & Gaesser. (2006). The epidemiology of overweight and obesity: Public health crisis or moral panic? *International Journal of Epidemiology, 35*(1), 55–60.

Carels, R. A., Burmeister, J., Oehlhof, M. W., Hinman, N., LeRoy, M., Bannon, E., Koball, A., & Ashrafloun, L. (2013). Internalized weight bias: Ratings of the self, normal weight, and obese individuals and psychological maladjustment. *Journal of Behavioral Medicine, 36*(1), 86–94.

Cooper, C. (2016). *Fat activism: A radical social movement.* England: HammerOn Press.

Crandall, C. S. (1994). Prejudice against fat people: Ideology and self-interest. *Journal of Personality and Social Psychology, 66*(5), 882–894.

Crandall, C. S., & Biernat, M. (1990). The ideology of anti-fat attitudes. *Journal of Applied Social Psychology, 20*(3), 227–243.

Crandall, C. S., & Martinez, R. (1996). Culture, ideology, and antifat attitudes. *Personality and Social Psychology Bulletin, 22*(11), 1165–1176.

Crandall, C. S., & Resser, A. H. (2005). Attributions and weight based prejudice. In K. D. Brownell, R. M. Puhl, M. B. Schwartz, & L. Rudd (Eds.), *Weight bias: Nature consequences and remedies* (pp. 83–96). New York: Guilford Press.

Crawford, R. (2006). Health as a meaningful social practice. *Health, 10*(4), 401–420.

Donaghue, N., & Allen, M. (2016). "People don't care as much about their health as they do about their looks": Personal trainers as intermediaries between aesthetic and health-based discourses of exercise participation and weight management. *International Journal of Sport and Exercise Psychology, 14*(1), 42–56.

Harjunen, H. (2016). *Neoliberal bodies and the gendered fat body.* New York: Routledge.

Henderson, M. E., Morris, L. L., & Fitz-Gibbon, C. Y. (1987). *How to measure attitudes.* Thousand Oaks, CA: Sage Publications.

Herek, G. M. (1986). The instrumentality of attitudes: Toward a neo-functional theory. *Journal of Social Sciences, 42*(2), 99–114.

Jutel, A. (2005). Weighing health: The moral burden of obesity. *Social Semiotics, 15*(2), 113–125.

Jutel, A. (2011). Does size really matter? Weight values in public health. *Perspectives in Biology and Medicine, 44*(2), 283–296.

Katz, I., & Stotland, E. (1959). A preliminary statement to a theory of attitude structure and change. In S. Koch (Ed.), *Psychology: A study of science* (pp. 423–475). New York: McGraw-Hill.

Lacroix, E., Alberga, A., Russell-Mathew, S., Mclaren, L., & von Ranson, K. (2107). Weight bias: A systematic review of characteristics and psychometric properties of self-report questionnaires. *Obesity Facts, 10*(3), 223–237.

Latner, J. D., & Stunkard, A. J. (2003). Getting worse: The stigmatization of obese children. *Obesity Research, 11*(3), 452–456.

Latner, J. D., O'Brien, K. S., Durso, L. E., Brinkman, L. A., & MacDonald, T. (2008). Weighing obesity stigma: The relative strength of different forms of bias. *International Journal of Obesity, 32*(7), 1145–1152.

LeBesco, K. (2011). Neoliberalism, public health, and the moral perils of fatness. *Critical Public Health, 21*(2), 153–164.

Lee, J. A., & Pausé, C. J. (2016). Stigma in practice: Barriers to health for fat women. *Frontiers in Psychology, 7*, 2063.

Lee, M., Ata, R. N., & Brannick, M. T. (2014). Malleability of weight-biased attitudes and beliefs: A meta-analysis of weight bias reduction interventions. *Body Image, 11*(3), 251–259.

Lewis, R. J., Cash, T. F., Jacobi, L., & Bubb-Lewis, C. (1995). Prejudice toward fat people: The development and validation of the Antifat Attitudes Test. *Obesity Research, 5*(4), 297–307.

Lupton, D. (2013). *Fat.* London: Routledge.

Lupton, D. (2015). The pedagogy of disgust: The ethical, moral and political implications of using disgust in public health campaigns. *Critical Public Health, 25*(1), 4–14.

Major, B., Eliezer, D., & Rieck, H. (2012). The psychological weight of weight stigma. *Social Psychological and Personality Science, 3*(6), 651–658.

Morrison, T., & O'Connor W.E. (1999). Psychometric properties of a scale measuring negative attitudes toward overweight individuals. *The Journal of Psychology, 139*(4), 436–445.

Morrison, T. G., Roddy, S., & Ryan, T. A. (2009). Methods for measuring attitudes about obese people. In D. B. Allison, & M. L. Baskin (Eds.), *Handbook of eating behaviors and weight-related problems: Measures, theory and research* (pp.79–113). Thousand Oaks, CA: Sage Publications.

Mueller, D. J. (1986). *Measuring social attitudes: A handbook for researchers and practitioners.* New York: Teachers College Press.

Murray, S. (2008). *The "fat" female body.* Melbourne: Palgrave Macmillan.

Nolan, L. J., & Eshleman, A. (2016). Paved with good intentions: Paradoxical eating responses to weight stigma. *Appetite, 102*, 15–24.

O'Hara, L., & Taylor, J. (2014). Health at every size: A weight neutral approach for empowerment, resilience and peace. *International Journal of Social Work and Human Services Practice, 2*(6), 272–282.

Pausé, C. (2017). Borderline: The ethics of fat stigma in public health. *The Journal of Law, Medicine & Ethics, 45*(4), 510–517.

Puhl, R. M., & Brownell, K. D. (2001). Bias, discrimination and obesity. *Obesity Research, 9*(12), 788–805.

Puhl, R. M., & Heuer, C. A. (2009). The stigma of obesity: A review and Update. *Obesity, 17*(5), 941–964.

Puhl, R. M., & Suh, Y. (2015). Health consequences of weight stigma: Implications for obesity prevention and treatment. *Current Obesity Reports, 4*(2), 182–190.

Robinson, B. E., Bacon J. G., & O'Reilly, J. O. (1993). Fat phobia: Measuring, understanding and changing anti-fat attitudes. *International Journal of Eating Disorders, 14*(4), 467–480.

Rogge, M. M., Greenwald, M., & Golden, A. (2004). Obesity, stigma and civilised oppression. *Advances in Nursing Science, 27*(4), 301–315.

Rosenberg, M. J., & Hovland, C. I. (1960). Cognitive affective and behavioural components of attitudes. In C. I. Hovland, & M. J. Rosenberg (Eds.), *Attitude organization and change: An analysis of consistency among attitude component* (pp. 1–14). New Haven: Yale University Press.

Rozin, P., Lowery, L., Imada, S., & Haidt, J. (1999). The CAD triad hypothesis: A mapping between three moral emotions (contempt, anger, disgust) and three moral codes (community, autonomy, divinity). *Journal of Personality and Social Psychology, 76*(4), 574–586.

Schvey, N. A., Puhl, R. M., & Brownell, K. D. (2011). The impact of weight stigma on caloric consumption. *Obesity, 19*(10), 1957–1962.

Seacat, J. D., & Mickelson, K. D. (2009). Stereotype threat and the exercise/dietary health intentions of overweight women. *Journal of Health Psychology, 14*(4), 556–567.

Stangor, C. (2009). The study of stereotyping, prejudice, and discrimination within social psychology. In Nelson, T. D. (Ed.), *Handbook of prejudice, stereotyping and discrimination* (pp. 1–22). New York: Taylor and Francis.

UConn Rudd Centre for Food Policy and Obesity. (2015). *Weight bias and stigma: Tools for researchers.* http://www.uconnruddcenter.org/weight-bias-stigma-tools-for-researchers

Vartanian, L. R., & Porter, A. M. (2016). Weight stigma and eating behaviour: A review of the literature. *Appetite, 102,* 3–14.

Weiner, B., Perry, R. P., & Magnusson, J. (1988). An attributional analysis of reactions to stigma. *Journal of Personality and Social Psychology, 55*(5), 738–748.

World Health Organization. (2014). *Obesity and overweight* (Fact sheet No 311). http://who.int/mediacentre/factsheets/fs311/en

4

LANGUAGE, FAT AND CAUSATION

Kimberly Dark

These are facts: my Body Mass Index is over 40. This is the highest classification of the BMI, level three obesity. Those who use this scale call me "morbidly obese." In my culture, I am embodied as something morbid. How easy it was for language to take my life and turn it toward death and disease. And it is not so easy to re-language myself back into full life. Let me bring this to the level of sensation: when I type or say that I am morbidly obese, something occurs in my body that was not happening just a moment before. My pulse quickens and my head throbs. Sometimes I feel panic and I want to cry. I feel like I need to take a deep breath, clear my lungs. I have been handling the themes and language of embodiment for decades and this is still my experience with the language. It is not like I'm dealing with a sudden diagnosis that brings a fear of the unknown. It is not like when someone says: you have cancer. There is no disease in my body, no illness and yet, according to the BMI, my existence is morbid. This statement is brought to describe an everyday experience in a body that does live, and act and make love and experience joy. I'm affected by this classification and language and I carry the classification in the body. I feel my stress level increase just so I can tell you this – and there will be effort involved in bringing this anxiety back to neutral.

There is nothing neutral about being fat in the United States of America.

It is great that we want to talk about health, and yet, we dwell on things that may be germane, but are not decisive to the issue. Let me say this another way. Numbers may be factual and still not tell the truth. We are not separate from the social sea in which we swim. Physical outcomes cannot be isolated to bodily circumstances alone.

I am walking up a hill a few paces behind my best friend. We are teenagers coming home late from a party. It is ten past ten p.m. and we are walking back to her house where I will stay the night. Our curfew is ten and she picks up her pace to one I cannot match. This is not the first time she has done this, nor will it be the last. She often walks at a formidable speed! I am working to match her stride but my feet hurt and I am tired. I wonder, as I have always wondered, if this is simply the pain I deserve for being too fat, for not exercising more. I want to keep up and I am simultaneously angry at this desire. She should respect me and my limitations. I am sweating out this anger. Is it excess sweat because fat people sweat more? Or is it because I am unfit or because I am angry, anxious and then, as she leaves me behind, turns the corner ahead of me for the final quarter mile home, I am also afraid. It is ten past ten pm and it is dark and before she left me behind she said she wanted to honour her mother's request that she be on time. And off she went, sort of trotting along the dark street. Perhaps I could keep up, but I do not even try now. I am seething with anger at this stupidity, this humiliation, and the fear that some ill could befall me, alone, in military-base part of town. I want to be as brave as she, but I also think she is stupid. Why would her mother prefer her arriving home alone at ten past ten rather than the pair of us arriving with apologies at twenty past the hour? But I am also not sure whether I deserve humiliation. I steel my demeanour and decide that I will not accept humiliation, whether or not I deserve it. In those last five minutes of the walk, I consciously slow my breathing and work on the comments that will let me save face upon entry, which will re-construct a sturdier self-image, one that is not worthy of derision, of being left behind.

When I come into the house, sweaty seething angrily behind a cool exterior, there sits my friend, leafing through a magazine on the sofa. Her mother sits nearby. Do I imagine a look of irritation on her face for my tardiness? Does her mother think it strange that we did not come in together? I do not know, and I do not show my feelings. I hide them, as practiced, and deliver the lines I have constructed in the dramaturgy of social life. I take the role I have been handed and play it as best I can, as all young people do. I discuss a lot of life's joys and pains with my best friend, but not this one. She is one of the unwitting perpetrators of oppression in this regard. And I know she loves me. No, I will not discuss this.

The experience and effect of stress on the fat body cannot be discussed independently from the stress of social interactions while fat. Down to the subtle sanctions of one's most supportive best friends, there is stress. Does the fat person experience more discomfort during physical exertion because of the biological impact of fat on the body, or because of the fear of not keeping up, being thought less than, seen poorly, fearing injury, having shoes or clothes that do not fit well or simply can never look "right." How does one weigh the fear of simply not being allowed to participate with "normal" people again? Moving easily through one's day as a respectable social participant has everything to do with health.

And what happens when fear becomes experience again and again, when fear becomes memory? How does childhood memory embed the cells of the stigmatized body? Being looked at, laughed at, sneered at, barely tolerated, not tolerated (and left behind).

According to the BMI, I am morbidly obese. This is a fact, though it is not necessarily true. The truth of how I inhabit this body is complex. It includes the duress of stigma and the joy of movement and creation. The research says that being too fat is unhealthy – "the research" – that unified thing that everyone quotes, sans specificity. Height and weight ratios can indeed serve as a proxy for body fat percentage – it is not terribly reliable in describing a person's life and health, but the process can yield data that can be factual based on specific parameters. The truth of living is complex and adaptive. I am a storyteller in part because the truth never sits still. It dances, slumps, rolls in the dirt and comes home after curfew. I help people understand how their particular positions and training influence what comes to be seen as truth or fiction, immutable or changeable.

Sometimes, a form of hatred and scapegoating can become so imbedded in the public discourse, it becomes laudable; science seems to support it. The popularity of eugenics science comes to mind, along with the obesity epidemic as examples of how science is part of culture and vice-versa. When I was a kid, I did all the same things that my slender friends did – all of them. I swam and biked and walked up hills late at night on my way home from parties. Sometimes I had a great time, though overall, I was more recalcitrant in the pursuit of physical activity in the company of others. I felt fearful and pressured and I did not compete well. If you would argue – because I am fat, that I did not sustain the same "health benefits" from those activities that my friends did, you must be arguing that it was because of the stress of derision, or other as yet uncharted factors. There was not as much joy in my walking, my bike riding, my

horseplay – this I can report. I was fearful that I would not look at home in these activities, not be welcomed and not be entitled to live a full life in the body I have. This I can report. Stress affects my body. We are never separate from the social sea in which we swim. The social world, and its science, are complex and intricate. We can want many things at once and it is hard to tell what caused which outcomes. I turn to stories as one way to make sense of the world.

So, how will I recover the emotional neutrality I lost when I used the language that associates my very being with death and disease? How do I move on comfortably? Luckily, an awareness of how language and derision affect well being can itself be a call to healing. When we take the time to really hear what causes us pain and ill health and oppression, then it is much easier to know that something requires redress. That is the first step: awareness that we are living in a time of fat hatred and that the stigmatized body requires particular care. A lot of people have stigmatized bodies – fat is just one form. Second I remind myself that the injury of stigma is not about me. It is separate from my body, my actions, and my life. I remember that I live in a culture that does not promote health; it promotes conformity. It is not personal. And I have the power to promote my own health, and to help others. That instantly makes me feel more alive.

The medicine for healing stress is within us. Body awareness, conscious relaxation and a will to help others are powerful health promoters. As we come together, we can begin to remind one another that health is also complex. We can look for and promote healing and we can construct systems and language that promote understanding, rather than just creating facts. And in doing so, we can become allies. Many who "look well" are not healthy. We can each bring our gifts and help each other toward greater vibrancy.

When I think back to my angry teenage self, trudging uphill behind my friend, feeling miserable and alone, I appreciate her most for this: she did not accept a simple story. Though she doubted her worth, she re-scripted a narrative in which her own dignity was central. She honed her power to change perception. She learned to level her breathing and she continued practicing joy when she could, without taking on negative labels as the truth of her identity. Her fortitude and savoir-faire constructed the person I am today. Through my storytelling, I have seen others develop the ability to re-script their own well being, to become positive actors in their own health rather than victims of morbid narratives. The language we use to describe our bodies can illuminate pathways to good or ill health. We do well to keep looking for what serves, what heals, what connects. We do well to name those things. And tell the truth about them in as many ways as we can find.

5

MY LIFE IS INTERSECTIONAL, SO MY COACHING HAS TO BE

Here is why this is a good thing

Tiana A. Dodson

The current culture of health coaching leads us to assume that there is a "right" way for a health coach to look because there is a "right" way to be healthy. However, this is a false assumption that both ignores the spectrum of what health can look like for individuals when the socioeconomic determinants of health are taken into consideration and tends to alienate certain groups of people. This is especially true for those who are more marginalized such as black and indigenous people of color, those who identify as queer, transgender, or non-binary, disabled, neuro-divergent, and fat individuals. Though there is a movement in our culture focusing on the inclusion of more marginalized individuals, there still remains a difference in the depth of service that can be provided by someone identifying as an ally versus someone with actual lived experience. In this chapter, I challenge assumptions about health and health coaching in general, while making the case for the value of providers with different lived experiences.

As defined by The Institute for Integrative Nutrition, a Health Coach is a supportive mentor and wellness authority who helps clients feel their best through food and lifestyle changes by tailoring individualized wellness programs to meet their needs. Health coaches ask the deeply probing questions that help you get to the bottom of why you struggle to eat vegetables, drink enough water, and exercise. They will help you overcome these struggles using simple practices because they have overcome these struggles themselves. And though most people who are drawn to health coaching do it because they want to help people and are well-intentioned, they too often, simply become agents who perpetuate the healthist and weight biased culture of dieting. Thus, the general expectation for what a health coach looks like is someone: blonde, white, skinny, and healthy. It is no wonder many people are initially skeptical when they learn that I am a health coach.

I am not blonde.
I am not white.
I am not skinny.

And I do not look like the ideal of "health" because I am a fat, multiracial woman with brown skin when the prevailing thought in our healthist and dieting-obsessed culture states that fat people cannot possibly be healthy because healthy people are not fat. So, who am I to be coaching anyone when it comes to learning how to be healthy? Well, the truth is that this supposed "disadvantage" makes me the perfect health coach for those who need it most.

Here is why: Fatness knows no boundaries.

People are fat across class, across race, across gender, across sexuality, across education level. Fatness is a great equalizer. It seems that the only things that keep some people from fatness are genetics and/or fanatical lifestyles focused on food restrictions and over-exercise, and even those things are no guarantee. To be focused on *absolute fatness* – a term I use to describe those people who are at all times, in all circumstances, by all people, judged as fat – means that you absolutely have to also be aware of how fatness can intersect with other marginalized identities.

Because bodies do not exist in a vacuum. If you worry about someone's weight without also considering their access to equitable health care, sufficient nourishing food, clean water and air, safety and security, wealth creation, bodily autonomy and sovereignty, support for their different ability levels, and equal rights under the law, you really do not care about them at all. You cannot truly advocate for fat people without also advocating for everyone, including non-binary, non-gender conforming, trans, and other identities that do not conform. As Civil Rights Activist Audre Lorde said, "There is no such thing as a single-issue struggle, because we do not live single-issue lives" (Blackpast, 2012, para 14).

This is why fat people, especially fat people of color, need their own health and wellness specialists. This is where I come in. Because when it comes to overcoming body hatred, yo-yo dieting, and the difficulties of navigating a fat phobic culture, I have been there, and my work is based in my own journey.

So, when a person tells me how hard it is for them to even be at the gym because of how other people look at them, I get it. I get it when someone says they really want to order dessert at a restaurant but are deterred by the thought of the dreaded eyebrow raise that says, "it looks like all you ever eat is dessert". I get the way that judgment can result in ordering foods that are less desirable to them but more acceptable to others. I get it when they say that they are dreading going home for the holidays because they had to buy pants in a larger size. I get it because I am fat, too.

When we then layer in how the experience differs for people of color, we also have to talk about the systemic oppression that routinely disenfranchises black, brown, and indigenous bodies. This is incredibly difficult to hold space for and truly empathize with if you have never experienced being othered. Recommending kale salad to someone who has limited funds or access to fresh produce who has no cultural context for kale salads makes it unrealistic for said person to integrate kale salad into their normal diet. If you have no relationship with cultures outside of what is dominant or "ideal" as a provider, you will not be able to offer an appropriate strategy or options for your marginalized clients.

Additionally, the inherent trauma of our recent ancestors who had little to no agency over their lives or bodies has lasting psychological consequences on our present day lives. So, it is also necessary to address this historical trauma as a potential source of resistance. This is a lens a provider will not have if they lack awareness or experience of such realities.

The experiences of being both a fat person and a person of color mean that when you enter a space, you tend to be strapped down, packed in. You are likely going to great lengths to present a version of yourself that is going to be palatable to that space. But this means that you do not get to show up as yourself. You show up as your representative. Maybe, given time, empathy and acceptance, that real you can come out. But that is a whole lot of effort, labor, and wasted energy before you can actually show up as you and get the health care and attention you need.

So, when a client comes to me looking for guidance on how to improve their health, I can easily put myself in their shoes because their experiences are so familiar to me. And experiential knowledge can never be outpaced by theoretical knowledge, no matter how many fat people a skinny health coach has worked with.

I have done – and am still doing – the work personally, so I know what it is like to go through the steps, to experience the back slides, and to overcome the hurdles again and again. The most well-intentioned ally can never be more than just that – an ally.

But when your health is on the line, you do not just need an ally. You need a peer. There is a wide chasm separating the affirmation of someone witnessing you through binoculars from a distant cliff, and someone walking with you hand-in-hand on a familiar road.

This of course does not mean that fat black people can only be well served by fat black coaches. Shared experience is not a prerequisite for empathy, where it is rendered respectfully, responsibly, and well. It does mean, however, that I have experiences that set me apart from some people and form a commonality with others, making it possible for me to provide a different experience – one that might make the difference between yet another failure or success.

References

Blackpast. (2012, August 12). *(1982) Audre Lorde, "Learning from the 60s"*. Blackpast. https://www.black-past.org/african-american-history/1982-audre-lorde-learning-60s/

Institute for Integrative Nutrition. (n.d.) *Nutrition and health coaching – the health coach*. https://www.inte-grativenutrition.com/health-coaching

PART 2

Theorizing fatness

Part 2 considers ways of theorizing fatness. Which, from a fat studies perspective, presents an inherent conundrum. Fat people and their experiences are not a monolith, and no singular theory can fit them all. In the chapters in this section, each author considers a different framework for theorizing fatness. Each of these frameworks are both generative and fraught, and the authors make this explicit. There is no framework that fully invites the multiplicity of fat existence at the intersections of geography, subject and identity, and yet scholars and activists in the field of Fat Studies know that these frameworks give shape and contextualization to some of the most salient aspects of fat lives. Ideally, Fat Studies will continue to trouble the prevalence of Western theories of fatness by exploring the vast communities of fatness and raising them to the center of exploration.

Amy Farrell opens Part 2 with her chapter on feminism and fat. Farrell presents an overview of how feminisms have provided a framework for theorizing fatness; intersectional feminism, black feminism, queer feminism, and more. Farrell suggests that while this framework has been rich and generative, it has also produced many tensions, especially between scholars and activists. Even with these tensions, Farrell notes "the fat queer body means opposition/resistance/a rejection of normative boundaries and expectations, and often a celebration of the abject" (p. 55).

As Farrell theorizes fatness through feminisms, Sofia Apostolidou theorizes fatness through the lens of modern Western culture. In their chapter, they consider the role that Greek cultural perspectives can play in disrupting what is considered uniform modern Western culture. By highlighting the unique and often contradictory relationship Greek culture has with fatness they disrupt the narrative of a singular Western lens by which fatness is understood. Exploring the Greek film, *To Klama Vgike Ap' Ton Paradiso,* Apostolidou uses the main character Djella to illustrate how fatness "blurs, complicates and intervenes for the Greek modernisation narrative" [and] "can be traced to the problematics of the Greek narrative, and its complicated relationship with linearity and transition to modernity, inclusion into Western-ness, and the relationship with colonialism" (p. 61).

Argentinian activist Laura Contrera's chapter, "Does that mean my body must always be a source of pain?" explores how the experience of fatness constricts the allowable narratives of fat sexual assault survivors and often furthers to victimize them. Contrera illuminates how fatphobic myths create harm and invisibilise the experiences of survivors. Narratives coupling fatness and desirability reinforcing notions that fat people and fat women specifically cannot be sexually violated are pervasive and impact everything from whether a survivor will disclose their assault to whether or not a court of law will presume them a "worthy" victim. In this chapter the reader is reminded that

> Even feminism has been mistaken about its approach in this point—in a wide range going from Orbach to Despentes, the idea that fat little girls get fat to avoid being further abused and that that unbearable weight is a way of performing our suffering.
>
> *(p. 64)*

This approach ties fatness to pathology while reasserting the false premises that fatness renders one's body inherently undesirable and that sexual assault is a function of desirability rather than a dynamic of power and control. Contrera uses this chapter to disrupt these mythologies that serve as obstructions to fat survivors' healing.

Hannele Harjunen explores the impacts of neoliberalism on how society engages the fat body through a review of the literature and set of considerations and inquiries in her chapter. Harjunen puts forth a definition of neoliberalism as the liberal economic free market system rooted in profit, productivity, and privatization that currently governs most of the Western world. In such a system, the fat body becomes a project of individual failure that hampers the ultimate aspirations of the framework: productivity and profit. Under neoliberalism, notions of health are inseparable from morality and virtue, rendering the fat body an amoral body and through individualism encouraging citizens to self-police the body as a means of performing "good" citizenry. The intersections of fatness, gender and race further cast specific fat bodies as "outlaws" to the goals of a neoliberal society. Hannele concludes the chapter by offering, "Indeed, the notion of fatness and the fat body as something diseased, costly, immoral, ugly, and above all, a symbol of individual failure, would probably not have such an impact were it not produced and maintained, at the same time, in so many spheres – discursive and otherwise. This is the power of neoliberal governmentality" (p. 74).

In the chapter "Fat and trans", Francis Ray White examines how fatness and trans identity have or have not been considered in relationship in activist and Fat Studies research and writing. White also considers how the field might reconcile this absence and thereby strengthen the discourse of both areas and those who live at the intersection of these identities. In reviewing the literature, White highlights how Fat Studies scholars historically have written about trans identity and fat identity from the "compare and contrast" perspective which fails to explore how trans identity impacts fat bodies and how fatness can disrupt or make legible the trans body. White offers the concepts of fluidity and liminality as potential starting points for understanding the embodied dance between fat and trans identities, positing:

> Rather than bemoaning fat people's inability to do gender, a fat/trans approach to Fat Studies could help 'de-exceptionalize' trans experiences of doing gender by revealing the embodied processes by which any/all gender is assumed thus destabilizing not only binary gender, but also the cis/trans binary.
>
> *(p. 85)*

Ultimately, White's work in this chapter seeks to, "chip away at the assumption that 'fat people' and 'trans people' are discrete groups; be that in order to acknowledge the existence of fat/trans people, or to recognize the role of fat in both cis and trans gender (un)intelligibility" (p. 85).

April Herndon's closing chapter, "Fatness and disability", considers whether theorizing fatness through a frame of disability is useful, appropriate, and a path to social justice. Herndon suggests that, "thinking through fatness as a disability still offers personal and political possibilities for justice and an important means of thinking through lived experiences using an intersectional model" (p. 88–89). Herndon also acknowledges the potential struggles with building alliances across fatness and disability as a result of dynamics of both ableism and fatphobia and emphasizes that:

> a field like Fat Studies [cannot] simply 'add and stir' class or disability. The frameworks must be renegotiated; the field must pull back from tightly focusing on a single issue to see the entire landscape. The social and legal models of disability – and even our medical understandings – must be expanded in ways that offer a finer grained image of how fatness and disability can and do come together in discourse, laws, and lives.
>
> *(p. 98)*

6

FEMINISM AND FAT

Amy Erdman Farrell

Feminist theories and fat

Feminism, in its most capacious sense and in all its manifestions as social movement, as theoretical perspective, as political theorizing and activism, concerns itself most fundamentally with personhood, with the right of every human to be identified as a person, as a citizen, as a being with full recognition. And, because the body connotes meaning, because it *signifies*, because it confers status, identity and power, all feminist thinking – from the radical, socialist, queer and edgy to the most liberal, narrow, and consumer oriented (not that edgy cannot be consumer oriented, or narrow socialist), from the early thinking of Elizabeth Cady Stanton and Sojourner Truth to the contemporary musings of Judith Butler and Patricia Hill Collins – concerns itself with the problem of the body. The problem of the *female body* has been the way it marks its bearer as a partial person, a "second" sex, to paraphrase Simone de Beauvoir, or, dependent upon its additional markings of age, nationality, and color, as a non-person entirely.

The problem of the *fat body* is this: within a Western context, fat is *irreconcilable* with personhood. Instead, fat works as a sign of a degenerate, primitive body, a state incommensurate with selfhood. A ubiquitous example of this are diet ads that portray a thin person emerging from a fat body. Described by feminist fat activist Ragen Chastain (2015), a 2015 ad, portraying a marble statue of a woman's figure, for instance, clearly portrays this. The figure appears to be white, youthful, with small breasts that certainly do not need the sports bra she is wearing to provide their perkiness; flowing, silky hair; extraordinarily well defined abdominals; a chiseled nose and cheekbones; forearms that reveal every bone and tendon; a half smile and look of deep concentration on her face. She chips away at the fat that encases her, immobilizes her, from the waist down. She is emerging a *person* from within that dimpled, thick fat that is falling, in chunks, unwanted, discarded, at her feet. Chastain bristles at this image, writing, "What's wrong [with this image] is telling fat people that we should think of ourselves as thin people covered in fat, a before picture, a perpetual potential future thin person, anything but a fully realized authentic person" (para. 7). As cultural critic Le'a Kent (2001) argues "The self is never fat. To put it bluntly, there is no such thing as a fat *person*" (p. 135).

Feminist analysis of Western dualistic thinking allows us to understand this antagonistic relationship between *person* and *fat*. As Susan Bordo (2003) explains,

> the constant element throughout [Western] historical variation is the *construction* of body as something apart from the true self (whether conceived as soul, mind, spirit, will, creativity, freedom…) and as undermining the best efforts of that self. That which is not-body is the highest, the best, the noblest, the closest to God; that which is body is the albatross, the heavy drag on self-realization.
>
> *(p. 5)*

Feminist thinkers have identified this mind/body dualism, this paradigmatic understanding of the world, as fundamentally destructive for women, as female bodies are always already identified and over-identified with physical matter, with the body, with that which "is not" mind. At best, the body is simply that which supports the mind, necessary but not "of" it; at worst, as Bordo explains, the body is a destructive "drag" on all that is connected to personhood. And so it goes for women, then, within this fundamental dualism: at best women can be the helpmate to men; at worst, they are the tempter, the seducer, the reminder and sign of the body's connection to the murky and mucky elements of life, or what feminist philosopher Julia Kristeva calls the abject, that which must be disavowed and rejected in order to claim subjectivity (as cited in Kent, 2001, p. 135). Feminist theories that analyze this mind/body split, then, are extraordinarily useful for a critique of the fat/person dialectic, as they help to explain why fatness – as a bodily, physical trait – would be so readily recognized and understood within Western culture as incommensurate with personhood, as the "drag" on all that is spirit, rational, and human.

Intersectional feminist theory provides a particularly strong lens through which to understand Western denigration of fat and the body. While scholar Jennifer Nash (2008) importantly points out that as a theoretical concept, "intersectionality" has multiple and sometimes conflicting meanings, two of its major strands are markedly useful for thinking though fat stigma. Coined by African American feminist legal scholar Kimberlé Crenshaw in 1991, the concept of intersectionality illuminates the complexity of identity and oppression within the context of daily life and real institutions and social contexts. Neither gender nor race, Crenshaw argued, were variables that could be isolated as demanded by most social science research or legal discourse; rather, as the lives of African American women demonstrate, race and gender "intersect" in powerful and inextricable ways. Far earlier than Crenshaw, other African American feminist thinkers had made this argument in other contexts, from Sojourner Truth's famous 1851 "Ain't I a Woman?" speech to Frances Beale's 1970 "Double Jeopardy: To Be Black and Female" and Deborah King's 1988 "Multiple Jeopardy, Multiple Consciousness" (as collected in Guy-Sheftal, 1995). This theoretical perspective about the intersectionality of identities and oppressions is fundamental to understanding how fat identities and discrimination against fat people work, as an integral and interlocking attribute of the person's other identities and characteristics. As activist Johnnie Tillmon wrote in a 1972 issue of *Ms.* magazine,

> I'm a woman. I'm a black woman. I'm a poor woman. I'm a fat woman. I'm a middle-aged woman. And I'm on welfare. If you're any one of those things, you count less as a person. If you're *all* of those things, you just don't count, except as a statistic.
>
> *(p. 111)*

Intersectional feminist theory, then, clarifies the ways that fatness as both an identity and as a category of discrimination and stigma must always be understood *in context* and *in relationship to* other forms of identity and oppression.

Black feminist thinking and intersectional theories also provide particular insight into how fat denigration works in tandem with the history of gender and racial oppression. In particular, it illuminates the way that the originating Western philosophies that articulated the mind/body split (and its attendant understanding that the masculine was linked to the mind and the feminine to the body) simultaneously articulated concepts of race that constructed "whiteness," "blackness" and theories of degeneracy and racial hierarchies. As Janell Hobson explained in detail in her pathbreaking work *Venus in the Dark* (2005), the emergence of scientific racism in the eighteenth and nineteenth centuries "sought to 'order' the natural world," "assigning to diverse plants, animals, and people a hierarchical position that supported the supremacy of European masculinity" (pp. 20–21). Emerging simultaneously with the international outcry for abolition, the discourse and institutions of scientific racism supported and then supplanted the workings of empire and the trade in enslaved people, providing "evidence" of the hierarchy of civilization and humanity. And, very important for understanding how this relates to the feminist analyses of fat, that "evidence" resided, as Hobson explained, in the body. The most well-known example of this is in the work of the French scientist Georges Cuvier, whose name is still celebrated in Paris, inscribed at the base of the Eiffel Tower and designating a street that runs all the way alongside the Jardin des Plantes on the Left Bank of the Seine. His 1816 autopsy of the enslaved woman Sara Baartman (also known as the Venus Hottentot) served as "proof" of the unevolved nature and unbridled sexuality of African people. And, as I have argued elsewhere, it was not only her large buttocks that served as evidence, but also the presence of fat throughout her body, on her knees, thighs, stomach and breasts that Cuvier cited as proof of her lowly status. Fat, then, served as a signifier of degeneracy, of the primitive, and became a deeply rooted and widespread idea, one that continues to flourish today (Farrell, 2011, pp. 63–67).

Queer feminist theories have also been crucial to explaining both fat denigration and the possibilities for new ways of centering, experiencing, and understanding fatness. As Jackie Wykes explains in the collection *Queering fat embodiment*, queer theory allows us to understand how "heteronormativity operates as a regulatory apparatus which underwrites and governs the discourse on—and management of—the fat body" (Wykes, 2014, p. 4). Queer, feminist fat activists outside the academy have been writing, organizing and performing in ways that illuminate and challenged the stranglehold of compulsory heterosexuality, to draw from Adrienne Rich's term, on fat people. In *Fat activism: A radical social movement* (2016), Charlotte Cooper describes queer fat feminism this way: "Queer rhymes with sneer and has an anti-normative, anti-assimilationist and punk streak to it … [moving] fat people beyond a discourse of shame to reclaim the messy, disobedient aspects of ourselves" (pp. 192–193). Queer feminist theory not only rejects the split between fat and self, but also challenges the very concept of the mythical civilized person, as Katie LeBesco points out in *Revolting bodies* (2003). Importantly, many queer, feminist fat activists articulated a politics that merged queer and fat politics long before the world of academic queer theory, which was relatively slow to pick up on the centrality of fatness to queer theory. In addition, as scholars such as Jason Whitesel (2014) and Marcia Millman (1980) have demonstrated, male queer cultures are not inherently fat friendly, as the male gaze generally enforces a thin aesthetic, whether that desiring gaze emanates from straight men toward women or from gay men toward other men. Likewise, lesbian communities often enforce a toned, athletic body ideal. Nevertheless, many feminist and lesbian queer communities and perspectives have been a comparatively generative location for articulating and experiencing fat acceptance and activism, as the work of scholar activists such as Charlotte Cooper, Kath Read, Sonya Renee Taylor, Substantia Jones, Allyson Mitchell and Virgie Tovar demonstrate.

Feminisms and fat activism

As feminist philosopher Susan Bordo (2003) explains,

> mind/body dualism is no mere philosophical position, to be defended or dispensed with by clever argument. Rather, it is a *practical* metaphysics that has been deployed and socially embodied in medicine, law, literary and artistic representations, the psychological construction of self, interpersonal relationships, popular culture, and advertisements—a metaphysics which will be deconstructed only through concrete transformation of the institutions and practices that sustain it.
>
> *(p. 13)*

In other words, the ideology that the mind is superior to the body, that spirit trumps the physical, is not simply a belief system but a set of practices, historically rooted and enacted on a daily basis that ensure the continuation and success of the ideology. Many of these practices often appear "normal," natural even, and freely chosen, from patriarchal naming practices to compulsory heterosexuality to rape culture, and, particularly relevant to this discussion, diet and weight loss regimes. Feminism challenges these normative practices, illuminating both the political aspects of "personal" life and the ways that patriarchal cultures threaten violence and rejection to those who break their mandates. As Karen Jones wrote in "Fat women and feminism" (1974), "Stripped of the benefits of male chivalry, the condition of fat women reflects the true position of women in our society. We must not be silent any longer; for as long as fat women are oppressed, no woman can be liberated!" (Jones, 1974, p. 147). To put this into contemporary perspective, Jones's argument would suggest that the kind of vitriolic rhetoric and actions that rain upon fat women – from the ubiquitous "No Fat Chicks" bumper stickers to the horrific language used against Heather Heyer, the protestor who was killed by a KKK and Nazi sympathizer after the 2017 Charlottesville, Virginia, rally, are not the actions of deranged individuals but rather the authentic feelings of a white, patriarchal culture that demonizes women who fail to conform and that perceives women, in scholar Sylvia Federici's (2004) terms, as resources to be colonized. Fighting fat denigration, then, is fundamental to feminism.

Limits to feminist challenges of fat denigration

Historically, feminist thinkers – again, in the most capacious sense of that word – *chipped away* at the idea that the body itself did *signify*, that it did *mean something*, eliminating certain characteristics that were irrelevant: the uterus, upper body strength, the weight of brains. Feminists of color challenged the significance of dark skin. But none of the eighteenth-, nineteenth- and early twentieth-century Western feminists fundamentally disavowed the idea that certain aspects of the body *did* signify, that it could be read for signs of status, intelligence, willpower, for signs of being "civilized" or a "throwback" to some earlier, less evolved state, that it could, in other words, tell you *something* about the humanity of that body. One of the major untouched areas of body meanings was *fat*, particularly for those feminists whom I will term "achievement feminists."

By "achievement feminism" I gesture to a theoretical perspective and a set of practices that is most similar to what has been identified as liberal feminism. Liberal feminism refers to thinkers and activists who generally articulate an agenda that focuses on the law as the locus for change, emphasize individualistic approaches, and seek incremental reforms rather than radical upheaval (Brown, 2003; Eisenstein, 1986; Tong, 2009). As Zillah Eisenstein explains in her now canonical work, *The radical future of liberal feminism*, however, even liberal feminism potentially creates sufficient change to cause significant and fundamental repercussions for patriarchy and capitalism. "Achievement feminism," in contrast, seeks to gain power and upward mobility explicitly within the systems already in place. Interestingly, one might identify aspects of achievement feminism within many different theoretical and activist approaches to feminism. And, generally, when achievement feminism blossoms, fat stigma and the belief that fat is incommensurate with personhood continues to flourish.

We see this particularly well in the activism of nineteenth- and early twentieth-century U.S. and British suffragists. During the campaigns for suffrage, anti-suffrage propaganda lampooned white suffragists as old, manly, and fat; many of their mocking cartoons drew from the stock portrayals of Irish and Black people, portraying suffragists with oversized lips, bulging eyes, and red or black skin. Significantly, however, prominent white feminists did not challenge the meaning of those attributes; they concurred that Black, fat, old and manly were all negative characteristics, signifying "ugly," "degenerate," and "uncivilized." Elizabeth Cady Stanton, who herself had mocked Daniel Lambert, the fat man who took part in the London curiosity circuit, as hardly "distinguished for any great mental endowments," (Farrell, 2011, p. 106) hated the fact that she had become fat as she aged, signing up for time in weight loss sanatoriums. The predominant visual defense suffragists used in their propaganda were images of suffragists as white, youthful, and *thin*.

It is not only white women who traded in fat phobia, however. Despite the prevalent belief that African American cultures are immune to fat denigration, the reality is that fat stigma weaves its way throughout the history of African Americans' campaigns for full equality and rights. Indeed, Black women's investment in thinness must certainly be recognized as a strategy to navigate a deeply racist, white supremacist society whose aesthetic preferences included the norm of thinness. In what was likely one of the first public speeches by an African American woman about women's rights, for instance, Maria Stewart in 1832 took up the "evidence" that African American women, with their strong, thick bodies, were obviously not made for thinking, for education, for full rights. In a fascinating passage, she makes clear her argument, not that a strong, thick body could think as well as a thin one, but rather, that it was the labor that had hidden, and defaced, the true slender and delicate person within:

> Most of our color have dragged out a miserable existence of servitude from the cradle to the grave. . . . O, ye fairer sisters, whose hands are never soiled, whose nerves and muscles are never strained, go learn by experience! Had we the opportunity that you have had, to improve our moral and mental faculties, what would have hindered our intellects from being as bright, and our manners from being as dignified as yours? … And why are not our forms as delicate, and our constitutions as slender, as yours? Is not the workmanship as curious and complete?
>
> *(as cited in Guy-Sheftal, 1995, p. 32)*

In other words, the real person, inside the body of an African American laboring woman – whether enslaved or free – was a delicate and slender person. Labor and drudgery had simply overlaid a false facade. And this belief – that the real civilized *person* was thin – manifested itself by the early part of the twentieth century in African American professional women's lives as a very robust culture of exercise and dieting to lose weight and maintain a slender figure, as the historian Ava Purkiss (2017) has demonstrated in her finely argued article, "Beauty secrets: Fight fat." In other words, among African American middle class women, among those who considered themselves professional, concerned about the uplift of their race and their sisters, fat was never "accepted," but rather was a trait that might be understandable (the result of drudgery and over-work) but certainly needed to be controlled and eliminated if a woman were to be seen as "fit" for citizenship. Interestingly, we can see the same focus on weight loss and a slender figure in contemporary versions of the professional Black women who Purkiss describes, namely Oprah Winfrey and Michelle Obama. Both women represent and advocate for women's place in public life, in women's economic opportunities, in women's reproductive rights and freedoms, and for Black equality and achievement in general. And, for both, weight loss and a slim figure are key: First Lady Michelle Obama launched her Let's Move! campaign in 2010 to "combat the epidemic of childhood obesity" because the "security of our nation is at stake" (Let's Move! Campaign, 2014). She even appeared – twice! – on the long-running television show *The Biggest Loser*, working out with Bob Harper in the White House, demonstrating how to do jumping pushups (*Politico*, 2014). Likewise, for media mogul Oprah Winfrey, fat is the betrayer, the curtain of shame and excess that envelopes and smothers the real, fit person who resides inside. As she said in a video piece announcing her 10 percent ownership of Weight Watchers (which sent the stock price soaring), "Inside every overweight woman is a woman she knows she can be" (Hines, 2016). For Michelle Obama, the fat body connotes an unfit citizen, a danger to the nation; for Winfrey, it's a loss of potentiality, a threat to self-actualization, the result of behaviors – overeating, feigning injury – that are understandable but ultimately defeating (Dowd, 2016).

This, of course, brings us to what is probably evidence of the most fraught relationships feminism has with fat, Susie Orbach's 1978 *Fat is a feminist issue: A self-help guide for compulsive eaters*, followed in 1982 by *Fat is a feminist issue II*. In the introduction to the 1978 text, Orbach wrote, "Fat is a social disease, and fat is a feminist issue" (pp. 6–7). She continued,

> For many women, compulsive eating and being fat have become one way to avoid being marketed or seen as the ideal woman: 'My fat says "screw you" to all who want me to be the perfect mom, sweetheart, maid and whore. Take me for who *I* am, not for who I'm supposed to be. If you are really interested in *me*, you can wade through the layers and find out who I am'.
>
> *(p. 9)*

In other words, for Orbach, who described herself as deeply involved in the feminist movement, a fat woman – whether unconsciously or consciously – became that way as a form of resistance to oppression, a protective and angry layer of defense *and* offense covering the real woman, hidden inside. It was an understandable, though ultimately destructive strategy, a "social disease." For Orbach, as for Stanton, Stewart, Obama, and Winfrey, the real person is by definition the thin person; the fat person does not exist, but is rather a thin person covered with fat. This is an important genealogy for us to follow, for it illuminates the fact that, although feminist theories generated the awareness that the body/mind split is at the heart of both gender oppression and fat oppression, many activists, particularly when primarily focused on "achievement feminism," have, even as other ideas about body signification have been challenged, maintained and propagated the idea that fat denotes either a failed person or a pathological response to stress and oppression.

Fat feminisms

Of course, this is not the only genealogy available of feminism and fat; there is also a generative relationship, powered by the underlying premise of feminism that the personal is political. Depending upon how generously one defines feminism, it might actually seem that all fat activism is feminist; this is not actually true, however. The frequently identified "first" feminist fat activist group in the United States, for instance, the Fat Underground, was founded in 1973 by women (Summer-Vivian Mayer, Judy Freedspirit, Gudrun Fonfa, Sara Gold Bracha Fishman, and Lynn Mabel-Lois) who broke off from the more conservative and heterosexually-focused Los Angeles based National Association to Advance Fat Acceptance. The first line of their "Fat Liberation Manifesto," reprinted in Esther Rothblum and Sondra Solovay's *The fat studies reader* (2009) signaled their critical understanding of how, historically, personhood had been inscribed as incompatible with fatness: "We believe that fat people are fully entitled to human respect and *recognition.*" Rather, they saw fatness as an oppressed identity, one allied with the struggles of "other oppressed groups against classism, racism, sexism, financial exploitation, imperialism and the like" (p. 341; Fishman, 1998). Throughout the 1970s, Sharon Bas Hannah and Vivian Mayer wrote and collected fat feminist essays, which eventually became the 1983 anthology *Shadow on a tightrope: Writing by women on fat oppression*, edited by Lisa Schoenfielder and Barb Wieser. If *Fat is a feminist issue* is the most explicit example of a feminist perspective on fat as incompatible with full, healthy, personhood, *Shadow on a tightrope* is a particularly rich text illuminating a different perspective, one connecting unruly bodies, beauty, nature, and fat liberation. A fundamental thread running through *Shadow* is the belief that fat was natural, and thus was part of authentic personhood. As the writer Joan Dickenson (1983) put it,

> A woman is not a two-fold thing, a mind and a body – nor is the body a prison for the mind. We *are* our bodies. Hating *them* is hating *us*. Fat is not trivial issue. The reducing diet is as American as Thanksgiving turkey, and both are symbols of conquest, of the rape of a people.
>
> *(p. 37)*

Throughout the 1970s and 1980s, fat feminism emerged in feminist periodicals, in the first editions of the Boston Women's Health Collective *Our bodies, ourselves*, and even in the U.S. based National Organization for Women, which in 1988 passed an ordinance against size discrimination and began a body image task force. In the same year, activists Françoise Fraïoli and Anne Zamberlan founded Allegro Fortissimo in Paris (Allegro Fortissimo, 2018). While not explicitly feminist, Allegro Fortissimo provided the closest thing to fat feminism within French culture, a context that was, and is, extraordinarily fat phobic, as Gabrielle Deydier has outlined in her 2017 book on what she terms "grossophobia" in France (Marsh, 2017). Guyanese-British poet Grace Nichols's *The fat Black woman's poems* came out in the early 1980s, with its powerful statement in one of the poems, "This fat Black woman ain't no Jemima" (as cited in Farrell, 2011, p. 153). British activist Mary Evans Young began the International No Diet Day in 1992, which became an international celebration the year after. By the 1990s, zines had supplanted small periodicals as the media of choice for young, North American feminists, and numerous fat feminist publications resulted, including the Canadian group Pretty Porky and Pissed Off's *Double Double*, Marilyn Wann's *Fat!So?: For people who don't apologize for their size* (which later became a book), Nomy Lamm's *I'm So Fucking Beautiful* and the San Francisco collectively produced *Fat Girl: A zine for fat dykes and the women who want them.*

It's crucial to note that this predominantly white, North American genealogy is a historiographical result rather than a reflection of reality. That is, feminists of color have consistently articulated resistance to fat oppression, as illuminated by Johnnie Tillmon's 1972 *Ms.* Magazine quotation and the work of Grace Nichols in *The fat Black woman's poems*. Their activism, however, is part of a multi-faceted resistance to white patriarchy, rather than a laser focus on fatness. African American spoken word artist Sonya Renee Taylor's organization, The Body Is Not An

Apology, is a formidable example of this intersectional approach, with its focus on so many categories in which people experience "body terrorism" – weight and size, skin color, disability, gender, race, sexuality, age. Problematically, however, scholars within the academy have often failed to trace this multifaceted lineage of fat feminism, which has resulted in a picture of fat feminism that is incorrectly painted white.

Ongoing dilemmas

As with any social and intellectual movement, there are many ongoing dilemmas and debates both implicit and explicit within fat feminisms. The concept of the *natural* is a particularly vexing one. One of the most fundamental feminist arguments against fat oppression is that fatness is *natural* and that attempts to control or eliminate it are actions of an oppressive culture and society. We can trace a version of this back to the clothing reforms of the nineteenth century, when feminists like Amelia Bloomer fought for the right to eliminate restrictive corsets and allow their bodies free movement in trouser-like undergarments. Interestingly, not only did proponents of the new clothing style endure mocking and harassment when they ventured into public, they also received editorial censure from writers who abhorred the "Turkish pants," for "ruining" women's figures, meaning that the body was allowed to expand (Farrell, 2011). By the 1960s and 1970s, much of U.S. second wave feminism emphasized the body and the oppression of the beauty industries. Feminists across the spectrum (radical, liberal, cultural, socialist, African American, lesbian) and in various formats (*Ms.* magazine, Combahee River Collective, Redstockings, the protests against the Miss America Pageant) argued that the beauty industries exploited women financially, sapped their energy, turned them into objects for male pleasure, and hurt their bodies and souls (Farrell, 1998). There was an attempt by many to strip away the oppressive aspects of a beauty culture that hurt women, to locate a *more authentic and natural state* – thus the refusal to shave body hair, the decision to let one's hair grow into an Afro rather than using straightening products. This focus on the politics of the body and the beauty industry was particularly salient for fat women, who, as one activist put it, "replaced the Amazon warriors of feminism with our own image of enormous, soft earth mothers" (Farrell, 2011, p. 152). The writers in *Shadow on a tightrope* were particularly invested in concepts of the natural, seeking a language – "source of life, natural process, natural physical manifestation, enormous soft earth mother" – to claim the beauty and the integrity of their own bodies, to describe a place free of physical, emotional, cultural, medical and economic brutality that had been wielded against their bodies, against their *selves*. If dominant culture has historically understood fat as a sign of a primitive body, one that was uncivilized, uncultured, and outside propriety, this anecdote suggests that when fat feminism emerged it did not necessarily reject the earlier configuration of weight, it just reversed the meaning. Nature was now good, as it meant women could love each other and love fat. While the example I use here is the 1980s *Shadow on a tightrope*, this idea is alive and well, I would argue, informing both the position of the Health at Every Size paradigm to the protagonist in Sarai Walker's dynamic and riveting novel *Dietland* (2015), whose pivotal epiphany that her *real life* is a fat life happens when she spies a pubic hair, "black and spindly as a spider's leg," on the toilet seat—another sign of a natural body unconstrained by the dictates of commercial, patriarchal culture (p. 148).

While many fat feminists have drawn – and continue to draw – on the ideas of nature and biology to resist what they saw as colonizations of patriarchy, racism, technology, and corporate greed *into and onto* their own bodies, other fat feminists have challenged the use of the natural. Indeed, the concept of naturalness has been resoundingly criticized by feminist, queer, and postmodern critics who challenge the notion of any "authentic" or "real" existence. Rather, these theorists argue, experience, perception and identities are continually and fundamentally shaped by culture and discourse. Crucially, these arguments continue, this evocation of the "natural" also reinforces essentialist, and usually white, ideas about womanhood and femaleness, ones based on the tyranny of the binary, compulsory cis-femininity and heterosexuality. Queer and trans feminisms often emphasize the *choice* to be different from however "nature" intended the body to be, the decision to *defy* normative expectations, to willfully, defiantly, reshape and play with the body. Interestingly, though, the fact of bodily signification remains intact: the fat queer body means opposition/resistance/a rejection of normative boundaries and expectations, and often a celebration of the abject. This, however, produces yet another quandary: for opposition/resistance/rejection to exist, the opposed and resisted must *also* exist – thus the "normative" is evoked with every act of rejection. And perhaps more theoretically troubling, as Katie LeBesco (2014) has challenged in her provocative work, what separates fat people's desire for body modification (i.e. dieting, thinning regimes, and surgery) and trans people's desire for body altering surgery and hormone treatment? The struggles of fat people and trans people cannot be conflated, of course; the cultural punishments are not the same for fat and trans people, nor are there the same kind of pressures to perform the "right" body for fat cis-gendered people as for transgendered fat or thin people. Nevertheless, LeBesco raises questions that complicate theoretical and practical concerns about body modification and transgression.

There is yet another perspective voiced by some fat feminists that suggests a way out of these quandaries – eliding the body/self split, the naïve evocation of the natural, and the limiting claim to the oppositional. Sojourner Truth spoke to this in her 1851 speech when she exclaimed, "Look at my arm! I have ploughed, and planted, and gathered into barns, and no man could head me! And a'n't I a woman? I could work as much and eat as much as a man – when I could get it – and bear de lash as well! And a'n't I a woman? (as cited in Guy-Sheftal, 1995, p. 36). In other words, the body is not a trustworthy signifier of identity or status. Substantia Jones, in her mesmerizingly engaging photography, plays with these lines consistently, challenging and blurring and questioning the boundaries among the "natural," the "contrived," the "beautiful," the "queer," the "norm." Sonya Renee Taylor, in her poetry and her website "The Body is Not An Apology," tells us what the body in all its manifestations and attributes (size, color, gender, age) is *not*, an apology, an "I'm sorry" for not meeting cultural standards necessary for full citizenship and belonging. And in refusing that apology (echoes of Marilyn Wann here), she refuses that split between body and self. Like Jones, however, she leaves more ambiguous what the body does signify: Beauty? Pain? Confusion? Joy? Delight? A shifting repertoire of experience and meaning? But nothing that would signify anything less than status as a full human being.

One final note is relevant to the discussion of fat and feminism is the growing body positivity movement. In a context where many countries have extraordinary rates of anorexia and body dissatisfaction among girls and women, in which 80 percent of those undergoing weight loss surgery are women, despite even rates of fatness among men and women, and in which the "war on fat" often translates to a war on women and children, it would at first seem that any attempts – from the Dove Beauty Campaign to body positivity blogs and sorority-sponsored Fat Talk Free Weeks – to challenge this pervasive fat stigma would be good (Herndon, 2014; Ward, 2015). As *Bitchmedia* writer Evette Dionne (2017) has noted, however, body positivity that focuses solely on fashion and feeling good about one's body, one that emphasizes the joy of spending and that fits squarely within a capitalist market, has little ability to challenge institutional discrimination, to champion disability rights, or to identify and resist the ways that fat stigma intersects with racism, patriarchy, and growing economic inequalities. Fat feminisms have the potential and the power to articulate a vision of justice and equality far greater than a slender body positivity or a narrow achievement feminism.

Acknowledgement: The author wishes to thank Kayleigh Rhatigan, Dickinson College '19, for help in completing the formatting and citations.

References

Allegro Fortissimo. (2018). Présentation. http://www.allegrofortissimo.com

Beale, F. (1995). Double jeopardy: To be black and female. In B. Guy-Sheftal (Ed.), *Words of fire: An anthology of African-American feminist thought* (pp. 146–156). New York: The New Press.

Bordo, S. (2003). *Unbearable weight: Feminism, western culture, and the body*. Berkeley, CA: University of California Press.

Brown, L. S. (2003). *The politics of individualism: Liberalism, liberal feminism and anarchism*. Montréal: Black Rose Books.

Chastain, R. (2015, November 9). The thin woman inside lie. *Dances With Fat*. https://danceswithfat. wordpress.com/2015/11/09/the-thin-woman-inside-lie/

Cooper, C. (2016). *Fat activism: A radical social movement*. Bristol: HammerOn Press.

Crenshaw, K. (1991). Mapping the margins: Intersectionality, identity politics, and violence against women of color. *Stanford Law Review, 43*(6), 1241–1299.

Dickenson, J. (1983). Some thoughts on fat. In L. Schoenfielder, & B. Wieser (Eds.) *Shadow on a tightrope: Writings by women on fat oppression* (pp. 37–51). San Francisco, CA: Aunt Lute Books.

Dionne, E. (2017, November 21). The fragility of body positivity: How a radical movement lost its way. *Bitchmedia*. https://www.bitchmedia.org/article/fragility-body-positivity

Dowd, K. E. (2016, April 10). Oprah Winfrey says Weight Watcher opportunity "felt like an intervention from on high." *People*. http://www.people.com/article/oprah-winfrey-talks-weight-watchers-body-image-super-soul-sessions

Eisenstein, Z. (1986). *The radical future of liberal feminism*. Boston: Northeastern University Press.

Farrell, A. E. (1998). *Yours in sisterhood: Ms. Magazine and the promises of popular feminism*. Chapel Hill, NC: University of North Carolina.

Farrell, A. E. (2011). *Fat shame*. New York: New York University Press.

Federici, S. (2004). *Caliban and the witch: Women, the body and primitive accumulation*. Brooklyn, NY: Autonomedia.

Fishman, S. G. B. (1998). Life in the fat underground. *Radiance, Winter*(5). http://www.radiancemagazine. com/issues/1998/winter_98/fat_underground.html.

Guy-Sheftal, B. (Ed.) (1995). *Words of fire: An anthology of African-American feminist thought*. New York: The New Press.

Herndon, A. M. (2014). *Fat blame*. Lawrence, KS: University Press of Kansas.

Hines, R. (2016, March 11). Oprah unveils her weight loss transformation, talks "best body" in O. *Today*. https:// www.today.com/health/oprah-unveils-her-weight-loss-transformation-talks-best-body-o-t79376

Hobson, J. (2005). *Venus in the dark*. New York: Routledge.

Jones, K. (1974). Fat women and feminism. *Connecticut NOW Newsletter*, October–November. Fat Liberation Archives. http://www.eskimo.com/~largesse/Archives/CTNOW.html.

Kent, L. (2001). Fighting abjection: Representing fat women. In J. E. Braziel, & K. LeBesco (Eds.), *Bodies out of bounds: Fatness and transgression* (pp. 130–150). Berkeley, CA: University of California Press.

King, D. K. (1995). Multiple jeopardy, multiple consciousness: The context of black feminist ideology. In B. Guy-Sheftal (Ed.), *Words of fire: An anthology of African-American feminist thought* (pp. 294–319). New York: The New Press.

LeBesco, K. (2003). *Revolting bodies? The struggle to redefine fat identity*. Amherst, MA: University of Massachusetts Press.

LeBesco, K. (2014). On fatness and fluidity: A meditation. In C. Pausé, J. Wykes, & S. Murray (Eds.), *Queering fat embodiment* (pp. 49–60). Burlington, VT: Ashgate.

Let's Move! Campaign (2014, October 1). Learn the facts. http://www.letsmove.gov/learn-facts/epidemic-childhood-obesity

Marsh, S. (2017, September 10). Gabrielle Deydier: What it's like to be fat in France. *The Observer*. https://www.theguardian.com/society/2017/sep/10/gabrielle-deydier-fat-in-france-abuse-grossophobia-book-women

Millman, M. (1980). *Such a pretty face: Being fat in America*. New York: Norton.

Nash, J. (2008). Re-thinking intersectionality. *Feminist Review, 89*(1), 1–15.

Nichols, G. (1984). *The fat black woman remembers*. London: Virago Press.

Orbach, S. (1978). *Fat is a feminist issue: A self-help guide for compulsive eaters*. New York: Paddington Press.

Orbach, S. (1982). *Fat is a feminist issue II: A program to conquer compulsive eating*. New York: Berkeley Books.

Politico. (2014, October 2). Michelle Obama works out on *The Biggest Loser*. http://www.politico.com/multimedia/video/2012/04/michelle-obama-works-out-on-the-biggest-loser.html

Purkiss, A. (2017). "Beauty secrets: Fight fat": Black women's aesthetics, exercise, and fat stigma, 1900–1930s. *Journal of Women's History, 29*(2), 14–37.

Rich, A. (1980). Compulsory heterosexuality and lesbian existence. *Signs, 5*(4), 631–660.

Rothblum, E., & Solovay, S. (Eds.) (2009). *The fat studies reader*. New York: New York University Press.

Schoenfielder, L., & Wieser, B. (Eds.) (1983). *Shadow on a tightrope: Writings by women on fat oppression*. San Francisco, CA: Aunt Lute Books.

Stewart, M. (1995). Lecture delivered at the Franklin Hall, Boston, September 21, 1832. In B. Guy-Sheftal (Ed.), *Words of fire: An anthology of African-American feminist thought* (p. 32). New York: The New Press.

Tillmon, J. (1972). Welfare as a woman's issue. *Ms.*, Spring, 111.

Tong. R. (2009). *Feminist thought: A more comprehensive introduction*. Boulder, CO: Westview Press.

Truth, S. (1995). Woman's rights. In B. Guy-Sheftal (Ed.), *Words of fire: An anthology of African-American feminist thought* (p. 36). New York: The New Press.

Walker, S. (2015). *Dietland*. Boston, MA: Houghton Mifflin Harcourt.

Ward, B. (2015, April 29). Why do obese men get bariatric surgery far less than women? *UC San Diego Health*. https://health.ucsd.edu/news/releases/Pages/2015-04-29-men-less-likely-to-have-bariatric-surgery.aspx

Whitesel, J. (2014). *Fat gay men: Girth, mirth, and the politics of stigma*. New York: New York University Press.

Wykes, J. (2014). Introduction: Why queering fat embodiment? In C. Pausé, J. Wykes, & S. Murray (Eds.), *Queering fat embodiment* (pp. 1–12). Burlington, VT: Ashgate.

7

BIG, FAT, GREEK MODERNITIES

On fatness, Western imperatives and modern Greek culture

Sofia Apostolidou

In this chapter, I explore the relationship between Westernisation imperatives and the representation of fatness by looking at what I describe as the liminal cultural space that forms modern Greek national identity. In order to help untangle the complex web of national narratives and how they relate to fatness, I examine a film from the early 00s, seminal in how it represents Greek imaginings around modernity and embodiment. I argue that the representation, and thus stereotypes, oppression and embodiment, of fatness is closely tied with cultural specificity. I mean this not in the general sense of different cultural approaches, but instead, with the very mechanisms that produce national narratives of identity in the Western world. As a fat researcher from Greece, utilising work mostly from the English-speaking paradigm, I have frequently found my own experiences tugging at the corners of the theory I am using; they fit, but not exactly. My research applies current fat scholarship to the Greek paradigm with a twofold aim. On one hand, I aim to destabilise the popularised idea of a dichotomy that places fatphobia in supposedly uniform West and fat appreciation in a nebulous Rest. On the other, I am trying to demonstrate how an identity so complex, situated and fluid as fatness can be explored in order to illuminate and nuance not only itself, but also a series of broader concepts and categorisations.

Why Greece?

Greece is positioned within a nefarious loop of indistinguishable origins. The narrative that wants Greece as the motherland of Western civilisation was offered by the dominant powers of the eighteenth-century West to the agents of the nascent Modern Greek State. As Anastasia Karakasidou (1998) explained, "In a sense, the nation of the Hellenes, is a conceptual entity entirely distinct from the citizens of Greece" (p. 26). Greek national identity is as much the result of the imaginings of the West as anything else. This produces a never-ending circle that feeds Western fantasies about Greece, and Greek fantasies about itself. Michael Herzfeld (2009) talked about "the curious paradox of Greece, at once the collective spiritual ancestor and a political pariah in today's 'fast-capitalist' Europe" (p. 345). This peculiar positioning of Greece within the dominant Western imagination produces interesting anomalies in how fatness is viewed and experienced within the Greek context. However, what I aim to show with this analysis is that these anomalies are not necessarily Greece-specific. I am using Greece as a specific example of a paradox: simultaneously the *cradle* and the *backwaters* of modernity, to illustrate how situated understandings of fatness are, and how closely connected they are to narratives of modernity and Western-ness.

What is fat (Baby don't hurt me)

As a budding Fat Studies scholar, I spent a significant amount of time trying to define what fatness exactly is, in an effort to situate this embodiment outside of personal shame, and into a collective political identity. As someone whose experiences and even native language did not necessarily exactly match that of the scholarship available to me, attempting to crystallise fatness into a coherent concept was particularly important. Fatness however, intense as it might be as a personal embodiment, proves to be rather elusive in definition. For Charlotte Cooper (2010), fat is "a fluid subject position relative to social norms, it relates to shared experience, is ambiguous, has roots in identity politics and is thus generally self-defined" (1020). Marilyn Wann, on the other hand, described how, "in a fat-hating society everyone is fat. Fat functions as a floating signifier, attaching to individuals based on a power relationship, not a physical measurement" (p. xiv).

This ambiguity, often necessary when analysing fatness, is also found in Samantha Murray's work (2016), in which she warned against situating the mind as the center of political change, as a continuation of a problematic mind/body split and an individualist perception that the main intention of fat liberation is the ability to *personally* change the way we view ourselves. Dismantling the idea that one's embodied experience can simply shift by exercising mind over matter perception, Murray turned to Merleau Ponty to remind us of the "fundamental ambiguity that marks our lived experience in the world, where we are subjects 'in ourselves' *and* 'subjects for others'". What is often neglected in the individualist politics of the Size Acceptance movement then, is the "irrevocability of intersubjectivity in our being in the world. We understand the world through our bodies and through our interactions with others, and we make meaning from these constant encounters" (Murray, p. 6). Following this perspective of how intensely interconnected the ways fatness is experienced and viewed are, I would like to explore how embodied ambiguities can arise when approaching representations of fat embodiment that do not come from the dominant, English speaking paradigm. While the area of my analysis, Greece, is still part of the West, belonging to the same cultural and political paradigm as scholarship and representation from the English speaking world, I hope to demonstrate how, on one hand, even slight cultural shifts can have a big influence on how fatness is perceived and experienced, and on the other, how local perspectives can destabilise what we think of as a uniform West.

Greece is then seemingly a part of the uniform "Western" society, but simultaneously a place where "Westerness," "Europeaness," or "modernity" are not seen as historically unchallenged identities but are instead entangled in a complicated web of cultural debt and initiative. In a first attempt to untangle this complicated relationship, I will analyze a specific cultural object that, in embracing Murray's ambiguity, portrays feminine fatness as simultaneously oversexualised and desexualised/ridiculed. I argue that this ambiguity not only has a lot to say about Greece and its specific geo-cultural formation, but has a lot to offer to fat scholarship and activism, by complicating the extremely different embodied experiences one can have even in the perceived "West."

Big fat Greek modernities

As several authors have demonstrated, the current Greek national narrative is as constructed as it is ambivalent (Karakasidou, 1997; Gourgouris, 1996). In "The Nation Has Two Voices" Tzanelli (2008) has examined the construction of the Greek national narrative as something which, in its *diforia*, "informs and is informed by the emergence of imagined communities through the private construction of historical autobiographies" (p. 505). *Diforia*, the split meaning of utterance and performativity in public, is a characteristic of nations with *crypto-colonial* encounters. *Crypto-colonialism* then is "a claim to national independence grounded in an idiom of cultural and territorial integrity largely modeled on Western exemplars . . . and restricted by the practical needs and intentions of the Western colonial powers. These claims, moreover, generated subordinate forms of colonialism" (Herzfeld, 2009).

How is one to speak about fatness within a Greek context, when the word *Greek* is loaded with contradictory signifiers? I analyze a scene in the popular Greek film *To Klama Vgike Ap' Ton Paradiso* (2001), which parodies popular tropes of the 1960s, the so-called golden era of Greek cinema.[1] Following the tradition of Cultural Analysis, (Bal & Gonzales, 2006), I use this film not as an example or a case study, but rather as an interactive illustration. The film itself unfolds its meaning under the scrutiny of theoretical examination, while, at the same time, my theoretical framework shifts and is informed by the analysis of the film.

One of the main characters of *To Klama*, Djella Dellafrangka, a depraved, rich, Westernised woman, frequents a *koutouki*[2] in order to satisfy her fetish for working-class men. Dellafrangka's character is a reference to the main character of a film shot in the 1960s, with one significant difference: the original character, portrayed by Mary Chronopoulou was thin, while Mirka Papakonstantinou, the actress portraying Djella, is fat. Clad in a red dress, Djella dances a seductive tsifteteli, singing about the boy that lit a fire within her. After every verse, the choir of the men in the *koutouki* hopefully ask Djella "Is it me?" Djella saucily rejects them. The "boy" in question plays the bouzouki, exchanging looks with Djella as she hypnotises the crowd with her bosom, ultimately causing the men to fall from their seats, with a series of well-aimed, bosom-centered dance moves. Djella's excessive, red hot femininity has turned the place upside down.

At first, Djella's fatness is the butt of a fatphobic joke: it is "funny" that slender, waifish Chronopoulou has been replaced with round, curvaceous Papakonstantinou. Yet, there is something undeniably celebratory about the way she is portrayed. As the scene progresses, her influence on the male characters gets more and more comical; the joke is no longer on her but the on the male population and its complete surrender to Djella's power. I want to examine this paradoxical coexistence of Djella's fatness as simultaneously ridiculous to sexualise and also directly sexualised. Greek narratives, I argue, unknowingly treat thinness as part of the state's Westernisation/modernisation initiative, in which case fat femininity is an all too visible threat to the Nation's "private construction of historical autobiographies" (Tzanelli, 2008, p. 505). At the same time, oversexualising fatness as part of this tradition can coexist with the thin modernisation initiative, in what Tzanelli (2006/2008) described as "oscillation between subordination to European demands and resistance to them" that is "often typical of anti-imperial nationalism" (Tzanelli, 2006, p. 34).

Dellafrangka's femininity is the operating field of a fatness that renders her both transparent and opaque to the desires of the Nation. Several points are projected on the abundance of her red-clad embodiment: Isn't it hilarious, the narrative implies, that the embodiment of modernisation has been replaced with this jolly fat woman? Doesn't she remind you of these times we've left behind? Isn't it funny how she's playing the object of desire, instead of ridicule? But, oh, what times they were, in their tradition of merriment and excess!

It is not by accident that Djella dances a *tsifteteli*, a popular, sexual Greek dance heavily influenced by Ottoman and Arab traditions. Stavros Stavrou Karayanni (2007) has analyzed the politics of *tsifteteli* and the discomforts caused by its "Oriental associations", which:

> hark back to the Ottoman occupation of Greece that lasted nearly four centuries—a chapter in the nation's history that is recounted as the most bitter and hurtful—yet they

also relate to the fervent desire for a modern Greek identity that is completely uncon-
nected with the Orient and firmly identifies, instead, with European civilization.

(p. 122)

It is highly indicative of the convoluted sense of self intrinsic to the Greek national narrative
that the very agent of modernity in this scene, Djella, dances a particularly Ottoman dance. In
the particular way that Greece cannot firmly situate itself within the either/or of modernity
and Western-ness, fatness and its representation follow suit. Caught in the oscillation between
differently coded signifiers, Greek fatness, especially fat femininities, emerge as a field of familiar contestation. The decision to put fat femininity and *tsifteteli* together in the same scene is
thus informed by a series of complicated motives. As if a second layer of discomfort must be
anticipated and dispersed, the fat lady and the oriental dance lend each other credibility as well
as ridicule, creating a cinematic experience that allows its Greek audience to both relish the
depiction of the "good old times" *and* to ridicule them, thus reaffirming a right to Western
claims. Utterance and performativity seem to dance their *diforic* dance alongside Djella, constantly swapping roles: is the utterance "Westernised" fatphobia and the performativity "tradi-
tionalist" appreciation, or the other way round?

The manner in which Djella's fat embodiment blurs, complicates and intervenes for the
Greek modernisation narrative can be traced to the problematics of the Greek narrative, and its
complicated relationship with linearity and transition to modernity, inclusion into Western-ness,
and the relationship with colonialism. I suggest that Djella's fatness is situated at the center of
such a diforic act of self-narration, with its contradictory meaning being directly connected to
the Greek attempt to claim its position in a Western narrative of Europeanness and modernisation, while at the same time retaining a narrative of national pride, authenticity, and historical
linearity. Thus, exploring fat embodiment and its representation not only illuminates fatness
itself and its subsequent oppression, but also complicates our understanding of wider concepts
such as modernity and Western-ness.

Notes

1 Featuring a star ensemble cast and written/directed by Thanasis Reppas and Michalis Papathanasiou.
The title is a parody of *To Ksilo Vgike Ap' ton Paradeiso* (1959).
2 Traditional, usually working-class frequented spaces, offering food and entertainment.

References

Bal, M., & Gonzales, B. (2006). *The practice of cultural analysis: Exposing interdisciplinary interpretation*. Stan-
ford: Stanford University Press.
Camp, J., Piening, H., Primavesi, O., Brinkmann, V., Dreyfus, R., & Koch-Brinkmann, U. (2017). *Gods
in color polychromy in the ancient world*. München: Prestel.
Cooper, C. (2010). Fat studies: Mapping the field. *Sociology Compass*, 4(12), 1020–1034.
Gourgouris, S. (1996). *Dream nation: Enlightenment, colonization, and the institution of modern Greece*. Stanford,
CA: Stanford University Press.
Herzfeld, M. (2009). The absent presence. In D. Saurabh (Ed.), *Enchantments of modernity: Empire, nation,
globalization* (pp. 341–371). New York: Routledge.
Karakasidou, A. N. (1998). *Fields of wheat, hills of blood: Passages to nationhood in Greek Macedonia, 1870–
1990*. Chicago: University of Chicago Press.
Karayanni, S. S. (2007). *Dancing fear & desire: Race, sexuality, and imperial politics in Middle Eastern dance*.
Waterloo Ont.: Wilfrid Laurier University Press.
Murray, S. (2016). *The "fat" female body*. Basingstoke: Palgrave Macmillan.
Reppas, M., & Papathanasiou, T. (Directors). (2001). *To Klama Vgike Ap' Ton Paradiso* [Video].

Rothblum, E. D., & Solovay, S. (2009). *The fat studies reader.* New York: New York University Press.

Tzanelli, R. (2006). "Not My Flag!" Citizenship and nationhood in the margins of Europe (Greece, October 2000/2003). *Ethnic and Racial Studies, 29*(1), 27–49.

Tzanelli, R. (2008). The nation has two "voices". *European Journal of Cultural Studies, 11*(4), 489–508.

Wann, M. (2009). Foreword. Fat Studies: An invitation to revolution. In E. D. Rothblum, & S. Solovay (Eds.) *The fat studies reader* (pp. ix–xxv). NYU Press.

8

DOES THAT MEAN MY BODY MUST ALWAYS BE A SOURCE OF PAIN?

Sexual violence, trauma and agency in Argentinian fat activist spaces

Laura Contrera

Fat people who suffer from sexual violence face a double silencing: on top of the fear of not being a credible victim, they must also experience the anguish of being ridiculed for the size of their bodies. Both mass media and those in the health and judicial sectors reproduce a violent, discriminating and stigmatizing logic when they listen to the victims. There is even a certain kind of feminism that favours a tunnel vision of the phenomenon by not making room for fat voices. Fat activism spaces are a place where, through the narration of violence, trauma enters into the political arena. In Argentina, since 2015, the collective work on fat policies, partnering with other movements of body, gender and sexual diversity, flourished into forms of resistance and agency whose story deserves to be told.

I am a cisgender and bisexual woman who has survived sexual abuse. I was 20 years old and in therapy when I was first able to speak about my experience, because that is the way the device of feminization works – we are ordered to remain silent (Contrera, 2018a; Despentes, 2006). I had written about paedophilia and the consequences of sexual violence during childhood and adolescence in a fanzine I published for many years, but I was not able to actually put my fat body into words. I needed fat activism to come into my life so I could give voice to this intersection that exists in my flesh. The story I am telling is personal, but it is also the story of many other fat people around the world.

I have been coordinating workshops for fat people and giving talks for almost 10 years. Sometimes I do it on my own, but I currently prefer to do all this with the fat activism collective I am part of, "Taller Hacer la Vista Gorda". Among the multiple experiences of human rights violations we share in these spaces for reflection, sexual violence is perhaps the most frequent narrative. Apart from the pain and silence that are usually associated with the experience of abuse, there is also the fear of cruel derision and the stigmatizing inquiry by the police and those in the medical and judicial sectors, who should instead listen empathetically without discriminating. For instance, a girl who had reported she had been raped in a disco was exposed to public scorn in the mass media, where anybody was able to call her victim status into question, just for being fat. Because being fat is having a body that is guilty, failed and abject (Murray,

2008), diseased and deformed (Braziel, 2001). And we know that must mean being undesirable and incapable of being raped.

A court from Puerto Madryn, a city in the south of Argentina, decided to acquit a man accused of having raped his fat ex-partner. This sentence made the news thanks to the argument of the official lawyer for the accused, which revolved around the fatness of the victim and the supposed inability of the presumed perpetrator, who was much thinner, to take her leggings off. "Where are the leggings?" asked the lawyer, adding that, if the victim was really forced to take them off, they should have been ripped apart. The emphasis on the leggings as evidence – described as a quasi-medieval contraption, impossible to remove without consent – proves that certain bodies should not wear certain clothes if they do not want to be ridiculed or if they intend to be credible victims for the punitive state machinery. Beyond the analysis the sentence itself deserves, the most sinister thing about the lawyer's argument is that, beyond the farfetched imagination her formulation requires, it appeals to a violent, discriminating and stigmatizing sense that should not have any place in courtrooms (Contrera, 2018a).

There are no statistics that mention anything about this double silencing those of us who have survived sexual abuse as fat people suffer, but the marks of violence engraved on our flesh and of the "struggle to be believed" (Beety, 2013, p. 526) sting again. They remain like Chiron's wound which never heals and are constantly renewed in the face of every institutional and individual affront that puts our own body experience into question and jeopardizes it.

Violence, power, domination

Fatness automatically withdraws us from the market of hegemonic desire, pushing us to the margins of what is possible. We, fat bodies, are not saleable goods in the mainstream sexual market (Murray, 2008). But we must also take into account another fact of reality that is easy to check: we as fat people are also abused while being fat. Because rape does not have anything to do with desire, but with submission, even though the dominant sense insists on keeping both of those terms together, especially when fatness is involved.

I understand sexual violence as an act of power that utilizes sexuality to guarantee the perpetuation of relations of dominance and submission (Weeks, 2011). We may think along the lines of Ahmed (2004) that sexual violence involves forms of power that are visceral and bodily, as well as social and structural. Vulnerability is not a feature any more inherent to a particular kind of body, but rather an effect that serves to assure certain bodies occupy a defined position. The feminist perspective is accurate when it points out that the fear of a future injury works as a form of violence in the present (Ahmed, 2004), as a call to the hierarchical order of bodies.

Sexual violence against fat bodies is an urgent problem that has not been deemed worthy of thoughtful reflection outside activism or Fat Studies, by which I mean a reflection that avoids the traps of fatphobia and embraces the complexities and intersectionalities of bodies. Even feminism has been mistaken about its approach in this point – in a wide range going from Orbach to Despentes, the idea that fat little girls get fat to avoid being further abused and that the unbearable weight is a way of performing our suffering. That way, it seems we accumulate fat excessively because we are looking to create an armour to protect from mistreatment and the chance of new abusive encounters. Fat conceals us and separates us from the world of patriarchal desire. As female fatties, we are simply bound to the mechanism that limits us to being eternal suffering victims: first, by the abuse of the rest and then of our own calorie abuse. At some point, we are always responsible for our restrictions and guilty of our own unhappiness, just for having a weight that society considers to be excessive and harmful.

Generally, every stray from the feminine-hetero-cis norm, from hysteria to lesbianism, has been associated with a pathology. As Royce (2009) says, research that establishes the traumatic consequences of childhood sexual abuse and sexual assault is important. However, it is complicated to suggest that the fat body is only a pathology that emerges in the aftermath of male-perpetrated violence against children or women (Braziel & LeBesco, 2001). This discourse is based on the positing of the body as something symptomatic (Braziel & LeBesco, 2001) and is not the kind of feminism that actually accepts fatness as one of its issues. This discourse fails at reporting what it means to incarnate a fat body because it does not listen to the voices of fat people, as Cooper has rightly said (2016) when tracing back the roots of fat activism in other feminisms and radical social movements.

Royce (2009) points out that violence affects fat women in ways specific to their size, but also fat women are sometimes targeted for violence precisely because of their size. We must also take into account the experiences from other sexual and gender identities and geopolitical contexts, since it is clear that feminism does not stop at the "woman" subject that is heterosexual, cisgender, white, able, middle-class and from the Global North. Therefore, apart from qualitative and quantitative intersectional research (Royce, 2009), we need to provide more opportunities for fat people to share their truths, be they academic or not (Pausé, 2014).

Trauma, narration, agency

The "Encuentros Nacionales de Mujeres" are a key instance to understand the current Argentinian feminist scene considering its wide participation, visibility and renowned importance both regionally and internationally. These summits have been carried out since 1986 in a self-convened, horizontal, federal, self-funded, plural and democratic way. It is estimated that on the first summit 1000 people assisted, a number that has grown to more than 70,000 in 2017. In this year, a fat activism workshop took place for the first time in the history of the meetings. The inclusion of this space was not easy and required a great struggle from the activist collective "Taller Hacer la Vista Gorda", born in Buenos Aires in 2015. The struggle implied an end to being a subtopic within the body workshop and the creation of a specific space to debate issues related to the politicization of fatness (Contrera, 2018b).

In the massive workshops that ultimately took place in the Argentinian cities of Resistencia (2017) and Trelew (2018), cis and trans women, lesbians, bisexuals and non-binaries from all over the vast Argentinian territory, but also from neighbouring countries, shared countless experiences of violence and discrimination. We talked about cross oppressions that make our lives less bearable, by stopping us from accessing and enjoying fundamental rights: the right to health, to employment, to education, to housing, to transport, to the city, to the autonomy and integrity of the body, but also to public movement devoid of violence, even in the markets of affection and desire. What we passionately argued can be summarized in the combined aspiration to materialize the right to live a life free of violence and stigma with the bodies we currently have (Contrera, 2018b).

During the two days we came together in the workshop, the traumatic experiences of abuse were overwhelming. All types of sexual violence were presented right next to the long chain of violence which is common for physiques and identities disqualified on the basis of gender or sexual orientation, but also due to their ethnic or racial background, class, age, migration status or abilities: physical, psychological, symbolic, verbal and economic violence and stalking and harassment either by people from their intimate environment or strangers. On top of that, the humiliating treatment received when looking for therapeutic or institutional help was also present, an issue that has been discussed in the literature originating from Fat Studies (see Ernsberger, 2009; Saguy, 2013, among others).

To speak about those experiences meant bringing the wound and its implied history of damage into the political realm, to envisage a common horizon from that pain or, rather, from its translation into the public and shared space (Ahmed, 2004). The stories that were shared in the workshop, beyond their differences and peculiarities, were connected: "our pain is more than personal – it is social, it is political" (Hannah, 1983, p. 137). Towards the end of the first day, an emotional atmosphere settled in – the certainty that something had finally been said. And it had been said by us, in the first-person singular and plural. The fatal knot of silence had been untangled by establishing a connection between the persistent but indefinite "feeling bad" (Cvetkovich, 2003, p. 3) and the efforts from the bodily device (Costa & Rodríguez, 2010), colonialism and "lean neoliberalism" (Contrera & Cuello, 2016, p. 127), which depict us as failed subjectivities and unhappy or improper body styles.

A source of pain overflowing

The conclusions that were the outcome of the collective work in the workshop in 2017 read: "We shout: desire is not abuse; abuse is not desire. We, fat people, are also abused and our bodies are targets of violence" (Conclusiones Taller N° 71, 2017, p. 189). But the conclusions said many more things that refute the collapse of the fat body into the traumatized body that Braziel and LeBesco (2001) have rightly analysed. As such, the final document weaves political resistance propositions with reflections from the complexity of everyday life shared by the attendants of the Workshop, who said:

> We appropriate the word *fat*, we define ourselves as overflowing bodies, we choose to name ourselves dissidents and we consider our fights to be political weapons. We agree that there is a medical diet industry that profits from the pathologizing of fat bodies. We hold that body oppression does not occur equally in fat women and fat men, just as it occurs differently in cis people and trans people. We appropriate the insult and now "fat" is the name of our rebellion. We are no longer named by the social, medical and economic power. We name ourselves.
>
> *(Conclusiones Taller N° 71, 2017, p. 189)*

The productive and the collective resistance possibilities that arise when room is made for the congregation of bodies, where we can talk, cry, get angry and go through all the emotional repertoire that traumatic experiences of social injustice bring, giving a name and concept to the experiential narrative of fatness, are pure power. Our political emotions – plural, constantly disputed – and our politics make room for the promise of being part of a public culture around that trauma and stigma, which no longer involves medical diagnoses or (re-)victimizations (Cvetkovich, 2003), but is represented in networks of affinity, information circuits, discussion and action, regional agendas, alliances with other movements of body, gender and sexual diversity (Contrera, 2018b), such as the trans and intersex movements, in addition to intersecting with the demands expressed in the collective actions from feminism and the current Argentinian women's movement.[1]

What we experience in the rare massive intimacy of the workshop is that every experience matters: a personal story always has a place on a stage that is not strictly individual but social. Every experience matters as it can be read next to other stories that, though different, recognize a common origin in hierarchical forms of social relations, marked and produced in terms of gender, sexual orientation, class, age, ethnic and racial background and more, but also morphological and geopolitical. Maybe every story is at some point impossible to communicate, but that experience can be understood because there is a device that makes it legible and an activism that transforms it into action.

To those of us who have been prevented from talking and telling our traumatic stories for a long time, forgetting would mean a repetition of the violence (Ahmed, 2004). But to find one another also means that, even if the wound stings, our bodies must not always be a source of pain, as Bikini Kill's song goes. We are also a rebellion, a resistance overflowing and finding new canals for another possible world. One where, minimally, we, the victims, are believed without any need to fight.

Acknowledgments: I would like to thank Cat Pausé for inviting me to write about fat activism in the Global South. I thank all the people who have shared their stories and I celebrate us, because we have survived. An eternal acknowledgement to those who have not been able to.

Note

1   The manifestations of political mourning due to deaths at the hands of hetero-cis-patriarchal violence in Argentina, expressed in mobilizations of hundreds of thousands of people from 2015 on, acknowledge their genealogy not only in the women's movement, but also in the Mothers and Grandmothers of Plaza de Mayo and their relentless pursuit of memory, truth and justice, and movements for the human rights of LGBTQI people. I cannot address here the complexity of the intersections between local fat activism, feminisms and other movements given the text limits.

References

Ahmed, S. (2004). *The cultural politics of emotion*. New York: Routledge.

Beety, V. E. (2013). Criminality and corpulence: Weight bias in the courtroom. *Seattle Journal for Social Justice*, *11*(2:4), 523–553.

Braziel, J. E. (2001). Sex and fat chics: Deterritorializing the fat female body. In J. E. Braziel & K. LeBesco (Eds.), *Bodies out of bounds: Fatness and transgression* (pp. 231–254). Berkeley: University of California Press.

Braziel, J. E. & LeBesco, K. (2001). Introduction. In J. E. Braziel & K. LeBesco (Eds.), *Bodies out of bounds: Fatness and transgression* (pp. 1–15). Berkeley: University of California Press.

Conclusiones Taller N° 71, XXXII Encuentro Nacional de Mujeres (2017). https://drive.google.com/file/d/1RB6mLdvYshCDAWj3VWT04kl9SrmcKX6k/view?ts=5ba4d60f

Contrera, L. (2018a). Incogibles. *Las 12*. https://www.pagina12.com.ar/110905-incogibles

Contrera, L. (2018b). Una Resistencia que desborda: Apuntes afectivo-políticos sobre el primer taller de activismo gordo en el XXXII Encuentro Nacional de Mujeres cis y trans, Lesbianas, Bisexuales e identidades no-binarixs (Resistencia, Chaco, 2017). In D. Orosz (Ed.), *Libro catálogo Mercado de Arte Contemporáneo (MAC)* (pp. 21–25). Córdoba: Municipalidad de Córdoba y Fundación Pro Arte Córdoba.

Contrera, L. & Cuello, N. (2016). Neoliberalismo magro. In L. Contrera & N. Cuello, N. (Eds.), *Cuerpos sin patrones: Resistencias desde las geografías desmesuradas de la carne* (pp. 127–128). Buenos Aires: Madreselva.

Cooper, C. (2016). *Fat activism. A radical social movement*. Bristol: HammerOn Press.

Costa, F. & Rodríguez, P. E. (2010). La vida como información, el cuerpo como señal de ajuste: los deslizamientos del biopoder en el marco de la gubernamentalidad neoliberal. In V. Lemm (Ed.), *Michel Foucault: Neoliberalismo y biopolítica* (pp. 151–173). Santiago de Chile: Ediciones Universidad Diego Portales.

Cvetkovich, A. (2003). *An archive of feelings: Trauma, sexuality, and lesbian public cultures*. Durham, NC: Duke University Press.

Despentes, V. (2006). *King Kong théorie*. París: Editions Grasset et Fasquelle.

Ernsberger, P. (2009). Does social class explain the connection between weight and health? In E. Rothblum & S. Solovay (Eds.), *The fat studies reader* (pp. 25–36). New York: New York University Press.

Hannah, S. B. (1983). The human potential movement: Judging people's humanity by their looks. In L. Schoenfielder & B. Wieser (Eds.), *Shadow on a tightrope: Writings by women on fat oppression* (pp. 135–138). San Francisco: Aunt Lute Books.

Murray, S. (2008). *The "fat" female body*. New York: Palgrave Macmillan.

Pausé, C. J. (2014). X-static process: Intersectionality within the field of fat studies. *Fat Studies: An Interdisciplinary Journal of Body Weight and Society*, *3*(2), 80–85.

Royce, T. (2009). The shape of abuse: Fat oppression as a form of violence against women. In E. Rothblum & S. Solovay (Eds.), *The fat studies reader* (pp. 151–157). New York: New York University Press.

Saguy, A. C. (2013). *What's wrong with fat?* New York: Oxford University Press.

Weeks, J. (2011). *Lenguajes de la sexualidad*. Buenos Aires: Nueva Visión.

9

FATNESS AND CONSEQUENCES OF NEOLIBERALISM

Hannele Harjunen

Introduction

My aim in this chapter is to inspect how neoliberal economic policy and rationale are enmeshed with conceptions of body and health in the contemporary (primarily Western) cultural sphere and how they have been addressed in research literature, particularly concerning fatness and the fat body. The relationship between neoliberalism, fatness and the fat body will be examined in the light of feminist and Fat Studies scholarship (Guthman, 2009a, 2009b; Harjunen, 2017; LeBesco, 2011; Rothblum & Solovay, 2009).

Neoliberalism is a mode of economic liberalism and free market capitalism that has been the dominant economic policy since the 1980s, the logic, discourse and practices of which have been adopted globally (Harvey, 2007; Ventura, 2012). Neoliberal economic thinking underlines the free market, privatisation of the public domain, cost-effectiveness, productivity, and profit. As has been reported in recent years, social structures, institutions, and policies have been transformed by neoliberal policies around the world (Wrede et al., 2008).

However, neoliberalism does not only shape general structures, it influences our private lives and embodiment too (Guthman, 2009a; Harjunen, 2017). Patricia Ventura (2012) has suggested that the values and norms that are followed today are shaped by a neoliberal logic: people's everyday lives, including bodies, become organised and regulated according to its needs, values, and priorities.[1] Ventura refers to this organisation of social realities according to the neoliberal economic rationale as "neoliberal culture". My intention here is to discuss how fatness and fat bodies are understood and dealt with in neoliberal culture. My starting point here is that neoliberally attuned social institutions such as health care policies; or structures, such as health care systems; not to mention social, moral, and political orders of the day, all contribute to the shaping of acceptable bodies conceptually as well as physically.

In neoliberal culture the body is understood as an individualistic project one can choose and shape as one wishes. However, neither all choices concerning the body, nor all bodies, are seen as being as possible or legitimate as others. The embodied subject of neoliberal culture is supposed to replicate the core neoliberal values of freedom and choice. Neoliberal culture has its normative or "preferred" body, the norms of which are based on self-control, productivity, and individual morals. In order to become a successful neoliberal subject, ability to perform this ideal or preferred body is crucial. Achieving the preferred body requires self-monitoring or self-disciplinary behaviour and apparent failing in self-governing is interpreted as a social and moral failing that results in social sanctions.[2] In neoliberal culture, individuals are expected to constantly work on the body in order to prove themselves as responsible, productive and effective (Dworkin & Wachs, 2009; Gill, 2007, 2008; Heywood, 2007). Guthman (2009a, p. 193) has proposed that neoliberalism creates individuals who, through contradictory impulses of free choice and responsibility, become "hyper-vigilant of control and self-discipline". Brown (2003, p. 7) for their part has noted that in the neoliberal era people are "controlled through their freedom".

Although fatness has been regarded as an undesirable and stigmatised characteristic, and the fat body has been perceived as the unruly and excessive body for a long time (Braziel & LeBesco, 2001; Farrell, 2011; Huff, 2001; LeBesco, 2004), in neoliberal culture, fatness and fat bodies have become especially feared and reviled. The moral panic or the "fat panic" of the past two decades (Boero, 2012; Gard & Wright, 2005; LeBesco, 2010; Saguy, 2013) seems to suggest that the fat body has become emblematic of failure in the embodied performance of control and responsibility in today's society. Furthermore, in a society/culture that is organised by neoliberal ethos, the fat body is interpreted as a sign of (ir)responsibility in a broader context than an individual's personal life – it becomes a sign of whether or not one is a proper, deserving, and productive (neoliberal) citizen. It is almost as if the fat body is constructed as a kind of "anti-neoliberal" body.

Fatness and fat bodies have become a target of intensifying biopolitical control and neoliberal governing in the 2000s. This is illustrated in the way the need to "manage" or "govern" fatness is more and more justified by economic reasons. Fat people as a group are singled out as expensive. This costliness is constructed, for example, through the stereotype of fat people as ill, over-consuming, unproductive, and morally wanting. Fat people are seen as unproductive, ineffective and as a (public) expense. In public discourse the fat body is regularly used as a representation as well as a metaphor to represent and as a culprit of a "bloated" public economy, which is in need of cuts. Interventions that aim at changing the fat body are treated as analogous to interventions that are needed to fix the ailing public economy.[3] Even the terms used to discuss fatness come from the economic sphere such as a "risk", "surplus", "excess", "waste", and "burden".

While aiming to produce a certain type of controlled embodied subject, neoliberal rationale has added a new discursive layer to the theorisation of the body and fatness that focuses on productivity, individual responsibility, and morals. This not only has an effect on the way we think about bodies and how the body is experienced, but also on how certain bodies are selected to represent this culture while others are excluded or vilified (Wingard, 2013).

The obesity epidemic, healthism and governmentality

As is well known, the so-called obesity epidemic discourse has dominated reporting, research, and debate on fatness since the early 2000s. The obesity epidemic discourse relies on the bio-medical understanding of fatness as a curable disease-like condition that spreads uncontrollably and in epidemic proportions (Campos et al., 2006; Gard & Wright, 2005; Oliver, 2006). Besides constructing "obesity" as a pandemic, the obesity epidemic discourse has also promoted fatness as a social problem (LeBesco, 2011), a moral threat (Gard & Wright, 2005; Jutel, 2005), and an economic issue. Links between the obesity epidemic discourse and neoliberal economic policy have been observed in a number of studies (Ayo, 2012; Guthman & DuPuis, 2006; Harrison, 2012; LeBesco, 2011).

Governmentality, a term introduced first by Michel Foucault, refers to a regulatory form of power by which people are governed. Governmentality can take a number of forms and it can allude to a wide range of practices from political government, and biopolitical control to self-regulating practices (Foucault, 1991). According to Foucault, the purpose of governmentality is to increase the welfare of the population by "the improvement of its condition, the increase of its wealth, longevity, health" (Foucault as cited in Faubion, 1994, p. 217). Fatness is a target of intensive biopolitical governing, and in recent decades especially, repeated attempts to control and normalize the fat body have been made by public health officials and medical professionals in Finland, the UK, the USA, and Australia to name a few (Boero, 2012; Harjunen, 2017; Wright & Harwood, 2008).

While governmentality refers to the manner in which the welfare of the population is governed by the state, neoliberal governmentality refers to a style of governing that orientates itself to the market (Foucault, 1991; Lemke, 2001). This means, for example, that the tasks previously considered the responsibility of the state have been privatised or outsourced to the market. Neoliberal governmentality relies on the market to set the tone and to provide services, while at the same time emphasising the individual's own responsibility and control; i.e., the individual must be self-governing in this market environment (Guthman, 2009a). When governing becomes enmeshed with neoliberal capitalism, the individual's role becomes increasingly perceived as one of consumer and entrepreneur.

Thus, in the age of neoliberalism, biopolitical control too is neoliberal (Lemke, 2001). An illustrating example of this is that health is increasingly understood and discussed in terms of the economy whether we are talking about its structural, institutional, cultural, or individual aspects. Health has become economised and commercialised. Ideological kinship of healthism, tendency to understand health as one's primary task and individual's responsibility, and neoliberalism in particular have been observed (Ayo, 2012; Cheek, 2008; Crawford, 2006). The obesity epidemic discourse can be interpreted as a mode of neoliberal governmentality, which draws from healthism, "the ideology of individual responsibility" (Crawford, 2006, p. 409), and economisation and commercialisation of health and health care, all of which have been linked to neoliberal thought and policy.

In the context of healthism, health is understood as one's own responsibility and controllable. One is required to constantly "do" health. The latter demand would seem to fit particularly well with a neoliberal rationale in which the body is a target of intense self-discipline and self-governance and its value is measured by how effective and productive it appears. Via healthist thought and demands placed on the body, behaviour, and morals of the individual, neoliberal ideas can be transferred to the everyday personal management of the body. It could be said that the obesity epidemic discourse has been used to introduce neoliberal governmentality into thinking, living and experiencing the body (Guthman & DuPuis, 2006). This means all bodies, not just the fat body. By demonizing fatness, the obesity epidemic discourse has promoted fear and disgust of fatness and has thus promoted its stigmatisation further (Rail et al., 2010). At the same time people have been made increasingly responsible for their own health, despite many of the constituents of health such as social and economic factors that are often beyond the control of the individual (Sutton, 2010).

Fat, health, morals, and neoliberal economy

It could be argued that fatness and the fat body may be in the focus of such intense attention globally, because the effects of neoliberal culture become particularly visible and exploitable in the fat body (Guthman & DuPuis, 2006; Mäkelä & Niva, 2009) and in particular in its biomedical incarnation of "obesity", the diseased fat body. Markula (2008) claims that the roots of the obesity epidemic were economic. Guthman and DuPuis (2006) have put forth that neoliberalism is partly responsible for rising body weight of populations (widening income differences, cheap food low in nutrition, but high in calories etc.) and at the same time it produces it as a problem that needs to be dealt with. This would suggest that obesity as a problem is internal to the logic of neoliberalism. The neoliberal economic logic would encourage people to consume more, but at the same time it rewards those who are able to avoid what is interpreted as its physical signs. Paradoxically, the disciplining process would require further consumption (of health foods, exercise club memberships, diet plans, etc.). Harrison (2012, p. 331) has observed aptly that the diet industry turns "bodies into economic units from which profits can be reaped, despite its persistent failure to change bodies in the ways promised".

In the neoliberal economy, health care, social care, education, and welfare are all commodities that can be marketed, bought, or sold (Guthman & DuPuis, 2006). Consumption and one's role as a consumer are increasingly underlined even in the relationship between the citizen and the state. One becomes part of society first and foremost by being a good consumer and adopting an entrepreneurial approach to work, relationships and the body, and one's value to society increasingly depends on an individual's ability to produce and consume. If individuals are not capable of being productive enough (in market terms), or performing consistently as a consumer, their limited value and role in society is somehow justified.

In a society that is organised according to neoliberal principles, individuals need to adopt the logic of the market when they think about their health. Health is a value in itself, but it is also valuable in other ways. Health increases the (both symbolic and material) value of the body, which in itself is a product that can be created, sold, and optimised (Ventura, 2012). In neoliberal culture, health is therefore more than just about being healthy, it is considered to be an integral part of a highly performing individual. A healthy body is a condition for optimal productivity and cost-effectiveness. Certain bodies (whether they are deemed unhealthy, fat, aged, depressed, disabled or something else) prevent a person from achieving the optimal results that neoliberal citizenship requires, for example staying in the workforce for as long as possible, working as effectively (and as much) as possible, staying healthy through vigorous exercise and eating nutritiously, and needing as little social or publicly funded assistance as possible.

In effect, the value of an individual is based on an analysis of cost in which the logic of reverse thinking applies. The body is expected to be productive, cost-effective, and dynamic. The less the individual needs public services the more cost-effective and productive/profitable the individual appears from the state's point of view. However, the goal of neoliberal governmentality is not an individual who does not need or use any health care services. The goal is to create individuals who take responsibility over their health to such a point that they no longer feel the state has a duty to care for them. In this way, the entrepreneurial subject of neoliberal governmentality feels a moral obligation to manage one's own health.

Brown (2003) has observed that neoliberalism removes the barrier between morals and economics and creates a world wherein moral decisions are made through a cost-benefit analysis of what will affect the self. This relationship between economics and morals is embodied in the discussion concerning fatness, health and the economy. Bodies are evaluated as "good" or "bad" based on their apparent value (productivity) and/or their cost to society, which is based on their assumed health. Those bodies that are perceived as unhealthy are viewed as unproductive, expensive, and a burden to society, for their assumed costs to public health care. When people are categorised as expensive based on their personal characteristics, we are in effect evaluating people's status as socially acceptable citizens according to their cost to society.

Health has turned into a merit and a sign of moral and fiscal solvency. Responsibility is evaluated, not only as certain type of behaviour in moral terms, but also by one's estimated costliness to society that is read off the surface of the body. One's worthiness can be proven by morally virtuous behaviour. Those individuals/groups of people who are believed (or assumed) to take risks "willingly" or are seen as somehow "choosing" to make themselves ill by their irresponsible behaviour, do not get much sympathy.

Costs and investment

The need to battle the obesity epidemic is justified with the alleged financial cost that fat people cause in the form of public health expenses. Fatness features in neoliberal economics, not only via public sector health care expenses, but also via the consumption of a wide variety of commercial products and services. The catch in neoliberal health care is that whereas public spending on the care of individuals is calculated in terms of cost, their own spending on care and health is seen as an investment. The amount of money fat people spend in order to lose weight are one example of this kind of investment that individuals are supposed to make out of their own pocket. Harrison (2012, p. 321) notes that this construct of fat bodies as costly allows for corporations and governments to "exploit some for the enrichment of others while reaping economic benefit from activities that harm human health to do so in relative impunity".

Costliness and cost-effectiveness readily become moral terms when talked about in the neoliberal context of using public funds. Costing money to the state and "making other people pay for your allegedly bad choices" through taxation becomes a moral question. Consumption is the key here and the fact that health has become about consumption. When people buy health foods, diet supplements, diet meals, fitness, and health services from the private market, they are good consumers who *invest* in their own health. This is one of the paradoxes of the neoliberal logics when applied to bodies and health; there is a pressure that one appears to be in control and responsible, yet at the same time one should continue to consume as much as possible (Guthman & DuPuis, 2006).

The very same fat bodies that are labelled as immoral and costly in the public sector somehow become very profitable and perhaps even moral (for generating revenue in the market) when they relocate to the private sector as consumers. In a sense, the ideal neoliberal body and health subject is thus not so much the person that abstains from using health services, but one that "consumes" (and therefore pays for) as many health services as possible and for as long as possible.

Enforcing the idea of fatness as always unhealthy and as a "curable" disease, normalising the thin body, stigmatising fatness and connecting it to individual moral failing, guarantees that the market stays profitable. Engaging in the possibly never-ending project of weight loss makes fat people the best consumers.

Sustaining the problem status of fatness is beneficial to a number of actors. The obesity epidemic discourse has promoted fatness as a business opportunity for the dietary, pharmaceutical, fitness, biotechnology, food, news, and entertainment industries among others. The diet industry is an emblematic of some of the contradictions inherent in the present day economised and commercialised neoliberal health and body culture. By insisting that it is possible to both stay healthy, shorthand for thin, and thus fulfil the moral imperative of control and continue to consume, if not food, its services and products.

In the end, it seems that, paradoxically, fatness is in demand in the neoliberal marketplace. Not only does it provide an easy target and scapegoat for the ailing public health care sector, but it creates economic opportunities in the private sector. Guthman & DuPuis's (2006) claim that the neoliberal economy both creates fatness while at the same time condemns it seems to ring true here.

Intersecting gender, class and fatness in neoliberal culture

The effects of the economy on the body are varied and multilayered. The body is an effect of economic, social, and political power conditions that constitute it. It is at the same time a consequence of the material conditions and resources available to it, as well as a symbol of them. Bodies are not only shaped by their local circumstances; in the global neoliberal economy bodies are also locally affected by global flows in the economy, as demonstrated for instance by Brown (2003) and Sutton (2010).

The economy affects different bodies in a variety of ways. Fatness is commonly associated with other hierarchical intersections of power, such as gender, ethnicity, and socioeconomic class. The neoliberal discourse's emphasis on individual responsibility for the appearance of health means that socioeconomic effects are ignored, as are those of class and gender.[4]

It has been well documented that the stigma of fatness and normative body ideals are gendered (Harjunen, 2009; LeBesco, 2004). Furthermore, social class is gendered and embodied (LeBesco, 2007). The combined stigmas of fatness, being female, and being poor have been observed, for example, by LeBesco (2007).

Thinness is seen as a marker and prerequisite for high-class status (Guthman & DuPuis, 2006). Skeggs (2005) has noted that the fat female body has begun to signify the deviant, the ignorant, and the body of an underclass that represents the "moral opposite" of the middle class body and the "normal" middle-class values attached to it. Herndon (2005) has observed how fatness often works as an exacerbating additional stigma for people who are already being marginalised for some other reason. Thus, attempts to control fatness often target people who are already being controlled anyway. Power relations embedded in these social statuses are all part of the issue of fatness; not only how fat is presented, constructed, and experienced, but ultimately also how fat people are treated.

Because of the intersectional effect of gender and fatness, fat women, for example, are frequently discriminated against in the labour market. Body size is in itself an economic question for women, and a body size that is deemed "wrong" poses an economic risk for women in particular. A fat body may thus automatically assign a woman to a lower class status in spite of her qualifications (Kauppinen & Antila, 2005). At the same time, fatness and socioeconomic status are also intertwined in a vicious circle so that fatness produces lower socioeconomic status and likewise lower socioeconomic status produces fatness (Stunkard & Sorensen, 1993). In this respect, fat women are often paid lower salaries, their career paths are rockier, and they are more frequently unemployed than their thin counterparts (Härkönen & Räsänen, 2008; Kauppinen & Anttila, 2005). In fact, a Finnish study found that especially highly educated fat women were discriminated against in working life, and that there was actually a significant wage gap between fat women and their normative sized counterparts (Sarlio-Lähteenkorva et al., 2004).

Gendered body norms: fitness, fatness and neoliberal surveillance and control

The obesity epidemic discourse, healthism and neoliberalism are also gendering and gendered discourses of power. Women, and women's bodies in particular, are targeted and governed through the healthist, fat phobic, and commercialised health discourse (Dworkin & Wachs, 2009; Heywood, 2007; Markula, 2008). In the case of women, health is often equated with physical attractiveness and a normative looking body, especially in the context of commercialised and neoliberally charged discourses on health.

The neoliberal rationale behind the construction of femininity and female bodies in popular culture has been observed in women's magazines, television shows and wider popular culture by researchers (Gill, 2007, 2008; Kauppinen & Anttila, 2005). Dworkin and Wachs (2009) have examined the fitness media and Heywood (2007) the image of the female athlete as an endorsement to neoliberalism.

Gill (2007) claims that neoliberalism is gendered and women are constructed as its ideal subjects. Shel has examined what is known as postfeminism as a sensibility and claims that it is aligned with neoliberal values of individual responsibility, self-regulation and free choice. Dworkin and Wachs (2009) and Heywood (2007), in their respective works, have observed how the neoliberal rationale has an effect on the way gendered bodies are represented in the media, how they are interpreted, and the demands they place on the female embodied subject. In the neo-liberal era, monitoring and surveillance of the female body has intensified. Gill (2007) agrees and lists three ways in which this takes place. Firstly, there has been an increase in self-surveillance by women, accompanied by a denial of such regulation. Secondly, surveillance is extended over new spheres of life and even regards intimate conduct. Thirdly, there is a focus on the psycho-logical, with a need to transform oneself and "remodel one's interior life" (p. 155).

Heywood for their part notes that the marketing of women's sports' programmes seems to unite feminism and neoliberalism by "presenting sport as a space where girls learn to become the ideal subjects of a new global economy that relies on individuals with flexibility who are trained to blame their inevitable failures on themselves rather than the system their lives are structured within" (Heywood, 2007, p. 113). The fitness of the body becomes a code for equality that depends on the individual's effort. Dworkin and Wachs note that the body's appearance and thinness is an important goal, especially in women's fitness (2009). They say that in women's fitness magazines, the emphasis is more on achieving a thin body than toning it. Their conclu-sion is that the notion of a fit and healthy subject in women's fitness magazines depends more on how the body looks than on actually being healthy.

The ideal female body is expected to be healthy and fit, but most importantly because these two criteria will also ensure thinness. Controlling body weight is, in itself, a way to discipline the female body, but demanding that the body looks fit in a certain way at all times adds yet another level of control, and connects body control to neoliberal politics even more tightly, as fitness adds a moral element to a body that might already be thin anyway. In this respect, it would seem that neoliberal rationale has been either incorporated into feminist thinking concerning the female body, and/or feminist thought is being appropriated by neoliberal culture.

Conclusion

It seems evident that the neoliberal body is being constructed in a number of connected spheres at the same time. Regarding the fat body, neoliberal governmentality seems to fuse the interests of several actors in, for example, public policy, the market, the patriarchy, and the individual. The medicalisation and stigmatisation of fat bodies via the obesity epidemic discourse certainly benefits the market, but it also acts as a vehicle for neoliberal biopolitical governance, as the commercialisation of health services increases the need for the population to self-manage these aspects of their life.

Indeed, the notion of fatness and the fat body as something diseased, costly, immoral, ugly, and above all, a symbol of individual failure, would probably not have such an impact were it not produced and maintained, at the same time, in so many spheres – discursive and otherwise. This is the power of neoliberal governmentality. The fat body, or perhaps in this case the pathologised obese body, seems to be a particularly susceptible target for the different modes of neoliberal governmentality that I have presented in this book.

In a culture where neoliberal governmentality reigns, there is no need to coerce or discipline people, because people discipline themselves. While people make it their duty to become a self-governing subject, the act of doing so is often misinterpreted as a sign of superior morals and deservingness. In this way, this class of people not only differentiates itself from the "oth-ers", but also helps to dismiss them as being somehow in the "wrong" too. As individual body management and economic success within society become conflated, success in body manage-ment becomes the sign of a well-adjusted neoliberal citizen who has taken responsibility over their health and therefore society. Fatness then is interpreted not just as a sign of an individual's immorality, but also as not being a proper neoliberal subject.

Notes

1 Ventura focuses on the United States of America. However, neoliberalism and its effects are not limited to North America alone.

2 Discrimination based on fatness is prevalent in such central fields of life as health care, the labour market, and education (Härkönen & Räsänen, 2007; Owen, 2012; Puhl & Brownell, 2001; Sarlio-Lähteenkorva et al., 2004).

3 In turn, the language of dieting has been adopted in economic rhetoric. For example, then Finance Minister of Finland, Jyrki Katainen noted in a speech in 2010 that "the public economy needs to go on a diet" (YLE, 2010). Finnish EU Commissioner Olli Rehn for his part stated that the "overgrown public sector needs to be slimmed down to a size that the economy can maintain" (Höltta, 2013), while citizens are encouraged to "tighten [their] belt[s]" (Elonin, 2014), and negotiations concerning cuts to be made in the social and health sector are referred to in terms of training and exercise (YLE, 2015).

4 Dworkin & Wachs (2009) observed in their analysis of women's health and fitness magazines that health and fitness are often used to express normative feminine beauty and body ideals, rather than physical fitness, endurance, and strength per se. This normative understanding of femininity, for its part, draws from middle class aesthetics and values (Skeggs, 2005), as the white middle class female body is considered to represent the "normal" body that other bodies are compared to and what they should strive to be like.

References

Ayo, N. (2012). Understanding health promotion in a neoliberal climate and the making of health conscious citizens. *Critical Public Health, 22*(1), 99–105.

Boero, N. (2012). *Killer fat: Media, medicine and morals in the American obesity epidemic.* New Brunswick: Rutgers University Press.

Braziel Evans, J., & LeBesco K. (2001). *Bodies out of bounds: Fatness and transgression.* Berkeley: University of California Press.

Brown, W. (2003). Neo-liberalism and the end of liberal democracy, *Theory & Event, 7*(1). https://muse.jhu.edu/journals/theory_and_event/v007/7.1brown.html

Campos, P., Saguy, A., Ernsberger, P., Oliver, E., & Gaesser, G. (2006). The epidemiology of overweight and obesity: Public health crisis or moral panic? *International Journal of Epidemiology, 35*(1), 55–60.

Cheek, J. (2008). Healthism: A new conservatism? *Qualitative Health Research, 18*(7), 974–982.

Crawford, R. (1980). Healthism and the medicalization of everyday life. *International Journal of Health Services, 10*(3), 365–388.

Crawford, R. (2006). Health as a meaningful social practice. *Health: An Interdisciplinary Journal for the Social Study of Health, Illness and Medicine, 10*(4), 401–420.

Dworkin, S., & Wachs F. (2009). *Body panic: Gender, health, and the selling of fitness.* New York: New York University Press.

Elonin, P. (2014, Apr 4). Hallitus kirii maaliin myöhässä – vyön kiristys jatkuu vuosia. Valtiontalous on kohtuullisessa kunnossa vasta vuonna 2018. *Helsingin Sanomat.* https://www.hs.fi/kotimaa/art-2000002721672.html

Farrell, A. E. (2011). *Fat shame: Stigma and the fat body in American culture.* New York: New York University Press.

Faubion, J. D. (Ed.) (1994). *4 essential works of Foucault 1954–1984.* London: Penguin Books.

Foucault, M. (1991). Governmentality (Lecture at the Collège de France, Feb 1, 1978). In G. Burchell, C. Gordon, & P. Miller (Eds.), *The Foucault effect: Studies in governmentality* (pp. 87–104). Hemel Hempstead: Harvester Wheatsheaf. (Original work published 1978).

Gard, M., & Wright, J. (2005). *The obesity epidemic: Science, morality and ideology.* New York: Routledge.

Gill, R. (2007). Postfeminist media culture: Elements of a sensibility. *European Journal of Cultural Studies, 10*(147), 147–166.

Gill, R. (2008). Culture and subjectivity in neoliberal and postfeminist times. *Subjectivity, 25*(1), 432–445.

Guthman, J. (2009a) Neoliberalism and the constitution of contemporary bodies. In E. Rothblum, & S. Solovay (Eds.), *The fat studies reader* (pp. 187–196). New York: New York University Press.

Guthman, J. (2009b). Teaching the politics of obesity: Insights into neoliberal embodiment and contemporary biopolitics. *Antipode, 41*(5), 1110–1133.

Guthman, J., & DuPuis, M. (2006). Embodying neoliberalism: Economy, culture, and the politics of fat. *Environment and Planning: Society and Space, 24*(3), 427–448.

Harjunen, H. (2009). *Women and fat: Approaches to the social study of fatness.* Jyväskylä Studies in Education, Psychology and Social Research no: 379, 2009. The University of Jyväskylä.

Harjunen, H. (2017). *Neoliberal bodies and the gendered fat body.* London: Routledge.

Härkönen, J., & Räsänen, P. (2008). Liikalihavuus, työttömyys ja ansiotaso. *Työelämäntutkimus – Arbetslivsforskning, 6*(1), 3–16.

Harrison, E. (2012). The body economic: the case of 'childhood obesity'. *Feminism & Psychology, 22*(3), 324–343.

Harvey, D. (2007). *A brief history of neoliberalism.* Oxford: Oxford University Press.

Herndon, A. (2005). Collateral damage from friendly fire? Race, nation, class, and the "war against obesity". *Social Semiotics, 15*(82), 127–141.

Heywood, L. (2007). Producing girls: Empire, sport, and the neoliberal body. In J. Hargreaves & P. Vertinsky (Eds.), *Physical culture, power, and the body* (pp. 101–120). New York: Routledge.

Hölttä, K. (2013, Jul 19). Puheenaihe: Komissaari Rehn uskoo yhä talouskuriin. *Aamulehti.* http://m.aamulehti.fi/juttuarkisto/?cid=1194827113902

Huff, J. (2001). A horror of corpulence: Interrogating bantingism and mid-nineteenth-century fat-phobia. In J. E. Braziel & K. LeBesco (Eds.), *Bodies out of bounds: Fatness and transgression* (pp. 39–59). Berkeley: University of California Press.

Jutel, A-M. (2005). Weighing health: The moral burden of obesity. *Social Semiotics, 15*(2), 113–125.

Kauppinen, K., & Anttila, E. (2005). Onko painolla väliä: hoikat, lihavat ja normaalipainoiset naiset työelämän murroksessa? *Työ ja perhe aikakauskirja 2, Työ, perhe ja elämän moninaisuus II.* Työterveyslaitoksen julkaisuja.

LeBesco, K. (2004). *Revolting bodies: The struggle to redefine fat identity.* Amherst: University of Massachusetts Press.

LeBesco, K. (2007). Fatness as the embodiment of working-class rhetoric. In W. DeGenero (Ed.), *Who says? Working-class rhetoric, class consciousness, and community* (pp. 238–255). Pittsburgh: University of Pittsburgh Press.

LeBesco, K. (2010). Fat panic and the new morality. In J. Metzl & A. Kirkland (Eds.), *Against health: How health became the new morality* (pp. 72–82). New York: New York University Press.

LeBesco, K. (2011). Neoliberalism, public health and the moral perils of fatness. *Critical Public Health, 21*(2), 153–164.

Lemke, T. (2001). The birth of bio-politics – Michel Foucault's lecture at the Collège de France on neoliberal governmentality. *Economy and Society, 30*(2), 1–17.

Markula, P. (2008). Governing obese bodies in a control society. *Junctures: The Journal for Thematic Dialogue, 11,* 53–66.

Mäkelä, J., & Niva, M. (2009). Muuttuva syöminen – yksilön vastuu ja yhteiskunta. *Kuluttajatutkimuskeskuksen vuosikirja.* Helsinki: Kuluttajatutkimuskeskus. 45–60.

Oliver, E. J. (2006). *Fat politics: The real story behind America's obesity epidemic.* New York: Oxford University Press.

Owen, L. (2012). Living fat in a thin-centric world: Effects of spatial discrimination on fat bodies and selves. *Feminism & Psychology, 22*(3), 290–306.

Puhl, R., & Brownell, K. (2001). Bias, discrimination, and obesity. *Obesity Research, 9,* 778–805.

Rail, G., Holmes, D., & Murray, S. (2010). The politics of evidence on "domestic terrorists": Obesity discourse and their effects. *Social Theory & Health, 8*(3), 259–279.

Rothblum, E., & Solovay, S. (2009). *The fat studies reader.* New York: New York University Press.

Saguy, A. (2013). *What's wrong with fat?* New York: Oxford University Press.

Sarlio-Lähteenkorva, S., Silventoinen, K., & Lahelma, E., (2004). Relative weight and income at different levels of socioeconomic status. *American Journal of Public Health, 94*(3), 468–472.

Skeggs, B. (2005). The making of class and gender through visualizing moral subject formation. *Sociology, 39*(5), 965–982.

Stunkard, A. J., & Sorensen, T. I. A. (1993). Obesity and socioeconomic status. A complex relation. *New England Journal of Medicine, 329*(14), 1036–1037.

Sutton, B. (2010). *Bodies in crisis: Culture, violence and women's resistance in neoliberal Argentina.* New Brunswick: Rutgers University Press.

Ventura, P. (2012). *Neoliberal culture: Living with American neoliberalism.* Farnham: Ashgate.

Wingrad, J. (2013). *Branded bodies, rhetoric, and the neoliberal nation-state.* Plymouth: Lexington Books.

Wrede S., Henriksson, L., Host, H., Johansson, S., & Dybbroe, B. (2008). *Care work in crisis: Reclaiming the Nordic ethos of care.* Lund: Studentlitteratur.

Wright, J., & Harwood, V. (Eds.) (2008). *Biopolitics and the 'obesity epidemic': Governing bodies.* London: Routledge.

YLE. (2010, Feb 9). Katainen tekisi keskustan uudesta johtajasta myös pääministerin. *YLE.* http://yle.fi/uutiset/katainen_tekisi_keskustan_uudesta_johtajasta_myos_paaministerin/5506350

YLE. (2015, May 20). Sote-mallista ei vielä päätöstä – "Jumppa jatkuu". *YLE.* http://yle.fi/uutiset/sote-mallista_ei_viela_paatosta__jumppa_jatkuu/8005798

10

FAT AND TRANS

Towards a new theorization of gender in Fat Studies

Francis Ray White

Usually when the words "trans" and "fat" appear together the ensuing conversation will feature some serious hand-wringing about processed foods, cholesterol and the pros and cons of banning something. That is not the type of trans fat under discussion here, rather the aim of this chapter is to explore how and why bringing Fat Studies and Trans*gender* Studies together could produce new ways of thinking about gender in Fat Studies. On the face of it, Fat Studies and Trans Studies appear to have much in common; they are both interdisciplinary fields, both oriented towards anti-oppressive goals and they both have a common interest in elaborating theoretical accounts of non-normative embodiments. However, despite this shared ground the two fields have, as yet, rarely intersected and as I will argue, this has resulted in accounts of gender in Fat Studies which both exclude the experiences of fat transgender people and limit understandings of the relationship between fat and gender.

The chapter is divided into three main sections. The first will review the existing academic literature that deals directly with issues of fatness and transness. Despite its small size this work does offer some possible ways to conceive of the intersection of fat and trans. Key is the question of whether fat and trans are posited as separate states to be compared – how is the experience/treatment of being trans similar or different to that of being fat? – or whether identities/embodiments forged at the intersection of the two are considered. Identifying this tendency, alongside the strengths and limitations of existing approaches, is necessary in order to further theorize fat and gender as inextricably linked.

The second section will discuss a selection of writings in Fat and Trans Studies that deploy the tropes of fluidity or liminality in their attempts to account for the ambiguous, unfixed, ambivalent or monstrous construction of either fat or trans identities and bodies. Often drawing heavily on poststructuralist and/or queer theoretical perspectives these pieces invoke fluidity or liminality but overwhelmingly only in relation to *either* fatness *or* transness. By comparing the differing, sometimes contradictory, uses these tropes are put to my aim is to illustrate how a simultaneous consideration of fat *and* trans remains under-theorized, and a "single axis" approach that implicitly assumes all the fat people are cis and all the trans people are thin prevails. The final section returns to the question of gender within Fat Studies to ask what a trans perspective could bring to the way Fat Studies "does" gender. Taking on the implications of the previous two sections, the aim for the final discussion is to critique existing work in Fat Studies, not to castigate it, but to suggest that its cis-centrism precludes a full realization of fat's central role in the production and destabilization of binary gender.

Fat/Trans so far

Only a small body of literature specifically addressing the interrelationship of fat and trans has emerged thus far in Fat Studies. While there has been discussion in online and activist spaces, (for recent examples see Aprileo, 2018; Bay, 2017; Luna, 2018) and without wanting to draw a rigid binary between activist and academic discourse, the theoretical development of these debates has been limited. However, it is possible to outline three main directions the existing academic literature has taken: first there are the approaches that focus on trans and fat anti-discrimination law (Glazer & Kramer, 2009; Vade & Solovay, 2009); secondly there are discussions of trans participation and inclusion in fat activism (Cooper, 2012, 2016; Lampe, 2016; LeBesco, 2016; White, 2014); and finally there are the autobiographical/autoethnographic accounts of fat/trans authors (Barker, 2009; Bergman, 2009; Burford & Orchard, 2014; White, 2014; Zach, 2015). It is notable that the overwhelming majority of this work has been published in Fat Studies rather than Trans Studies; it is also dominated by white trans masculine authors and experiences.

Dean Vade and Sandra Solovay's "No apology: Shared struggles in fat and transgender law" (2009) was arguably the first significant attempt to bring together fat and trans analysis. In it they highlight how in discrimination cases claimants who are fat or trans are more likely to be favored by the courts, "as long as they show a strong desire to conform to societal gender and body norms" (p. 173–174), in other words if they apologize for their non-normativity. Vade and Solovay's rejection of this and call for the protection of "civil rights for everyone, not just those who fit in boxes" (p. 174) is vital, however, their approach to thinking about the "shared" features of fat and trans experience is limited. In their opening sentence, they refer to "people who are transgender, fat, or both" (p. 167), but in what follows, the "or both" option disappears and discussion is confined to people who are fat (and implicitly cisgender) or trans (and implicitly thin). They then discuss either fat people's failure to uphold *bodily* norms or trans people's failure to uphold *gender* norms, but not fat people's failure to uphold gender norms. In other words, they do not consider the extent to which gender normativity is predicated on the possession of a slender body. Thus, there is something of a gap, especially given how many (cis) fat writers attribute the failure to achieve a normative gendered embodiment to fat (see the final section of this chapter for a fuller discussion of this).

The tendency to compare and contrast fat and trans experiences in approaches such as Vade and Solovay's also has the effect of erasing the experience of those who are both fat and trans (see LeBesco, 2014 and Lee, 2014 for examples of this in different contexts). Happily this omission is beginning to be addressed, especially in relation to fat/trans participation in fat activism. Much of this work highlights the incommensurability of fat and trans political discourses, either around the malleability of the body (Burford & Orchard, 2014; White, 2014), narratives of identity origin (Lampe, 2016) or ideas about "body acceptance" and/or positivity (Burford & Orchard, 2014; LeBesco, 2016), resulting in what Lampe calls the impossibility of a coherent fat/trans subjectivity. Moreover, attempts to make visible "LGBT" contributions to the history of fat activism, often do not distinguish between LGB and T. Although examples exist in other contexts – Ingraham's (2015) discussion of size diversity in queer porn for example – in general, as Burford and Orchard note, "promises of inclusion fail to deliver. Indeed sometimes the 't' appears to be mere relish adorning and 'inclusifying' the main meal of lesbian and gay" (2014, p. 61).

One such example is Charlotte Cooper's "queer and trans fat activist timeline" (2012) which does valuable work gathering and archiving fat activist history, but does not provide explicit detail about whether and in what sense either the activists or the activism they engaged in was "trans". Cooper's (2016) longer work on the genealogy of fat activism features a high ratio of trans or genderqueer participants, five in her sample of thirty-one fat activists (p. 43), and although some details of their experiences as fat and trans do emerge (p. 149), they are not analyzed. Further, she notes that feminism's "struggles around race, imperialism, trans people, or class ... also reflect problems within fat activism" (2016, p. 102), but does not expand on what it might mean for trans participation in fat activism that significant US fat feminist networks were forged at/through the Michigan Womyn's Music Festival, a space which is notoriously trans exclusionary, particularly of trans women (p. 138, see also Davis, 2008, p. 114). Nor does Cooper explore what prompted NOLOSE to abandon its "women-only" conference policy in 2004 (p. 149). It is clear that further research into trans people's involvement in and/or exclusion from fat activism would be welcome, and may help to explain both the seeming absence of trans feminine voices in Fat Studies, and the presence/predominance of particular theorizations of gender.

The final strand of existing literature is the autobiographical or autoethnographic writing by people who are fat and trans or non-binary. Such authors often reflect on their experiences of moving through the world, or being read as, both fat men and fat women. S. Bear Bergman's descriptions of this in "Part-time fatso" (2009) are particularly evocative. They note how, "when I am taken for a man, I am not fat" (p. 139) whereas, "as a woman, I am revolting. I am not only unattractively mannish but also grossly fat" (p. 140). Zach (2015) similarly observes that, "I can always tell if I'm being read as male because people will never comment about my weight" (p. 94). Many stories in this genre bring up differences around food that are dependent on how the author is presenting or being perceived at the time. Sam Orchard notes how as a man dining at friends' houses, "I'll be offered more, and seconds without hesitation" (Burford & Orchard, 2014, p. 69, see also Barker, 2009). This and the availability of men's clothes in regular stores are used to exemplify the gendered natured of fatphobia and its disproportionate impact on women and those presenting/being read as female. Despite this, although a trans feminine perspective on this dynamic has been articulated in some online/activist writings (for example Burns, 2016; Mey, 2013) it has yet to feature in more academic Fat Studies analyses.

While these insights are undoubtedly fascinating, they do, in places, reproduce the "compare and contrast" approach, which assumes fatness is an attribute of a body that is already male or female (White, 2014). However, Bergman and Burford and Orchard begin to complicate this through their more detailed discussions of how the presence or location of fat on the body produces certain attributions (or not) of gender. Orchard describes how, "within transmasculine communities, I felt as though my weight was seen as feminine, or rather, as feminizing, as in: 'urgh, look at my curves'" (Burford & Orchard, 2014, p. 63). He also notes the general perception of fat as both a "failure" of femininity, and something which makes one, "too curvy to be seen as male" (p. 69). In different contexts though, Orchard notes, "there's something about bulk that can be read as a masculine indicator" (p. 69), which aligns with Bergman's admission that:

> It's my fat for which I am sometimes most grateful when I want the world to see me as a man ... this is an option for me because my natural physiognomy (mesomorphic musculature and masculine fat distribution) allows me to get read as a man.
>
> *(2009, p. 141)*

Bergman also mentions how "my girth and breadth allow my smallish breasts to be read as 'fat boy tits'" (p. 141). It is this type of attention to the gendering properties of fat which has potential for development in theorizations of gender within Fat Studies. It is to the gender producing/disrupting qualities of fat that I will turn in the following sections.

Fluidity

If the existing literature on fat and trans tends to maintain fatness and transness as discrete phenomena, the aim of the following discussion is to explore ways to bring them together via an examination of fluidity and liminality. These tropes have been invoked in both Fat and Trans Studies in the service of rejecting essentialist notions of embodiment and/or identity and retheorizing them as shifting and unfixed. However, fat and trans theorists have deployed ideas of fluidity and liminality in differing and sometimes contradictory ways. Thus, the following discussion asks how these deployments can be made to speak to one another in order to open up new possibilities for theorizing both fat/trans embodiment and gender within Fat Studies.

In "Situating fluidity" (2008), Erin Davis argues the concept of "fluidity" has been enthusiastically taken up by queer, postmodern theorists seeking to "destabilize gender categories rooted in biologically deterministic gender paradigms" (p. 98), and that trans folk have come to exemplify multiplicity and the social constructedness of binary gender, because they "have histories and bodies that do not reflect hegemonic expectations" (p. 98). However, Davis highlights how debates around trans fluidity have foundered over the desire of some trans individuals for precisely the kinds of coherent and stable identities fluidity is supposed to subvert. Davis's critique of this centers on the experiences of her trans research participants for whom "fluidity" or unintelligibility threatens social inclusion (p. 123, see also Wilson, 2002). Hence they "typically present themselves as a man or a woman" (p. 105), or adopt a "traditional feminine image" (p. 108) in order for their gender to be intelligible enough to get by. How might such an embrace or evasion of fluidity work in relation to fat (trans)gendered embodiment? The possibility of a "traditional" feminine/masculine image may not be available in the same way for fat people. Sam Orchard, for example, reports that as a (female-identifying) teenager, "my weight contributed to my feeling that I was 'failing' at being a girl" (Burford & Orchard, 2014, p. 69). Despite having a history that reflects "hegemonic expectations", here Orchard's gender is destabilized by his fatness, rendering it less intelligible and more fluid.

If fluidity, as Davis notes, "implies an escape from the constraints of gender assumptions and a refusal to stay within one category or another" (p. 101) to what extent is fat fluid? This question is addressed by Kathleen LeBesco (2014) in her "meditation" on fatness and fluidity. She proposes the concept of "size-fuck" (p. 52), a play on gender-fuck, as a way to critique the fat political orthodoxy that casts weight change, particularly intentional weight-loss, as a betrayal of fat activism/acceptance. Drawing explicitly on queer and trans uses of fluidity, LeBesco wonders whether Fat Studies could revalue fluctuations in weight in order to reject the fixity of the body and essentialist models of the self (p. 53). Thus, in the context of her own changing weight she notes, "like a genderqueer person, I like presenting an incoherent identity" (p. 53). "Size-fuck" is undoubtedly compelling, but ultimately LeBesco reproduces the "compare and contrast" model where fat and trans experiences are likened, but not thought to overlap. What if LeBesco was not just "like" a genderqueer person, but in fact "was" one? What if the distinction between gender fluidity and size fluidity was collapsed? What if we fully acknowledged that fat is central to securing gender "within one category or another"?

Sellberg and Sellberg (2014) offer an alternative reading of the fluidity of fat that helps elucidate these "what ifs". They discuss the literal fluidity of fat as a corporeal substance; "fat is a 'wobbly' substance, and a simultaneously substantial and insubstantial fluid" (p. 305). They argue that fat's presence in the body is not only excluded from anatomical representations throughout history, but from fat feminist analyses of fat which:

> Tend to focus on how fat as an *exterior addition* to the idea of the female body beautiful affects our sense of self, but seldom touch on how fat as an *interior part* of us always already functions within the continual constitution of said self.
>
> *(p. 305)*

As such, the Sellbergs question the notion of fat as something laid "on top of" some more solid sense of self and instead suggest that fat, in its fluidity, is "both outside and inside the body, but it is also both outside and inside the organs. It muddles the borders and defies classification" (p. 307). The question here is whether this "muddling" can be extended to gender? In a sense, yes it can: "Whether we look at a male or a female body" they say, "what is really striking about human corporeality is the contrast and juxtaposition between fluid and solid, muscle and fat" (p. 307). In which case, if gender is a configuration of muscle and fat, and fat, as Sellberg and Sellberg have noted, "defies classification" then the fluidity of both fat and gender is one and the same. Although Sellberg and Sellberg do not set out to attend to fat/trans embodiment, theirs might be the most usefully intersectional account of fat and gender in the existing literature, because it proposes a model that does not assume the fat body is not a trans one or vice versa.

Liminality

Davis, LeBesco and Sellberg and Sellberg all caution against an unreserved embrace of fluidity because not all bodies are capable of infinite or permanent weight or gender change; as Sellberg and Sellberg warn, "fats have both fluid and solid states" (2014, p. 311). One way around the tension between change and fixity that dogs theorizations of fluidity can be found in Katariina Kyrölä and Hannele Harjunen's (2017) model of fat liminality. Typically, liminal states are thought to be temporary periods of in-betweenness that are passed through on the way to somewhere more fixed. This is very much how Wilson (2002) takes up liminality in relation to the embodied experiences of her trans research participants, specifically to describe a phase, "which all people transgressing 'normative' gender boundaries will at some stage occupy ... it is a 'space' where genders are suspended and remodeling occurs" (2002, p. 431–432). For Wilson's participants, the liminal phase is a temporary, necessary evil to be endured in order to reach a more fixed end (2002, p. 432). Kyrölä and Harjunen, however, use the concept to capture the way their research interviewees related to fatness as a transitory phase, and desired to move through it, though many of them had been, and would likely remain, fat their entire lives (2017, p. 103). Embodying this type of liminal fatness meant, "nearly all of the women seemed to consider their 'real' body size to be thin, or saw it as a self-evident goal" (p. 103).

In "Monstrous freedom" (2015), Lesleigh Owen also discusses fat as a liminal state, not in terms of it being temporary, but in relation to its monstrosity. Owen describes fatness as, "that scary, liminal, shadowed place where certainties fizzle and boundaries fade" (2015, p. 2). In the context of dualistic constructions of biological/social, inside/outside, attractant/repellant, Owen argues fat cannot fully occupy either "side" and it is this which makes it ambivalent and "monstrous" – "fat bodies are scary and repulsive precisely because they throw cause and effect into question, blur supposedly sharp lines between seeming opposites" (2015, p. 2). This fear of indeterminate states is also echoed in Wilson's research where one participant states, "you can't be not one thing or the other. I don't know what you can be classed as, to me you are nothing" (2002, p. 438, see also Davis, 2008, p. 124). Wilson's argument, made in 2002, does not address what would now be known as genderqueer or non-binary people, who may absolutely desire to be "something" that is not one thing or the other. However, what is clear is that liminality for Wilson refers almost exclusively to gender, while the lines Owen's fat monsters "blur" do not appear to threaten the integrity of gender boundaries. Ironically, in a throwaway comment, Owen notes that, "monsters exist to scare us ... as cautionary tales to help scare good girls and boys into normalcy" (2015, p. 3). It may be more apt to say that as a monster, fat is a cautionary tale that helps scare us into *being* "good girls and boys" – the legibly gendered kind – lest we slip into liminality.

Given the different configurations of liminality Wilson, Kyrölä and Harjunen and Owen assign to trans and fat bodies, in what sense might a fat/trans body experience liminality? Sonny Nordmarken's (2014) experience of gender transition provides an interesting case study. Nordmarken describes starting to take testosterone and experiencing the liminal "in-betweenness" of gender illegibility (much as Wilson (2002) describes it), but as time passes he finds:

> My legibility as male (rather than female or "indiscernable") becomes clearer to others, my legibility as a person, as human, becomes clearer to others ... for the first time in my life, I feel how it feels to be seen as a "normal" male body. This is the shape, the articulation of gender normative.
>
> *(2014, p. 43–44)*

However, what if the extent to which Nordmarken's newly acquired gender normativity is predicated on his slenderness is considered? He describes his body as, "sinewy and wiry ... a leaping lizard type of body", referring also to his "waifiness" (2014, p. 42). Hence, it is clear that Nordmarken is not "fat" and although he remarks on the "hormones moving flesh in my body, shifting like tectonic plates, pushing fat deposits and muscle densities into new formations" (p. 42), the "configurations of fat and muscle", to echo Sellberg and Sellberg (2014), that emerge produce a non-liminal state uncomplicated by the type of fat liminality Kyrölä and Harjunen theorize. While testosterone can undoubtedly produce embodiments that are legibly male *and* fat, they would still not be the "normal" male body Nordmarken achieves because, as Owen (2015) notes, "fat bodies defy markers of averageness, that modern representative of 'normalcy'" (p. 8). If fat bodies are not "normal", does that push them into a liminal state? Wilson asserts that, "cultural gender texts inform a culture's members of how far the gender categories can stretch before stepping over into a problematic liminal state" (2002, p. 439–440). Could it be that it is not just the assumed temporariness of fatness that makes it liminal, but also its ability to "stretch" gender categories into in-betweenness?

Perhaps the bigger question here concerns the fantasy that liminal states are escapable at all. Even Nordmarken, with his newfound gender legibility, enters other states of illegibility and liminality in his embodiment as a "feminine sort of masculine being" (2014, p. 43) and as a queer man. Thus even for what Nordmarken calls "shape-shifters", as opposed to Kyrölä and Harjunen's "shape-unshifters", there is no truly "other side" to come out into, and the fantasy of gender transition is like the fantasy of weight-loss in that they both promise, but cannot deliver, some kind of fixed/permanent state of the type already deconstructed in theories of gender, and size, fluidity. As Kyrölä and Harjunen suggest, "the problem is not that corporeality is a mixture of persistence and malleability, of material and immaterial forces, but that the boundary between "essential" and "removable" corporeality becomes too fixed and unrelentingly managed" (2017, p. 113). This allows for analysis to be refocused on the construction and regulation of "fixed" versus "in-between" bodily states and enables fatness to be positioned as more involved in the production of supposedly "fixed" gender states than previously thought. It is this suggestion I will explore in the following section in relation to some examples of how gender has been made intelligible within Fat Studies.

Gender and fat trans-formed

There is certainly no shortage of gender analysis in Fat Studies. The aim of this section is not to provide a comprehensive review of that literature, but to draw out some of the assumptions underpinning it and how they could be re-theorized using the concepts of fluidity and liminality, as well as Trans Studies approaches. Work in Fat Studies has often positioned fatness as something which causes gender to "fail"; for Cecelia Hartley (2001), fat is "a reminder of all that a woman cannot and should not be" (p. 66). Jeanine Gailey (2014) similarly observes that fat (female) bodies, "tend to demonstrate characteristics associated with both masculinity and femininity" (p. 112, for further discussion see White, 2019). These theorists make valuable contributions to theorizing the experience of (cis) fat women, what they don't do is develop the implications of gender fluidity in their statements; nor do they consider women who are "failing" at normative femininity as in a potentially liminal state.

The same tendency appears even in queer Fat Studies work. In her analysis of the performance of fat, Stefanie A. Jones (2014) argues that in a heteropatriarchal model of gender, "the fat feminine body is ... necessarily expelled from the paradigm of heteronormativity, the fat body is regulated to the periphery, left in a no-man's land of desire" (p. 41). Fat bodies are queer for Jones in the sense they disrupt, "the current arrangement of fields" relating to desire (p. 41). However, she does not also consider how they might "queer" or disrupt the very categories of gender those desires are supposedly lodged in. Despite the notion of a "no-man's land" being tantalizingly close to that of a liminal state, Jones does not allow the category of woman to "stretch" (Wilson, 2002, p. 439) that far. Work such as this contradictorily keeps fat people within fixed gender categories whilst simultaneously asserting their exclusion from those same categories and thus implicitly adheres to a binary model that assumes gender is assured/fixed through some, usually unstated, bio-essentialist foundation.

This is problematic, not only because it reproduces cisnormativity, but because it precludes a fuller consideration of the active role of fat in producing a legibly gendered body in the first place. Michelle Green's (2015) discussion of the construction of fat women's gender is a case in point. She suggests that:

> Fat women do not find the 'doing' of gender as accessible as slim women, and therefore it is hard to 'undo' gender with the politicized force Butler claims. Fat subjects, and particularly fat women, find it harder to undo gender because they find themselves excluded from the practice of gender.
>
> *(p. 186)*

This implies that there is something, an already-gendered "doer", perhaps, behind fat women's "doing" of gender. Not only is this precisely the opposite of Butler's point that, "there is no gender identity behind the expressions of gender" (1990, p. 25), but it assumes that gender exists independently of fatness. Furthermore, if fat women are excluded from "doing" gender, or more accurately from doing heteronormative binary gender, then aren't they actually "undoing" gender? If, as Green implies, fat women are not fully able to access the category of woman, but they are equally not legible as men, then not only does this suggest some sort of other liminal option, but also that gender intelligibility is absolutely reliant on particular configurations of muscle and fat (Sellberg & Sellberg, 2014, p. 307), rather than on a pre-gendered doer.

The irony of Green's inability to recognize the "gender trouble" (Butler, 1990) fat women might cause is further compounded by invoking a direct comparison with trans people. Quoting Natalie Boero (2012), Green asserts that, "not unlike transsexuals learning the appropriate doing of gender as adults, fat people, particularly women, have often been excluded from normative patterns of gendered behavior, interaction and embodiment" (as cited in Green, 2015, p. 186). Neither Green nor Boero develop this analogy, and thus never interrogate how it is not just that this process is "like" the one trans people may experience, but it is that process. Davis affirms this when arguing that, "given mainstream assumptions of sex/gender congruence, transgendered individuals' gender claims are particularly precarious and subject to public dispute. Yet *all individuals* are held accountable to gender expectations and negotiate their self-presentations accordingly" (2008, p. 125, emphasis added). Rather than bemoaning fat people's inability to do gender, a fat/trans approach to Fat Studies could help "de-exceptionalize" trans experiences of doing gender by revealing the embodied processes by which any/all gender is assumed, thus destabilizing not only binary gender, but also the cis/trans binary.

Given the previous discussion, if the presence or absence of fat is central to gender legibility, then how might weight-loss (or gain) be understood through this lens? Already in the literature there are comparisons between weight loss and gender transition. Lee (2014) likens her desire for a thin(ner) body to those of an ex-partner who transitioned from female to male: "perhaps I related to a desire to change the body to fit your idea of who you are" (p. 93). However, she draws a distinction between the different political value attached to these two projects, saying, "his desire for change included shedding other people's expectations that he would conform to his allocated female gender and upbringing, whereas my desire for change was about conforming to what I thought a woman should be" (p. 93). Trans modifications are cast as transgressive, whereas the desire to be thin is mere capitulation to patriarchal notions of female embodiment. Framing the difference between these projects in this way alludes to debates around the ethics of body modification articulated by trans and fat rights advocates (see White, 2014 for a fuller discussion of this). However, it also precludes consideration of Lee's "transition" from fat to thin as a gender transition, even though it is clearly "about" gender. Green similarly discusses weight-loss as involving a "reassertion of heteronormativity" in the face of gender norms that "render this social group [fat people] less gendered, if not de-gendered" (2015, p. 186). If failing to conform with "what a woman should be" is "de-gendering" and thus places someone outside of binary gender, then the process of weight-loss as a means of bringing them back into the binary fold can arguably be conceived of as a kind of gender transition.

Conclusions: Fat as a gender-fluid

In this chapter I have attempted to offer a critique of some existing approaches to trans and gender more generally within Fat Studies, with the aim of suggesting how it might move beyond the additive or comparative models of fat/trans embodiment that currently dominate the limited literature that exists. Reconfiguring the tropes of fluidity and liminality might offer one route towards this end. My intention in drawing on these tropes was not to erase the different ways in which fat and trans people might relate to fluidity or liminality, but rather to chip away at the assumption that "fat people" and "trans people" are discrete groups; be that in order to acknowledge the existence of fat/trans people, or to recognize the role of fat in both cis and trans gender (un)intelligibility.

There may be definite benefits to this approach. Within current theorizations fat is presumed to exist as a layer on top of some pre-existing gender; it may cause that gender to "fail", but not in ways that ultimately bring its existence into question. This has tended to mean fat is viewed as having a negative effect on gender, or at least on the possibilities for social recognition within an economy of heteronormative binary gender. Entertaining the possibility that fat does not cause gender to fail, but edges it into a liminal state "between" binary genders, not only opens up space for the subversion of that binary, but also enables us to think about what fat "does" – the positive role it plays in producing legibly gendered bodies.

Admittedly, embracing liminality as a practical strategy, even in the hope of destabilizing binary gender, may be an unattractive option given the relentlessly negative tenor with which liminal states are regarded. Kyrölä and Harjunen's (2017) version of fat liminality is not experienced by their participants in particularly positive terms, whilst Davis's (2008) trans participants are similarly skeptical about gender in-betweenness. As Davis notes, "gender identities are ways to gain social recognition" (2008, p. 123), and the lure of that recognition when the alternatives may mean invisibility at best, and violent erasure at worst is understandable. However, an alternative approach can be identified in the shift from "liminal" to "monstrous" found in the work of Owen (2015) and Stryker (2006). Owen's enticing declaration that "there is a freedom in being a monster" (2015, p. 9) perhaps offers something other than liminality's literal "nothingness" with which to replace the certainties of social recognition. Stryker further endorses this approach arguing it will provoke "the establishment of subjects in new modes, regulated by different codes of intelligibility" (2006, p. 253).

I would like to conclude by suggesting a "new code of intelligibility" is what is required to develop a fuller account of fat/trans identity and embodiment. When we think from the position of fat/trans not only are the gaps in existing theories of fat and gender opened up, but more importantly new possibilities for theorizing gender emerge. This project is not about attempting to come up with a unified theory of "the" fat/trans subject position, because this position does not exist. Even aside from the multiple vectors of race, ethnicity, class, location, age and sexuality, fat/trans existence is shaped, literally, by volume and distributions of fat and by a spectrum of gender identities, and a range of bodily interventions or "transitions". As a necessarily unfixed location, then, fat/trans can perhaps operate as the juncture that reveals the unsustainability of separating gender and fat for anyone.

References

Aprileo, J. (2018). How fatphobia impacted my gender identity. *Comfyfat*. https://comfyfat.com/2018/03/22/fatphobia-impacted-gender-identity/

Barker, J. E. (2009). Transfatty. In C. Tomrley & A. Kaloski (Eds.), *Fat studies in the UK* (pp. 32–34). York: Raw Nerve Books.

Bay, K. (2017). The intersection of fatmisia and transmisia. *Medium*. https://medium.com/@kivabay/the-intersection-of-fatmisia-and-transmisia-78fb10f90551

Bergman, S. B. (2009). Part-time fatso. In E. Rothblum & S. Solovay (Eds.), *The fat studies reader* (pp. 139–142). New York: New York University Press.

Boero, N. (2012). *Killer fat: Media, medicine and morals in the American "obesity epidemic"*. New Brunswick, NJ: Rutgers University Press.

Burford, J., & Orchard, S. (2014). Chubby boys with strap-ons: Queering fat transmasculine embodiment. In C. Pausé, J. Wykes, & S. Murray (Eds.), *Queering fat embodiment* (pp. 61–74). Farnham: Ashgate.

Burns, K. (2016). My intersection with being trans and fatphobia. *Medium*. https://medium.com/gender-2-0/my-intersection-with-being-trans-and-fatphobia-6f77474bf6a2

Butler, J. (1990). *Gender trouble: Feminism and the subversion of identity*. London: Routledge.

Cooper, C. (2012). A queer and trans fat activist timeline: Queering fat activist nationality and cultural imperialism. *Fat Studies*, 1(1), 61–74.

Cooper, C. (2016). *Fat activism: A radical social movement*. Bristol: HammerOn Press.

Davis, E. C. (2008). Situating "fluidity": (Trans) gender identification and the regulation of gender diversity. *GLQ*, *15*(1), 97–130.

Gailey, J. (2014). *The hyper(in)visible fat woman*. New York: Palgrave.

Glazer, E., & Kramer, Z. (2009). Trans fat. *Hofstra University Legal Studies Research Paper, 09–11*, 1–31.

Green, M. (2015). Coming of age through weight loss: The fat woman as sexually amature in Margaret Atwood's *Lady Oracle*. In H. Hester, & C. Walters (Eds.), *Fat sex: New directions in theory and activism* (pp. 181–198). Farnham: Ashgate.

Hartley, C. (2001). Letting ourselves go: Making room for the fat body in feminist scholarship. In J. E. Braziel, & K. LeBesco (Eds.), *Bodies out of bounds: Fatness and transgression* (pp. 60–73). Berkeley, CA: University of California Press.

Ingraham, N. (2015). Queering porn: Gender and size diversity within SF bay area queer pornography. In H. Hester, & C. Walters (Eds.), *Fat sex: New directions in theory and activism* (pp. 115–132). Farnham: Ashgate.

Jones, S. A. (2014). The performance of fat: The spectre outside the house of desire. In C. Pausé, J. Wykes, & S. Murray (Eds.), *Queering fat embodiment* (pp. 31–48). Farnham: Ashgate.

Kyrölä, K., & Harjunen, H. (2017). Phantom/liminal fat and feminist theories of the body. *Feminist Theory, 18*(2), 99–117.

Lampe, M. C. (2016). *Identities without origins: fat/trans subjectivity and the possibilities of plurality* [Unpublished masters thesis]. University of Louisville, Louisville, Kentucky, USA. *Electronic Theses and Dissertations,* Paper 2425. https://doi.org/10.18297/etd/2425

LeBesco, K. (2014). On fatness and fluidity: A meditation. In C. Pausé, J. Wykes, & S. Murray (Eds.), *Queering fat embodiment* (pp. 49–60). Farnham: Ashgate.

LeBesco, K. (2016, June 29). *Genderqueer, trans, fluid, fat: Physical modification and the politics of acceptance.* [Conference presentation]. Fat Studies: Identity, Agency, Embodiment conference, Massey University, Palmerston North, New Zealand.

Lee, J. (2014). Flaunting fat: Sex with the lights on. In C. Pausé, J. Wykes, & S. Murray (Eds.), *Queering fat embodiment* (pp. 89–96). Farnham: Ashgate.

Luna, C. (2018). The gender nonconformity of my fatness. *The Body is Not An Apology.* https://thebody-isnotanapology.com/ magazine/the-gender-nonconformity-of-my-fatness/

Mey (2013). Fat, trans and (working on being) fine with it. *Autostraddle.* https://www.autostraddle.com/fat-trans-and-working-on-being-fine-with-it-168108/

Nordmarken, S. (2014). Becoming ever more monstrous: Feeling transgender in-betweenness. *Qualitative Inquiry, 20*(1), 37–50.

Owen, L. (2015). Monstrous freedom: Charting fat ambivalence. *Fat Studies, 4*(1), 1–13.

Sellberg, K., & Sellberg, A. (2014). Fluid fat: Considerations of culture and corporeality. *Interalia: A Journal of Queer Studies, 9*, 304–318.

Stryker, S. (2006). My words to Victor Frankenstein above the village of Chamounix: Performing transgender rage. In S. Stryker & S. Whittle (Eds.), *The transgender studies reader* (pp. 244–256). London: Routledge.

Vade, D., & Solovay, S. (2009). No apology: Shared struggles in fat and transgender law. In E. Rothblum, & S. Solovay (Eds.), *The fat studies reader* (pp. 167–175). New York: New York University Press.

White, F. R. (2014). Fat/trans: Queering the activist body. *Fat Studies, 3*(2), 86–100.

White, F. R. (2019). Embodying the fat/trans intersection. In M. Friedman, C. Rice & J. Rinaldi (Eds.), *Thickening fat: Fat bodies, intersectionality and social justice* (pp. 110–121). London: Routledge.

Wilson, M. (2002). "I am the prince of pain, for I am a princess of the brain": Liminal transgender identities, narratives and the elimination of ambiguities. *Sexualities, 5*(4), 425–448.

Zach (2015). Zach. In J. W. Shultz (Ed.), *Trans/portraits: Voices from transgender communities* (pp. 94–95). Lebanon, NH: Dartmouth College Press.

11

FATNESS AND DISABILITY

Law, identity, co-constructions, and future directions[1]

April Herndon

In 1997, Charlotte Cooper boldly asked the question "can a fat woman identify as disabled?". Cooper was arguably the first scholar in a field that would come to be known as Fat Studies to pose this question so directly. Influenced by Cooper and others, five years later, I wrote a piece that asked the same question; in part by examining my own experiences and the cases of fatness and deafness alongside each other, I came up with a similar answer to Cooper (Herndon, 2002). Yes, a fat woman can consider herself disabled. Now more than fifteen years out from my own piece, scholars and activists are still engaging with the question of whether or not fatness is a disability and how those two categories can be understood in tandem. From many people's perspectives, including mine and Cooper's, fatness can certainly be considered a disabling condition; those who are fat can arguably adopt the label of disabled for themselves personally and even legally. Yet, resistance remains to considering fatness a disability, among everyone from legal scholars to activists, with worries ranging from the mutability of fatness to frivolous claims and the fear that fat people will be further stigmatized by claims to disability.

Activists and scholars who feel fatness and disability are not mutually exclusive categories nor embodiments have continued to point out that whether or not those embodiments are mutable or not misses the point of protective legislation. Those who understand fatness as a bodily trait that can – at least sometimes – cause disability, argue that resistance to thinking of fatness as a disability is often born out of misguided healthism that has become part of a much larger neoliberal project that aims to make some bodies and people seem worthy and others seem unworthy. Similarly, others argue that there is now an urgent need to tie fatness and disability together because state violence against groups closely identified with those categories, such as African Americans, is often bolstered by fatphobia and ableism.

Thus, to be sure, there are complications and tensions around fatness and disability and still an ongoing conversation about the nuances of tying fatness and disability together and its possible consequences. In this chapter, I review the scholarship about fatness as a disability with the aim of showing that – twenty years out from her initial inquiry and fifteen years out from my own – fatness as a disability is still being explored by scholars in ways that raise important and challenging questions. From the perspective of many people in the scholarly and activist community, in a world where both people who are fat and people who are disabled (and perhaps especially people who live at the intersections of those identities and other marginalized social locations) are still positioned as social pariahs, thinking through fatness as a disability still offers personal and political possibilities for justice and an important means of thinking through lived experiences using an intersectional model.

The legal case for fatness and disability: the social model

Many scholars have suggested identifying as disabled under the law as a route to providing justice in cases of fat discrimination. Most notably, legal scholar Sondra Solovay's book *Tipping the scales of justice* (2000) took up the issue of weight-based discrimination and an examination of then current U.S. laws and cases, drawing the conclusion that disability claims were an appropriate avenue to justice. Influenced by Solovay's work and my own desire to find a path of justice for those suffering under fatphobia, I also took up this approach in my article, "Disparate but disabled: Fat embodiment and Disability Studies" (2002). In that piece, I aimed to explain the contours of how fat and deaf people each constitute relatively cohesive social groups through their shared intra- and inter-group experiences and how examining fatness and deafness alongside one another can help us understand that fatness shares a great deal of territory with deafness, a condition many people would never question as being disabling. In doing so, I argued that the *Americans with Disability Act (ADA)*, especially the prong that addresses those *perceived* as disabled, could offer a path toward justice for those facing fat discrimination. At its base, the "perceived as" prong of the *ADA* suggests that the person being discriminated against may or may not have a condition that affects one or more major life activities but may be *perceived* as being affected (United States Government, 1990). Using scholarship by key legal figures, I used an approach created in the 1970s by a group of disability activists in the UK called the "social model" (The Union of the Physically Impaired Against Segregation, 1997). This model "challenges the hegemony of the traditional 'medical model.' In contrast to the medical model, which defines disability in terms of individual biological defects, the social model focuses on barriers created by cultural attitudes and the built environment" (Mollow, 2017, p. 112). Later, this model was further developed by others in the field of Disability Studies who favored a focus on the social construction of disability.[2] I argued that it was primarily the "perceived as" angle that could be useful for situating fat people as a group who were being discriminated against based on stigma and built environments. More recently, other scholars have investigated fatness as a disability using various models and have come to similar conclusions – regardless of model. Toby Brandon and Gary Pritchard (2011) conclude that "fatness can in many respects be considered a disability, disability here being conceptualized further than traditional medical impairment to include elements of political, social, and positive personal identity" (p. 89). This approach is arguably the most common taken in Fat Studies scholarship and by activists in the community who aim to suggest that fatness can, in fact, be tied to disability through both self-identification and legal definitions. In her landmark article, "Can a fat woman call herself disabled?" Cooper (1997) plainly states, "I consider the experience of being fat in a fat-hating culture to be disabling" (p. 39). Cooper reaches this conclusion by charting out the multitude of ways that fat people are disabled by that "fat-hating culture," including an analysis of defining features like physical spaces that do not work for larger bodies and employment-based discrimination. As such, the social model approach also suggests that the "fix" is in the social realm rather than via people's bodies.

Recently, Mollow (2017) echoed Cooper, noting that "when analyzed through the lens of the social model, fatness *can* be understood as a disability" (p. 111). In fact, in a piece where she calls for disability scholars to "get fat," Mollow (2015) argues that doing so is necessary "because in the fatphobic cultural imaginary, fatness is inseparable from disability" (p. 199). Mollow's point is spot on in the sense that representations of fatness are almost always coupled with representations of physical disability. One need only think of the number of posts on websites such as

"People of Walmart" that regularly feature photos of large people using motorized carts and the comments that almost always center around fatness being the reason the person is using a cart to make the store accessible to be reminded of how tightly bound fatness and disability are in our cultural imaginary. Unfortunately, a number of photos are of fat people using motorized carts for accessibility. The comments very often center around claims that the person wouldn't need the motorized cart for accessibility if they would walk through the store without assistance. While on one level this suggests that those commenting do see fatness as a disability, the comments also suggest that the "blame" is with the individual and that people can lose weight – perhaps even a significant amount – by walking through Walmart.

Yet, resistance to understanding fatness as a disability under the law in the U.S. remains among activists, scholars, and citizens. Although it is beyond the scope of this piece to go into all reasons for resistance, suffice it to say that the biggest ongoing fear of the general public and many legal scholars is that of frivolous claims, a fear driven by fatness being seen as a moral short-coming and/or mutable. Arguably, the first time the issue of obesity meeting the legal definition of disability was addressed was in a 1981 case involving an employee of Union Pacific. In that case, the ruling was against the plaintiff, with the court ruling that "obesity was not a disabil-ity because it was 'not an immutable condition such as blindness or lameness'" (Vallor, 2013, p. 289). While a full review of all the legal cases involving obesity and disability claims is beyond the scope of this piece, it is fair to conclude that plaintiffs have had mixed results with lawsuits in which they attempted to use the *ADA* or other state based legislation to file discrimination claims using obesity as a disability. Currently in the United States, only the state of Michigan and few cities scattered here and there offer protections specifically for weight, so available legislation and recourse are sparse.

At the same time, Canadian provinces are also discussing weight as a disability. While the *Canadian Human Rights Act* does not include fatness per se, it does include disability and genetic conditions as protected categories (Government of Canada, 1985). Further, Canadian law has recognized in recent cases that some plaintiffs' obesity "[could] be characterized as a real or perceived disability" (Luther, 2010, p. 167). In November 2017 a bill was introduced in Mani-toba to prohibit size discrimination but was voted down due to claims that it would prove near impossible to enforce (Lambert, 2017). An activist group is currently lobbying again to have "physical size and weight" included in the human rights code, prohibiting discrimination against both people who may be described as fat and those who are of short stature (McGuckin, 2018).

In most cases, the strongest legal objections to considering fatness a disability tend to center around concerns that the condition is preventable and/or mutable (Kirkland, 2003, 2006, 2008; Luther, 2010; Vallor, 2013). Such interpretations, I would suggest, meet neither the letter of the law nor the spirit of the *ADA* in the United States (or most other legislation aimed at protecting people who are disabled). Anti-discrimination law around disability also does not focus on the cause of one's disability historically. For example, if one uses a wheelchair because of a congen-ital condition or a preventable injury (such as a drunk driving accident) is irrelevant in the eyes of the law because it is not supposed to be a moral decision about how one became disabled. Further, although an unpopular claim, let us imagine that weight is mutable – even if through life altering and life-threatening measures and even though weight loss may only be temporary. Regardless, the law does not itself require that one change one's body rather than claiming disability. Although there have been some cases in the U.S. where fat plaintiffs who have been injured while at work were asked to lose weight after filing for compensation as a requirement of their ongoing "treatment" for injuries,[3] for the most part disability law has recognized that changing one's body is not a requirement. I explored this issue of an "elective disability" in my piece on cochlear implants and noted that courts have not, as yet, forced people to adopt cochlear technology (Herndon, 2002, p. 128). As Regan Chastain (2014) succinctly states about the *ADA* in particular, "the *ADA* rules apply to the person standing in front of you who meets the definition right now, not the person you think they might be someday who would not." Using the law in these ways, however, has arguably sidestepped issues of impairments (Wendell, 1996), what would be considered physiological challenges of being fat, creating some notable tensions with the social model's focus on built environments and social attitudes. While the analysis the social model provides has been and remains invaluable for naming the problems that exist in societies rather than bodies, the social model – and perhaps what some would call an overemphasis on it – runs the risk of implying that fat people are *only* made disabled by attitudes or inadequate spaces. As a result of this emphasis, many scholars and activists have raised an uncomfortable and necessary point: what about people who are disabled by their fatness and not by the environment or other people's attitudes? Where do these people fit into such frameworks and what are the consequences if and when they don't?

Legal scholar Anna Kirkland (2006) is perhaps one of the most vocal legal voices about weight and disability, and, from her perspective, some people have celebrated the "regarded as" prong of *ADA* legislation precisely because they believe it turns attention to the social issues and away from medicalization. In short, Kirkland argues that using the *ADA*'s "regarded as" prong is mostly a reliance upon the social model of disability rather than necessarily tending to the medical issues that may accompany fatness. Kirkland (2006) goes on to note that "Fat activists would want fatness to be named a disability, but only if another model of disability were to eclipse the medicalized one that they understand the *ADA* to offer them" (p. 5). In short, Kirkland points out that relying on the "regarded as" prong as the main part of the *ADA* to be used to gain justice takes into account the problems with fat people being stigmatized as lazy or incapable, but that Fat Studies scholars and activists, by using that strategy, are also resisting the medical model. Without doubt, the medical model has been incredibly troublesome, and it should be resisted. As a frame for understanding fat and/or disability, the medical model has cast any problem that members of these groups face as a result of their bodies and/or conditions. In short, the medical model allows no room for engaging social issues that may create, cause or exacerbate fatness and/or disability. For example, under the medical model, lack of access to support services, proper nutrition, and medical care as conditions that might lead to someone becoming disabled or more disabled or becoming fat or fatter are irrelevant. But this resistance to the medical model comes with what are likely unintended consequences for some members of the fat community.

First, she argues that labeling obesity as a disability works *against* mainstream fat activism that aims to position fatness as a natural human variation like height. She writes, "Establishing obesity as a disability would contradict [National Association to Advance Fat Americans] identity concept by setting fatness apart from thinness or normalcy and acknowledging that it is an affliction rather than simply part of the variation of healthy bodies" (Kirkland, 2003, p. 27). Second, she argues that naming fatness as a disability under the *ADA* replicates the issue of individualizing fatness rather than offering group protection to fat people. According to Kirkland, what she names "managerial individualism" of the *ADA* legislation, means that the social dimensions of discrimination take a back seat in favor of accommodating a person based on their individualized needs. She writes that, under this rubric, "fat identity will not be assisted in its political emergence by gaining disability rights because they will operate managerially on fat people one by one, destabilizing opportunities for collective accounts of fat oppression" (Kirkland, 2006). In other words, fat people, as they filed claims, would be assessed one by one rather than fat people as a group gaining protections under the legislation as a politicized group. In the case of employment, for example, each person's fatness would be assessed as it affected or did not affect the person filing the claim's ability to perform the work with a reasonable accommodation, and then that "difference" would be managed accordingly. From Kirkland's perspective, this does little to really expand the rights of fat people as a whole because under this system "fatness would not be able to acquire the sort of politicized identity that may be necessary to compel other expansions of legal rights" (2006). In short, Kirkland is skeptical about the *ADA* as a mechanism for eventually gaining wholesale rights for fat people.

In fact, Kirkland argues that disability claims, which are most often successful when the litigant proves that he or she can perform a job with reasonable accommodation, which is often called "functionalism," do little or nothing to forward the underlying goals of fat activism: "because this concept of functionalism best accommodates fat people who function in the same way as their thinner counterparts on the measured criteria, it does nothing to promote difference or to unsettle antifat biases" (2003, p. 33). Ultimately, Kirkland maintains that if one of the tenets of Fat Studies scholars and fat activists is to dismantle fat discrimination, strategies that set up thin(ner) people who do not need accommodation as the norm.

Kirkland also notes that many fat activists themselves have not embraced the idea of using disability as a means to gaining protection from discrimination. In a series of interviews with members of the National Association to Advance Fat Acceptance, Kirkland (2008) noted palpable tension around the notion of fat people being disabled with her interviewees being sharply divided when she posed a question about whether or not employers should provide armless chairs as an accommodation for fat workers. She writes that "reactions varied, but most interviewees were either sharply negative about being considered disabled (even if it would secure more rights) or highly pragmatic about using the label *disabled*" (Kirkland, 2008, p. 420). Kirkland cites fat activist Marilyn Wann as saying "In the dark times you use whatever you have" (2008, p. 420). In the end, Kirkland (2008) summarizes her participants' responses as characterizing fatness as a bodily difference (larger people need larger chairs) that can be accommodated through universal design rather while still suggesting that they are uncomfortable labeling fatness in and of itself as disabling.

What's "health" got to do with it? The good fatty/bad fatty divide

Kirkland is not alone in her concern that what appears to be a refrain of "fat people are just like thin people" may provide short-lived justice – and only for a few members of the fat community. In fact, because of such concerns, some Fat Studies scholars and activists have begun to take on different approaches that step away from legal definitions of disability and seeking rights through identifying a disability as defined by legislation, with some, like Lucy Aphramor (2009), stating that she is not concerned with legal definitions but rather with "whether fatness should … be politicized as a disability issue" (p. 905). In other words, some Fat Studies scholars have, it seems, begun to step away from meeting legal definitions of the *ADA* as a mechanism for justice.

Part of the scholarly field and some activists have moved in different directions because they see claims that suggest fat people do not have health problems, such as the kinds of claims often made when the *ADA* has been invoked, as equally troubling. For example, Zoe Meleo-Erwin (2002) argues that strategies of normalizing fatness by claiming that fat people are always healthy sets up "health" as another kind of troubling norm to be met by anyone seeking justice. She writes, "the desire of some fat activists to bring fatness under the banner of 'normal,' particularly through attempts to link certain forms of fatness and health, is a losing battle" (p. 388). Fat Studies scholars and activists have long pointed out that within mainstream society there is a tendency to separate fat people into groups frequently referred to as the "good fatty" and "bad fatty" camps (Chastain, 2016). Explaining the camps, Regan Chastain (2016) notes those thought to be in the "good fatty" camp are fat people who "take care of themselves" by exercising and eating right, perhaps make attempts to lose weight, talk about their attempts to lose weight as a kind of confessional moment of their desire to be thin (i.e. "normal"), and so forth. Those in the "bad fatty" camp are fat people who do not engage in weight loss projects, do not apologize for their size, and who may very well be ill – either because of their fatness or may be fat because of an illness (good fatty bad fatty bs). Some of the worry with strategies that attempt to define fatness as "normal" and all fat people as "healthy" is that those who are not healthy are even further stigmatized.

And while Fat Studies scholars and many fat activists have positioned themselves as "bad fatty" rebels in the sense that they do not diet and disparage attempts at weight loss because they believe that health is not dependent on size, one criticism that has been leveled against them is that through a regular refrain of "we're totally healthy" scholars and activists have unwittingly engaged in healthism and ableism that are not, in fact, healthy. It is a process Kathleen LeBesco (2004) refers to as the "will to innocence," a process by which many different strategies, including references to feats of athletic performance and claims of health, are used to suggest that "despite their girth, [fat people] deserve to be treated well because their deeds make them healthy" (p. 112). Thus, arguments that attempt to position fat people as always healthy people who are never affected by their fatness run the risk of creating a category of fatness that is also exclusionary and setting up "health" as another moral standard by which people are judged worthy of protections (or not).

In particular the Health at Every Size Movement (HAES), which no one denies has done an incredible amount of positive work for fat people, has recently been implicated in setting up a subtle yet disconcerting divide between good fatties and bad fatties by working very hard to connect fatness and health – or at least to uncouple fatness from disease. The HAES movement has been key to helping spread the message that fatness, in and of itself, is neither disabling nor a disease. On their website, HAES notes that the organization "celebrates body diversity" and "values body knowledge and lived experience." As Aphramor (2009) encapsulates their message, HAES "problematizes institutionalized body hatred, not bodily difference, and recognizes the role and impact of oppression in scientific ideologies on health and outcomes" (p. 904). Like many other scholars, fat activists, and fat people, in the early development of my fat identity and my scholarship about fatness, HAES was thrilling and new and formative because it talked back to the medical establishment and made room for more conversations about the sociocultural constructions of fatness rather than just speaking about fatness as a medical pathology and/or fat people as always already diseased.

Yet, as time has gone on, many of us have begun to wonder about what happens to people for whom the idea and reality of "health at every size" doesn't ring true. Where is the room for such people within the theoretical frameworks and within the movement for fat justice? S. E. Smith (2014), in a piece called "Not your good fatty" says bluntly, "We need to talk about what it's like to *not* be healthy at every size." Smith's main concern is the "erasure of people with disabilities from the size acceptance movement" (2014). Mollow (2017), in her criticism specifically of HAES philosophy, expresses concerns that when disability is spoken about by Linda Bacon, one of the founders of HAES, it has sometimes been spoken about as a tragedy, noting that Bacon has claimed fatness does not "doom" people to a life of "disability" (p. 112). What is important to note here, again, is that Bacon likely made such a statement out of a desire to counter the medico-cultural narrative that constructs fatness *always* disabling and always doom and gloom. Yet, both Smith (2014) and Mollow (2017) have a legitimate concern regarding the word choice and discourse that emphasizes health and arguably catastrophizes disability. Further, Jennifer Lee and Cat Pausé (2016) argue that while HAES has many laudable goals, the very concept of "health" the framework relies upon is overdetermined. They write, "at times HAES is still often presented, especially in short-hand, in reaction to the current dominant health paradigm, hence only in terms of exercising and eating, and in terms of a notion that we are aiming, and should be aiming for 'health' without really addressing what 'health' is and is not and who is allowed to be considered 'healthy'" (p. 11). Thus, in the modern day neoliberal environment Pausé and Lee express deep and warranted concern that, at its core, HAES supports a notion of "health" as defined in ways that may be inherently problematic for some bodies and prohibitive of ever reaching "health."

What is lost in HAES and similar philosophies, according to these scholars, is a narrative and framework that allows for fat people who *are* disabled by their fatness and/or who are not healthy. Smith (2014) goes on to note that "hardline HAES advocacy [the insistence that fatness is never a health concern nor disabling] plays directly into the good fatty/bad fatty dichotomy that looms so large in the minds of many of us" (para. 9). In other words, within its own borders, the community of fat scholars and activists risks setting up a good fatty/bad fatty dichotomy around "health" and ability. And because fat people who experience their fatness as disabling and/or as a health concern understand that some parts of the fat community think respect and rights are more reachable within the "good fatty" framework, Smith (2014) goes on to talk about the pressure exerted by hardliners' demands that "we [fat people] must be healthy, happy fatties, and we cannot diverge from this mission, or we will be letting the side down." "Letting the side down" means being a bad fatty that society can point to as an example of fatness as a disabling trait brought upon one's self because of poor choices. What Smith gestures to is the pressure to perform a certain kind of fatness that has been constructed as politically useful: the good fatty who is healthy, able-bodied, and "just like thin people."

The pressure exerted by this need for politically useful narratives has been examined by other scholars and activists within the community. In some of her ethnographic work, Meleo-Erwin (2002) writes about a meeting called "The right to be ill: Queer hedonism and policing health" where participants in a New York based group called Queer Commons discussed how imperatives to health affected their lives. Meleo-Erwin (2002) notes that "some attendees discussed the difficulties of maintaining a fat positive attitude in the face of illness and impairment. Others acknowledged the challenges of avoiding good fatty/bad fatty trap within fat politics" (p. 398). It's fair to say that such criticism is reaching critical mass. Cooper (2016), in her book, *Fat activism*, notes that the "[focus on health] creates fat activism that quickly becomes intolerable and untenable for many people, including those who are superfat, unfit, unhealthy, or chronically ill" (p. 185). And, like it or not, these may be the very people who do experience and narrate their fat as disabling or at least contributing to their being disabled. If we are tending to the materiality of fat bodies as well as their cultural constructions, then there must be space to allow for people's stories of their own embodiments as becoming disabling or contributing to being disabled. For example, there is no direct evidence that being fat causes osteoarthritis of the knees; plenty of thin people also have the condition. However, for some people who have the condition, they may maintain that losing or gaining weight can affect their mobility and/or pain levels. For someone who is super fat, not being mobile primarily because of one's size is disabling. Thus, frameworks that can hold an account of fatness that is sometimes neutral in people's lives and may at other times represent problems seem especially important.

Fatness, disability, and the neoliberal project of being a good citizen

For some fat activists, the call to be "healthy" is seen not only as inaccurate but as yet another neoliberal project of proving one's self to be a good citizen through individual choices, leaving those who supposedly fail to make the appropriate choices to blame for their own conditions and as a drag on those who are choosing appropriately (Biltekoff, 2007; Herndon, 2006; McPhail, 2017). Cooper (2016) writes about the focus on health and citizenship in this way: "Healthist fat activism downplays important connections with disability politics because it does not regard disability, ill health, or impairment as a part of the project of becoming good citizens" (p. 187). And although she does not directly tie it to citizenship, Cat Pausé's (2018) blog "Why I don't care about health" expresses similar reservations about "health" becoming another means to respectability politics, "a term coined by Evelyn Brooks Higginbotham to explain the efforts made by black women to demonstrate they were good enough for white society to overlook their flaw of being black (and women)." Speaking bluntly, Pausé (2018) goes on to argue that "health is the latest form of respectability politics for fat people. And I want no part of it." In a powerful statement about why she sees health as a kind of ultimately bankrupt respectability politics for fat people, she writes:

> I am incredibly fat; death fat as we like to say in the Fatosphere. In this way, I may have learned earlier than others that emerging in respectability politics wasn't going to get me anywhere. It doesn't matter how much I exercise or am seen eating a salad, the world will perceive me as incredibly unhealthy and incredibly unworthy. It doesn't matter what my health status is, everyone, including healthcare providers, will treat me like a ticking time bomb that will, one day, implode and double-stomachedly take down public healthcare systems.

Thus, Pausé rejects the project of proving one's self as worthy of respect or protection via claims to "health" or being a "good fatty" because she sees this as an avenue not open to fat people in the first place because of how overdetermined the story of their embodiment is in fatphobic societies.

Furthermore, people should be protected from discrimination regardless of health status; to suggest otherwise is to engage in ableism that roots people's rights and protections in having a body that is never ill, infirmed, or disabled. Mollow (2017) writes, "This newer thread of fat studies scholarship makes the important anti-ableist observation that fat people deserve social justice regardless of whether they are 'healthy'" (p. 112). Thus, in resisting the turn toward the respectability politics of health, scholars and activists are also embracing those who may not diet or exercise, the superfat, those who are ill, and disabled.

Also refusing to engage in respectability politics and interested in bringing fatness and disability closer together in academic disciplines is Mollow (2015), who recently argued that fatness and disability need to be coupled in very direct ways by calling on Disability Studies, as a field, to "get fat." From her perspective, "getting fat" means adopting a kind of "sideways" identification with fatness, identifying *with* rather than as an "ally," through understanding and owning how similarly constructed fatness and disability are (p. 200). Yet, in the same way that there has been hesitation to name fatness as a disability, Mollow (2015) understands that Disability Studies scholars may also have hesitations. She writes, "to get fat is to risk losing a lot: notions of individual control, fantasies of superiority over subjects whose bodies are larger than yours, and faith in scientific 'facts'; all fall away when we get serious about getting fat" (p. 201). Her argument here is applicable to Fat Studies and Disability Studies as fields but also to people who inhabit the social locations those fields study and who are activists in the communities. Fat people and fat scholars and activists may feel the same tension with identifying as disabled. To identify as disabled has been thought to mean giving up that vision of fatness as always "normal" and never pathological and to embrace another identity that is also often seen as spoiled in mainstream America.

Future directions: why race, fatness, and disability

Yet identifying fatness and disability as co-constructed has gained a kind of urgency as these categories and the cultural narratives about the people in them are being used to bolster racism in the United States, in particular. Thus, there is an emerging call to closely identify fatness with disability on the personal level but also on the levels of our theorizing of identity-based categories and violence against members of those categories. As a field, Fat Studies has consistently expressed an ongoing commitment to ongoing intersectionality – in terms of discourse analysis and lived experiences. According to LeBesco (2011), "'the body' is never just a material reality but also the site of contested discourses about power, health, beauty, nature, *race*, class and a bevy of other possibilities" [emphasis added] (p. 99). And this site of contested discourses, particularly about race, is one of the places where thinking about fatness as a disability is most urgent. In Mollow's recent piece, "Unvictimizable: Toward a Fat Black Disability Studies" (2017), she analyzes the tragic death of Eric Garner, an African American man who died at the hands of police. In examining how Garner's body and death were described, both in official accounts, and in comments on the case, Mollow showcases how fatness and disability are inextricably tied, especially when it comes to black bodies in the United States and state sanctioned violence.

For many years, Fat Studies scholars have argued that fatness is at once invisible, in the sense that socio-medical constructions of fatness render people invisible as fully human agents, and hypervisible, in the sense that fatness is constantly portrayed in diet commercials and government documents as a scourge to be dealt with at any cost (Gailey, 2014). In our society, fatness functions as both an incredibly visible marker thought to indicate someone's moral character and health status but also a trait not to be acknowledged as important enough to be worthy of protections. In short, fatness exists in such a complicated matrix of signification that it often serves what seem like contradictory purposes. Mollow (2017) extends this analysis and argues that race and disability exist in a similarly and seemingly contradictory set of signifiers, meaning that when fatness and blackness converge in one body, fatphobia, racism, and ableism unite to make everything the fault of the individual. She roots this framework in the history of slavery in the United States, writing that the commonplace thinking was that

> black people were so prone to physical and mental disabilities that they could not survive without the 'protection' of their white owners – while at the same time maintaining that people of African descent possessed such inordinate strength that they didn't suffer from the abuses that their enslavers imposed upon them.
>
> *(p. 105)*

In the case of Garner and other African Americans, then, large bodies mark them both inherently disabled and simultaneously unable to be harmed. Thus, "black people—of all sizes, but fat black people in particular—are figured as innately disabled but also as invulnerable to disability, injury, or suffering" (Mollow, 2017, p. 105).

What results is a climate in which "fatphobia and ableism function as weapons of anti-black violence, allowing Garner to be blamed for his own death at the hands of police" (Mollow, 2017, p. 105). For example, Mollow (2017) notes that one Congressman, defending the police chokehold that killed Garner, specifically named Garner's fatness, asthma, and heart conditions as the true causes of his death and his size as what necessitated the chokehold in the first place (p. 105). Thus, on the one hand Garner was so morally weak he could not make good food choices and ended up being a "350-pound person" with asthma and a heart condition, but at the same time he was so powerful that he had to be put into a chokehold and eventually killed (Mollow, 2017, p. 105).

Mollow (2017) sums it up this way:

> One side of this double bind renders violence against black people inconsequential by suggesting that fatness is the root cause of all injuries inflicted upon them, while its other side depicts violence as the necessary response to the excessive physical power that black people, especially those who are fat, are imagined to embody.
>
> *(p. 105)*

Although she does not specifically name Marilyn Frye (1983) in her essay, this situation reflects what Frye wrote about as the very definition: "One of the most characteristic and ubiquitous features of the world as experienced by oppressed people is the *double bind* situations in which options are reduced to a very few and all of them expose one to penalty, censure, or deprivation" [emphasis added] (p. 2).

It is also important to note that, although she does not explicitly discuss it in the case of Garner, Mollow (2015) has written elsewhere that one of the key experiences that both fat people and disabled people share is not being believed about their symptoms or their narratives of their bodies (p. 206).[4] Tragically, Eric Garner repeatedly told the officers choking him that he could not breathe, which, under the *ADA* would qualify as a disability; yet, he was not believed. In fact, named in the "major life activities," any one of which the *ADA* says must be affected in order for an individual to be seen as disabled in the eyes of the law is breathing (United States Government, 1990). After Garner's death, the line "I can't breathe" became a rallying call among those seeking to end police brutality against African Americans (Gross, 2017). Here, then, it becomes clear again that fatness and disability are inherently tied and that frameworks must take them both into account, especially if the aim is to understand how state violence against African Americans in the United States is fueled by fatphobia and ableism in addition to racism: "fatphobia and ableism function as weapons of antiblack violence, allowing Garner to be blamed for his own death at the hands of the police" (Mollow, 2017, p. 105). Mollow (2017) argues that "because fatness and disability are inseparably linked in the cultural imagination it is impossible to adequately theorize antifat oppression without simultaneously attending to ableism" (p. 106). In other words, Mollow's (2017) claim is that fatness and disability cannot, in fact, be separated in any useful way. Given this, she declares that "we need … a methodology that takes measure of the deeply imbricated relationships among racism, ableism, and fatphobia" and suggests that a new field emerge, a field she tentatively names "fat black disability studies" (p. 106).

Several activists have already begun doing this timely and important work, taking seriously the notion that frameworks cannot simply "add in" new identities but must be intersectional from their inceptions. Speaking specifically about her time with Leroy Moore and Patty Berne, founders of the *Sins Invalid* project, Nomy Lamm (2015) writes about the vision of "disability justice" that Berne and Moore bring to life in their performances where she "witnessed some of the most radical work [she'd] ever seen or imagined" (para. 3) as she watched people of color and queer identified people with disabilities engage with assistive technologies and revel in their bodies on stage. Speaking to Berne about the work, Lamm (2015) realizes that the performance spoke to something she had noticed but never fully grasped about a good deal of disability activism: "it was single issue focused. It was dominated by whiteness, straightness, and maleness" (para. 4). Echoing the need to move away from a singular focus, in a keynote address Mia Mingus (2010) argued that intersectionality "is about moving beyond single-issue politics; it's about understanding the complexities of our lives. It is understanding that fighting for racial justice

IS queer; fighting for disability IS queer." In the same way, fighting for fat justice is fighting for disability justice, racial justice, and queer justice. These identities can no longer be cleaved from one another if we hope to move the field of Fat Studies forward in a way that recognizes and honors the richness and complications of people's lives.

Whether or not a new field emerges, there is no doubt more theorizing needs to be done about disability and fatness and how those categories interact with social locations around race and sexuality and class. More attention needs to be paid to how fat and/or disabled people experience their bodies. Legal frameworks and political frameworks need to take into account that the experiences of fatness and disability are wide ranging; in the same way that the monolithic account of fatness as always already diseased did not serve fat people well, neither will frameworks that suggest fat people are always healthy or that fatness is never a disabling condition nor ever contributes to disability. And all of this work must happen as we pay increasingly careful attention to race, class, gender and other categories that affect people's experiences of their bodies and how fatness and disability are constructed. And the way the field pays attention matters. Chandra Talpade Mohanty (2003) argued that fields of study cannot simply "add and stir" race (p. 519), nor can a field like Fat Studies simply "add and stir" class or disability. The frameworks must be renegotiated; the field must pull back from tightly focusing on a single issue to see the entire landscape. The social and legal models of disability – and even our medical understandings – must be expanded in ways that offer a finer grained image of how fatness and disability can and do come together in discourse, laws, and lives.

Notes

1   For the sake of focus, this article's scope is limited to primarily the United States and Canada, especially where legal approaches to fatness as a disability are concerned. I do, however, employ a wide range of theorists whose ideas have been key to the development of the field of Fat Studies.
2   The list of scholars here is almost too numerable to name because the social model has been so key to the field. As a start, the work of the following Disability Studies scholars is notable in this respect: Mike Oliver; Simi Lintin; Susan Wendell; Rosemarie Garland-Thomson; Lennard Davis; Harland Hahn. In addition to these scholars are a host of scholars who have worked with the social model to show its shortcomings, such as Tom Shakespeare and Liz Crow.
3   Anna Kirkland discusses these cases in her article, "Representations of fatness and personhood: Pro-fat advocacy and the limits and uses of the law." Using several different cases, she explains how plaintiffs have been legally found to either be responsible for their own injuries because they were fat at the time they happened and/or were found to be at fault because they later failed to lose weight when weight loss was prescribed as a treatment for something like back pain.
4   Inckle (2014) also writes about this in her work about gender politics and disability. She notes that in cases involving young girls who have learning disabilities, signs of sexual abuse are routinely understood within the medical realm as being part of their "condition" rather than a sign of sexual abuse. For example, she details one specific case where the sexual abuse of a young girl was questioned because no one could imagine someone wanting to have sex with her (397). I include this example here to show a pattern – across many kinds of disabilities and experiences – that suggests that, in general, people with disabilities aren't believed and it's often their conditions that are blamed – even when they are harmed by others.

References

Aphramor, L. (2009). Disability and the anti-obesity offensive. *Disability and Society, 24*(7), 897–909.

Biltekoff, C. (2007). The terror within: Obesity is post 9/11 U.S. life. *American Studies, 48*(3), 29–48.

Brandon, G., & Pritchard, T. (2011). Being fat: A conceptual analysis using three models of disability. *Disability and Society, 26*(1), 79–92.

Charlton, J. I. (2000). *Nothing about us without us: Disability oppression and empowerment*. Berkeley: University of California Press.

Chastain, R. (2014, Dec 19). Is "obesity" a disability? *Dances with Fat.* https://danceswithfat.wordpress.com/?s=is+obesity+a+disability&submit=Search

Chastain, R. (2016, Mar 15). Good fatty bad fatty bs. *Dances with Fat.* https://danceswithfat.wordpress.com/2016/03/15/good-fatty-bad-fatty-bs/

Cooper, C. (1997). Can a fat woman call herself disabled? *Disability and Society, 12*(1), 31–42.

Cooper, C. (2016). *Fat activism: A radical social movement.* Bristol: HammerOn Press.

Crow, L. (1992). Renewing the social model of disability. *Roaring Girl.* http://www.roaring-girl.com/work/renewing-the-social-model-of-disability/

Davis, L. (1995). *Enforcing normalcy: Disability, deafness, and the body.* London: Verson Press.

Frye, M. (1983). *Politics of reality: Essays in feminist theory.* Freedom, CA: The Crossing Press.

Gailey, J. (2014). *The hyper(in)visible fat woman: Weight and gender discourse in contemporary society.* New York: Macmillan.

Garland-Thomson, R. (1997). *Extraordinary bodies: Figuring physical disabilities in American culture and literature.* New York: Columbia University Press.

Government of Canada. (1985). *Canadian Human Rights Act.* https://laws-lois.justice.gc.ca/eng/acts/h-6/FullText.html

Gross, T. (2017, October 23). "I can't breath" examines modern policing and the life and death of Eric Garner. *NPR.* https://www.npr.org/2017/10/23/559498678/i-can-t-breathe-explores-life-and-death-at-the-hands-of-police

Hahn, H. (1985). Towards a politics of disability: Definitions, disciplines, and policies. *The Social Science Journal, 22*(4), 87–105.

Health at Every Size. (2018). Mission statement. https://haescommunity.com/

Herndon, A. M. (2002). Disparate but disabled: Fat embodiment and disability studies. *NWSA Journal, 14*(3), 120–137.

Herndon, A. M. (2006). Collateral damage from friendly fire? Race, class, nation, and the "war on obesity." *Social Semiotics, 15*(2), 127–141.

Inckle, K. (2014). A lame argument: Profoundly disabled embodiment as critical gender politics. *Disability and Society, 29*(3), 388–401.

Kirkland, A. (2003). Representations of fatness and personhood: Pro-fat advocacy and the limits and uses of law. *Representations, 82*(3), 24–51.

Kirkland, A. (2006). What's at stake in fatness as a disability? *Disability Studies Quarterly, 26*(1). https://papers.ssrn.com/sol3/papers.cfm?abstract_id=920485

Kirkland, A. (2008). Think of the hippopotamus: Rights consciousness in the fat acceptance movement. *Law and Society, 42*(2), 397–432.

Lambert, S. (2017, Nov 2). Manitoba government rejects bid for human rights protection for the obese. *CBC-News.* https://www.cbc.ca/news/canada/manitoba/manitoba-obesity-rights-bill-rejected-1.4384627

Lamm, N. (2015, Sept 2). This is disability justice. *The Body is Not an Apology.* https://thebodyisnotanapology.com/magazine/this-is-disability-justice/

LeBesco, K. (2004). Fat politics and the will to innocence. In K. Lebesco, & J. Braziel (Eds.), *Revolting bodies: The struggle to redefine fat identity* (pp. 111–124). Amherst: University of Massachusetts Press.

LeBesco, K. (2011). Epistemologies of fatness: The political contours of embodiment in fat studies. In M. J. Casper, & P. Currah (Eds.), *Corpus: An interdisciplinary reader on bodies and knowledge* (pp. 95–108). New York: Palgrave Macmillan.

Lee, J., & Pausé, C. (2016). Stigma in practice: Barriers to health for fat women. *Frontiers in Psychology, 7*, 1–15.

Lintin, S. (1998). *Claiming disability: Knowledge and identity.* New York: New York University Press.

Luther, E. (2010). Justice for all shapes and sizes: Combatting weight discrimination in Canada. *Alberta Law Review, 48*(1), 167–188.

McGuckin, A. (2018, Oct 18). Manitoba group wants size discrimination protection included in Human Rights Code. *Global News.* https://globalnews.ca/news/4534399/manitoba-group-wants-size-discrimination-protection-included-in-human-rights-code/

McPhail, D. (2017) *Contours of the nation: Making obesity and imagining Canada 1945–1970.* Toronto: University of Toronto Press.

Meleo-Erwin, Z. (2002). Disrupting normal: Toward the "ordinary and familiar" in fat politics. *Feminism and Psychology, 22*(2), 388–402.

Mingus, M. (2010, February 25). "Intersectionality" is a big fancy word for my life. *Leaving Evidence.* https://leavingevidence.wordpress.com/2010/02/25/%E2%80%9Cintersectionality%E2%80%9D-is-a-big-fancy-word-for-my-life/

Mohanty, C. T. (2003). "Under western eyes" revisited: Feminist solidarity through anti-capitalist struggles. *Signs, 28*(2), 499–535.

Mollow, A. (2015). Disability Studies gets fat. *Hypatia, 30*(1), 199–216.

Mollow, A. (2017). Unvictimizable: Toward a Fat Black Disability Studies. *African American Review, 50*(2), 105–121.

Oliver, M. (1983). *Social work with disabled people*. London: Macmillan.

Oliver, M. (1990). *The politics of disablement*. London: Macmillan.

Pausé, C. (2018, April 3). The HAES files: Why I don't care about health. *International Society of Critical Health Psychology*. https://ischp.info/2018/04/03/the-haes-files-why-i-dont-care-about-health/

Shakespeare, T. (2013). *Disability rights and wrongs revisited*. New York: Routledge.

Siebers, T. (2018). *Disability theory*. Ann Arbor: University of Michigan Press.

Solovay, S. (2000). *Tipping the scales of justice: Fighting weight-based discrimination*. New York: Prometheus.

Smith, S. E. (2014, Jun 2). Not your good fatty: HAES and disability. *Disability Intersections*. http://disability intersections.com/2014/06/453

United States Government. (1990). *Americans with Disabilities Act*. https://www.ada.gov/pubs/adastatute08.htm

The Union of the Physically Impaired Against Segregation. (1997). *Fundamental Principles of Disability*. https://disability-studies.leeds.ac.uk/wp-content/uploads/sites/40/library/UPIAS-fundamental-principles.pdf

Vallor, J. (2013). Gut check: Why obesity is not a disability under Tennessee law and how the legislature can address the obesity epidemic. *Tennessee Law and Society, 9*(2), 265–326.

Wendell, S. (1996). *The rejected body: Feminist philosophical reflections on disability*. New York: Routledge.

PART 3

Fat in the institution

Part 3 highlights how for many, fatness is personal. It is about identity, embodiment, agency. But fatness is not a state that is simply for an individual to experience and navigate. Fatness is socially constructed, and those constructions are (re)produced through social institutions, such as education, industry, healthcare, government, and the media. Chapters explore fatness, the fat body, and the lived experience of being fat, within the context of these institutions.

Katariina Kyrölä invites us to consider the role of the media in shaping our understandings of what constitutes a normal – a good – body, and how this reinforces negative ideas of fatness. She notes, "Among the most powerful ways of making fat embodiment appear threatening and in need of urgent intervention are the so-called 'factual' discourses in the media"(p. 107) raising to awareness media narratives that portend to be realistic representations of fat life, while employing sensationalistic perspectives by which to view fat life. Through illustrating examples of scholarship in this area, as well as examples of fat representations in the media, Kyrölä urges the reader (and future Fat Studies scholarship) to consider the role of affect in the media production and consumption of bodies, especially fat bodies.

Amena Azeez discusses the pervasive friction that exists between the fat body and the fashion industry. By recounting her experience as a life-long lover of fashion, fashion blogger, and chubby Indian woman, she illuminates how she charted her pathway to activism at the intersection of an incredibly fatphobic industry. She shares,

> Growing up as a fat girl in India I had no fat role models to look up to. Even when I started blogging there was no Tess Holliday or Ashley Graham or Gabi Gregg in India to seek inspiration from. I had to become my own role model.
>
> *(p. 117)*

It was through her choice to become her own role model that she began carving out a new space for fat fashion in India. Azeez reminds the reader that existing in a space that has vehemently denied one access is a powerful act of rebellion and political resistance.

Erin Cameron and Connie Russell, the scholars who brought us *The fat pedagogy reader* (2016), revisit their Fat Pedagogy Manifesto in their contribution to the Handbook. After briefly reviewing the history of fat pedagogy, and the literature in the field, the duo reflect on – and revise – the Fat Pedagogy Manifesto they produced for the Reader. These revisions include updates and new awareness related to power, praxis and focus. One such example is around an originally stated need for activists and scholars to better "meet" each other in their work. The authors reflect that it may be more productive

> to think of fat pedagogy not as a "two-way street" but as an intersection where multiple roads crisscross. Thus, not only are accessible research and evidence-informed practice important aspects of fat pedagogy, so too is learning about, from, and through fat activism.
>
> *(p. 123)*

The chapter is structured to represent the ways they have learned (and unlearned) in the preceding years in their hope that others may take up this manifesto to fatten their own educational ideas and practices.

Stephanie von Liebenstein's chapter provides an international perspective on the questions of weight and the law. Von Liebenstein presents an overview of weight discrimination in the law, and in Fat Studies scholarship, noting that very little has been done on the latter. She considers whether following a similar path that disability activists have trod could be an economical solution for those who wish to see legislation protecting individuals from discrimination based on their body size. She offers,

> none of them acknowledge the fact that even the social model of disability needs an impairment as a prerequisite to be applicable. And it is this prerequisite that many fat activists and fat studies scholars, especially those who do not experience their fat bodies as diseased or impaired in any way, feel uncomfortable with.
>
> *(p. 138)*

Consideration is also given to whether adopting the framework of protecting people under "physical appearance" legislation, as in France or Belgium. Von Liebenstein concludes that much more scholarship in this area is needed and provides suggestions for future scholars to follow.

May Friedman examines the key considerations present in Fat Studies scholarship at the exploration of parenting, pregnancy, and fatness. Friedman presents how fatness renders the pregnant body a site of danger in social discourse, positioning fat pregnant people as suspects. She states, "When people become pregnant, all behaviour is open to a heightened degree of surveillance and condescension" (p. 152). Fat pregnant people are subjected to even higher scrutiny and bias. This scrutiny is often undergirded by the use of fields like epigenetics, which positions fat pregnant people as potentially "passing fatness on" to their foetus. Friedman also discusses the intersection of mother blame and fatness, reminding us, "At the centre of mother blaming arguments is a deep value-laden belief in the notion of worthiness, and of fat people as intrinsically unworthy" (p. 157). Ultimately, Friedman finds opportunity in Fat Studies to push back against narratives of fat pregnancy and parenting as a location of inevitable unhappiness by elevating new, diverse, politicized stories of fatness and family, expanding to other arenas of theory such as Motherhood studies. It is in this that the field can be broadened and the narrative expanded to hold the fullness of fat family lives.

In the final chapter, Natalie Ingraham considers whether Fat Studies and Public Health can find common ground in promoting health for those in fat bodies. Building on an earlier article in the *Fat Studies Journal* (Santinsky & Ingraham, 2014), Ingraham's chapter extends beyond her earlier analysis of existing conflicts and contradictions between the two fields; in this offering, she suggests Health at Every Size as a bridge that can connect the two and allow for a field, or at least subdiscipline, of fat public health. She notes,

> While it is unlikely that public health will ever shift to being fully weight neutral, the field has shifted its views of obesity and fatness over the last 20 years. The work of the Rudd Center and individual scholars in HAES, critical obesity/weight studies, and fat studies continue to push for health interventions and health policy that reduces fat stigma and improves the lives of fat people across the globe.
>
> *(p. 172)*

Ingraham proposes that in making both small changes (such as using size affirming language) and large changes (shifting public health campaigns away from using fat stigma as a tool), there is room to create something new that will promote the health and well-being of fat people.

References

Cameron, E., & Russell, C. (2016). *The fat pedagogy reader: Challenging weight-based oppression through critical education*. New York: Peter Lang.

Satinsky, S., & Ingraham, N. (2014). At the intersection of public health and fat studies: Critical perspectives on the measurement of body size. *Fat Studies, 3*(2), 143–154.

12

FAT IN THE MEDIA

Katariina Kyrölä

In feminist and other critical media studies, scholars have long been interested in the role that media imagery plays in deeming some bodies desirable, acceptable, or "normal," others threatening, shameful, or excessive. Most bodies we see in the media are slim or normatively sized. Many classic studies on how gendered body norms and beauty ideals take shape and transform in and through the media have focused on just that, what we mostly see: norm-abiding, idealized, dieting, or eating disordered bodies (e.g. Bordo, 1993; Wolf, 1991). However, the categories of "normal" or "desirable" are at least as much produced through what constitutes their outside, what is understood as "excessive," "too much," or "over" – all things that fat is claimed to be. When we examine images of fatness and fat people in the media, we are therefore not only analyzing fat but also the very boundaries of corporeality and "normalcy" overall. Thus media images of fat unavoidably entangle with the production of gender, sexuality, class, race, and ability, while they also deserve to be a research focus in their own right.

Fat bodies are relatively invisible in the body-scape of popular culture (e.g. Kent, 2001; LeBesco, 2004). When fat bodies do appear, they tend to appear in rather specific contexts: in particular genres and modalities (Kyrölä, 2014). Why does fatness appear so often in comedy, reality television and so-called "trash TV" (Raisborough, 2014), but much more rarely in televisual or cinematic drama? What characterizes news publicity around fatness, and what is fat's appeal in pornography? Even though the cultural limitation of fat bodies to certain genres rather than others is a testament to how fat people are still not seen as being capable of representing the whole spectrum of humanity, these genres are not without subversive potential to challenge, or even unravel, body normativities.

In scholarship about fat in the media, fat bodies' relationship to "normalcy" has been a fraught one. On one hand, scholars and activists have called for a broader range of roles and characteristics for fat actors, so that they would not have to be limited to being defined first and foremost through their fatness, or to the roles of, for example, funny sidekicks or emotionally damaged binge-eaters (Jester, 2009; LeBesco, 2004). A call for "normalcy" in fat representation in the media is, at the same time, a call for fat people to be seen as fully human, good as well as bad, complicated as well as superficial, sympathetic as well as annoying, exciting as well as boring (Cooper, 1998; Mosher, 2001). On the other hand, Fat Studies scholars have also seen subversive, revolutionary potential in the excess and indeed the abjection that fat has come to signify in western culture (Braziel, 2001; Kent,

2001; Kyrölä, 2014; LeBesco, 2004). Why aim for normalcy, when the whole category of the "normal" is already so oppressive? A better strategy might be to refuse and dismiss the notion of "normalcy" altogether and embrace the excess and danger to bodily boundaries that fat has come to stand for, similarly as queer theory aims to do with the concept "queer" (LeBesco, 2004, p. 5; Kent, 2001, pp. 136–137).

Media images furthermore participate in producing understandings of what counts as "normal" or fat overall, how we are expected to feel about such definitions, and how other categories of difference, such as gender and race, intersect with fat. In contemporary Hollywood, actors are considered "fat" at much lower sizes than in the surrounding world, and such standards easily seep into everyday lives. Sensationalistic celebrity journalism observes actors' bodies in minute detail, and weight-gain as well as weight-loss are targets of keen and fully normalized speculation. Actors' weight fluctuations for roles are praised as signs of dedication, but otherwise strictly condemned. For example, American actress Reneé Zellweger as Bridget Jones (*Bridget Jones's Diary*, 2001; and *Bridget Jones: The Edge of Reason*, 2004) may have looked simply average-sized in the role, but her "incredible" weight gain was still highlighted, as well as her difficulties losing the weight. Many celebrities, such as Oprah Winfrey, Britney Spears, and Monica Lewinsky, have also fluctuated in weight repeatedly, and have thus come to embody the fraught relationships between weight, wealth, race, sexuality and gender in the public eye (Farrell, 2011, pp. 121–127).

Given the key role of media in defining and redefining fat, it is not surprising that many Fat Studies writers have addressed the media at least in passing. Academic writing on fat bodies in the media has become a rich field during the 2000s and 2010s, addressing images of fatness in particular genres (for example, Hole, 2003; Kipnis, 1999; Kulick, 2005; Raisborough, 2016; Stukator, 2001); mediums such as television, magazines and zines, or digital media (e.g. Feuer, 1999; Mosher, 2001; Braziel, 2001; Snider, 2009; Pausé, 2016; Lupton, 2017), or the significance of fatness for the celebrity personas of fat actors (e.g. Rowe, 1995; Bernstein & St. John, 2009; Moon & Sedgwick, 2001; Ulaby, 2001). At the time of writing this chapter, there are only two book-length studies about fat across genres in the media, Kathleen LeBesco's *Revolting bodies? The struggle to redefine fat subjectivity* (2004), and my *The weight of images: Affect, body image, and fat in the media* (2014). Both draw on feminist and queer theories of the body and critiques of "normalcy" in order to map out the jarring and revolutionary potential of mediated fat, while LeBesco's key framework is theorization of subjectivity, and my focus is on the affectivity, the emotional appeal of fatness in the media. The media sphere that attracts most research interest in fat media studies currently is digital media, blogs and social media as well as other online spaces, where the meanings and lived realities of fat are under constant renegotiation.

It's the appearance and disappearance, the persistence and transformability of fat that have made it into a highly emotional and charged bodily quality in the media. Questions of affect and emotion have also been at the forefront of many feminist studies about fat and its popular cultural representations, particularly how fat connects to shame (for example Farrell, 2011), disgust (for example Kent, 2001; LeBesco, 2004), and pride (for example Murray, 2008; Taylor, 2018). Although it may seem like media images of fat bodies largely tend to marginalize, induce anxiety around and represent fatness as undesirable, this is also a matter of where we look and how we look. In the contemporary media culture, radical fat activist politics are gaining more ground, even if this development is fraught with controversies. This chapter challenges Fat Studies scholarship to focus not only on analyzing media representations, and how body normativities are constructed in and through them, but also on what their affective appeal is, what they invite viewers and readers to feel – and what kind of (fat) politics they call for.

"Factual" fat: news and reality television

Among the most powerful ways of making fat embodiment appear threatening and in need of urgent intervention are the so-called "factual" discourses in the media. These tend to focus on fatness as a health problem – news, documentaries and reality television (which, of course, is partly scripted, yet which involves people in real life). Many Fat Studies scholars have indeed studied and made important interventions in the discourses of the "war on fat" and the "obesity epidemic." They have shown that while these discourses claim to be factual and merely present "neutral facts," their neutrality can be contested – which is obvious in the popular metaphors of war, natural disasters and epidemics (e.g. Farrell, 2011; Herndon, 2005; Kyrölä, 2014, pp. 31–60; LeBesco, 2004; Saguy & Riley, 2005; Raisborough, 2016). One of the most obvious paradoxes is "anti-obesity" campaigners' claim that fat has not been condemned strongly enough in the media, since people are not getting any slimmer statistically. At the same time, research in the US (Saguy & Riley, 2005), Finland (Kyrölä, 2014) and Sweden (Sandberg, 2004) has shown that the vast majority of all news addressing fat present it as a health problem, and that the amount of such news articles has multiplied from the 1990s to the 2000s.

Fat bodies become visible as problematic or dieting bodies not only in the news discourse, but also habitually on reality TV. While weight-gain and weight-loss stories and advertising as well as various kinds of makeovers have long been the basic stuff of newspapers and magazines (Farrell, 2011), the upsurge of reality TV programming in the 2000s drew extensively on the cultural appeal of both dieting and the makeover. One of the most famous reality TV dieting makeover shows is *The Biggest Loser* (2004–2016), an American format show which has been broadcast worldwide and made into local versions in about 30 other countries, reaching hundreds of millions of people around the world.

Even if news discourse and reality TV shows both utilize fat bodies mainly to require their "un-becoming" (Murray, 2008), as in the removal of fat, their narrative and visual representation of fat people is quite different. News representations tend to dehumanize and abstract fat. The most common visuals involve fat as statistics and numbers, not bodies, abstracting the lived experience of fat embodiment into something calculable, costly and threatening. Occasional images of fat people in news articles are most often example-like, nameless, only vaguely situated in place and time, and strikingly often headless – to the extent that fat activist Charlotte Cooper (2007) has coined the term "headless fatty" to describe the phenomenon of literally cutting off the head of anonymous fat people illustrating the "obesity epidemic". Such images have ended up as the bulk of images of fatness in stock photo depositories such as Getty images which news agencies often use with little or no criticism, and often the "headless fatty" photos have been taken without the permission of people appearing in them.

In contrast, even though weight-loss makeover shows such as *The Biggest Loser* also portray fat as unequivocally unhealthy, they enable fat individuals to become visible as people with depth and complexity, making space for identification and empathy with fat experience in a sizeist society, as Jayne Raisborough (2014, 2016) argues. Furthermore, even though the shows themselves end in the predictable moment of (happily ever) "after" – claims of health and happiness through weight-loss – the contestants' stories have often continued in other media, including social media, revealing their "after the after" struggles with eating disorders, weight re-gain, and the whole ideology of dieting after the show (Hass, 2017). In news discourse, there is little space or interest for fat experience (Raisborough, 2014, p. 156) – the focus on "facts" does not consider experiential knowledge "real" knowledge, with potentially devastating consequences (Kyrölä & Harjunen, 2017).

In my own research (Kyrölä, 2014, pp. 31–60) about the representation of fatness in public health policies and the largest Finnish newspaper, *Helsingin Sanomat*, I found four interrelated strategies of constructing fat as a "factual" threat. The first of the strategies is the massive rep-etition of one-sided views from expert authorities, often white, slim, middle-aged men that represent either government agencies or the medical community. Second, the threatening entity, fat, is made into an abstract, floating, measurable but vague entity in the visual language of news, represented either as graphs or as "headless fatties," utterly separated from living and feeling fat bodies with personhood. Third, the "factual" threat functions through temporality, an orienta-tion towards the threatening future presented as knowable, more ill and heavier than the present, even if there is no evidence of increase in people's experience of illness now. This temporal orientation towards the future concretizes also in the language of "weight management" which, although meant as a more subtle alternative to dieting, expands the threat into a potentiality that concerns all bodies, not only those visually or measurably marked as fat in the now (see also Coleman, 2012).

April Herndon (2005) connects the policing of fat bodies in the news to policing of racial-ized and national boundaries, linking the on-going "war on terror" to the "war on obesity" in America. The "war on obesity" was officially launched by the government and declared by the Surgeon General during the aftermath of the 9/11 terrorist attacks in late 2001. Herndon sees the temporal and linguistic overlaps between these two "wars" as yet another sign of a national-istic project propelling moral, even religious, policing of corporeal boundaries, managing race through fat and fat through race (Herndon, 2005, pp. 130–131). Furthermore, the very same discourse which declares fat people powerless targets of warlike action demands them to change themselves – a task often referred to as "easy" and "simple." Herndon argues that, like in the war against AIDS and in the war against poverty, it is impossible to separate the problem from the people who suffer from it or have come to embody it in public (Herndon, 2005, p. 129). Jeannine Gailey (2014) has reflected on the consequences of the metaphors of wars and epidem-ics particularly for fat women by using the concept of "hyper(in)visibility": fat women become hypervisible as objects of concern and intervention within the "obesity epidemic" discourse, while their subjectivities, experiences and bodies remain largely invisible.

In contrast, the general atmosphere of reality TV dieting shows builds on promise, not explic-itly on threat. (Kyrölä, 2014, pp. 69–84). The structure of promise builds on a linear narrative which moves from a body and a life marked by shame and disgust into a body marked by pride and happiness. The structure of before and after, of emergence from shame to pride, is massively repeated and normalized in reality TV series such as *The Biggest Loser* – even though the affective appeal of the promise of weight-loss has also been contested and complicated, as contestants have told their "after the after" stories of regaining the weight or being propelled into eating disorders (Hass, 2017). Reality TV dieting shows also enable great visibility for fat bodies, otherwise rel-atively invisible in the media, although fatness tends to be made into a visual and affective spec-tacle through images of eating in close-up, crying, laughing, shivering, grinning, and sweating, stomachs bouncing in slow motion, hidden skin exposed for measuring, flesh changing shape. Audience research shows, however, that these shows invoke widely varying responses from their viewers, from empathy towards fat individuals and anger towards the shows' humiliating struc-tures to complicity with their broader weight-loss ideology (Holland et al., 2010).

What kind of relationship between the body and the self, then, is at stake in such "factual" representations? The procession from the "before" to the "after" and the pain-staking journey in between involve a shift from lived, subjective corporeality to suddenly seeing one's body as an object, something one inhabits, owns, and molds, not something one is. In news articles on the threat of fat, treating bodies as objects is a key part of producing and distributing supposedly neutral information which has nothing to do with fat people or their stigmatization. In dieting narratives, the spotlight is on the very relation that is hidden in news articles: on the self's relation to the body, on the body's relation the world, and on the transformation of both. The "true" and "healthy" self, however, is always slim in factual media discourses.

In the quest of peeling out the "true self" in reality TV, fat appears to exist in an impossible space of being concretely under one's skin but socially and culturally forbidden from the material self and the core of one's being. This paradox is manifested in a representation of fatness as a shell from which to hatch or which needs to be peeled off to find the core self underneath (Kent, 2001, pp. 134–135). Fat is thus only "surface," not an identity, and dieting is seen more as a revelation of the "true" self in all its glory, slimness, and moral redemption. The rhetoric, or indeed imperative, of personal and individual-driven transformation obscures how societal and cultural power structures nevertheless condition people's lives and bodies in asymmetrical ways. As Cheryl Thompson (2015) points out, such an individualistic approach to fatness and self-transformation does a particularly apt job in hiding racialized, classed and gendered power structures. Thompson analyzes media images of dieting or dieted Black women in Hollywood – Oprah Winfrey, Queen Latifah, Jennifer Hudson and Octavia Spencer, who all have appeared in advertisements for dieting programs such as the Weight Watchers and Jenny Craig – arguing that they are emblematic of how middle-class Black women now have access to and success as self-disciplined and moral subjects, but only through distancing themselves from working class, presumably "out of control" Black women (Thompson, 2015, pp. 805–807).

The "hatching" of a slim body out of a fat body can further be compared to "coming out as fat": both involve something previously hidden becoming visible, but they are each other's polar opposites in terms of the fat body's relationship to visibility. Queer theorists Michael Moon and Eve Kosofsky Sedgwick ([1991] 2001, p. 305) famously draw a parallel between the closet of sexuality for gay men to the closet of size for fat women, looking at levels of secrecy: fatness can be downplayed with clothes and posture, but it can never be hidden. The stigma of fatness is simply the stigma of visibility. Epistemologically, the problem is not that the one inside the closet of size knows more than the outside world, as in the case of closeted gay people, but that other people think they know something about a fat woman she presumably does not. Surely if she knew, she would have done something about her fatness. According to the logic of the closet of size, her body proves a certain "self-delusion" which reality TV dieting shows, of course, promise to heal. But to Moon and Sedgwick, coming out as fat means instead expressing one's knowingness about one's fatness, embracing it and rejecting others' derogatory views. The "factual" media discourses around fat do not offer any possibilities for coming out *as* fat, only coming out *from* fat. But in other genres and modalities, such as comedy, there are more possibilities for coming out as fat, unruly, unashamed and unapologetic.

Funny fat (suits): film and television comedy

Comedy is perhaps the only popular cultural arena where fat women and men not only have made notable appearances but also have had continuing and widespread success and fame. Anne Hole, in her research on fat female comedians, has even claimed that the fat body is so common to comedy that it is considered almost innately funny (Hole, 2003, p. 315). Successful fat comedians span from early classical Hollywood slapstick star Oliver Hardy (1892–1957) of the Laurel and Hardy thin man/fat man pair; to the 1970s and 1980s American camp sensation, drag queen Divine; from the American "everyman" Drew Carey, who starred as a beer-drinking office worker in his own TV sitcom, *The Drew Carey Show* (1995–2004); to loud-mouthed American comedian Roseanne Barr, whose fat working-class femininity has been a source of outrage for conservative commentators and celebration for feminist researchers until rather recently (Bernstein & St. John, 2009; Rowe, 1995); and to contemporary women of color comedians such as Mo'nique and Margaret Cho who have explored the intersections of size, race and gender. Today's perhaps biggest fat comedy star is American actress Melissa McCarthy (1970–) who was Hollywood's third best paid actress in 2016 and 2017 (Elkins, 2018). She came to fame by starring in the TV sitcom *Mike and Molly* (2010–2016) and the film *Bridesmaids* (2011), in the latter as a crude-talking but kindhearted friend of the bride. From *Bridesmaids* to *Tammy* (2014) – the latter of which was a big box-office success but slammed by critics – most of McCarthy's characters have been unstylishly dressed, white, lower-class women whose sexual appetites, ability to push through tough situations, and confidence have nevertheless been rather intact (see Meeuf, 2016).

Feminist scholars of media and popular culture have passionately examined the relationship between fat women and laughter for over two decades (for example, Feuer, 1999; Hole, 2003; Kyrölä, 2014; Meeuf, 2016; Rowe, 1995). While many renowned fat comedians have turned their fat bodies into an asset and a trademark, comedy is also a field in which size norms are reinforced. Fat jokes abound, and non-normative bodies regularly become laughingstocks. How to judge when fat and otherwise non-normative bodies are displayed only for cheap laughs versus when they pose a threat to ideas around "normalcy" overall? Under what circumstances can laughter become a revolutionary force, and when is it also a powerful tool of policing bodily boundaries?

Particularly in mainstream Hollywood films of the 1990s and early 2000s, fat comedic roles were most commonly played by slim people in fat suits, as in body prosthetics and makeup that make one appear fat. In the 2010s, fat suits seemed to have lost some of their popularity – possibly due to the critique that they have received. However, fat suits have been and are still regularly used on TV, especially to indicate former fatness and temporary fatness, such in the Netflix series *Insatiable* (2018–), where a slim actress (Debby Ryan) plays a former fat girl who loses weight and decides to get back at her bullies, in *Friends* (1994–2004) in flashbacks to Monica's (Courteney Cox) youth as a fat girl, and in *Mad Men* (2007–2015) for Betty Draper's (January Jones) temporary weight gain. Earlier popular fat suit characters in films include Mrs. Doubtfire (Robin Williams) in *Mrs. Doubtfire* (1993); Sherman Klump (Eddie Murphy) in *The Nutty Professor* (1996) and its sequels; Big Momma (Martin Lawrence) in *Big Momma's House* (2000) and its sequels; Fat Bastard (Mike Myers) in *Austin Powers: The Spy Who Shagged Me* (1999) and *Austin Powers in Goldmember* (2002); and Rosemary (Gwyneth Paltrow) in *Shallow Hal* (2001) (see also Mendoza, 2009; Wykes, 2012). In contrast, melodramatic content, for example films *What's Eating Gilbert Grape?* (1993), *Precious: Based on the Novel Push by Sapphire* (2009), have featured actual fat performers (Darlene Cates and Gabourey Sidibe). Why aren't fat characters always played by fat actors? Why are fat suits so popular in comedies? Do fat suits give permission to joke more viciously about fatness than if a real fat person were playing the role, or do they perhaps unwittingly protect actual fat persons from the potential harm of being laughed at? Whatever the case, fat suits have become an established way for popular comedy actors to show their "range" without actual weight fluctuation.

The situation with fat suits, however, can be compared to the tradition of white people acting in blackface, redface, brownface, and yellowface (LeBesco, 2004; Mendoza, 2009). Whites have been perceived as generically representing "people," capable of performing a wider range of roles than non-white actors, since whiteness is usually not understood as a race or an ethnicity. Similarly, slim or even thin people represent just "people" whose dressing up as marginalized is coded comedic. Protests against fat suits may not differ greatly from earlier protests against blackface, which argued that it is degrading not to consider a social group worthy, capable, or powerful enough to represent itself (compare to Shohat & Stam, 1994, p. 190). On the other hand, fat suit comedies have also shed light on fat oppression and provided images of fat people as resourceful, successful, and valid love interests.

Fat suits relate to the common comedic film theme of cross-dressing or passing for some-one else. The theme of switching gender has been particularly popular, but its comic effect seems to work mostly one way: men playing women, the dominant playing the marginalized, is funny; but women playing men rarely provokes laughter. A similar logic applies to fat and slim. Fat-to-slim dieting narratives are romantic and dramatic stories about self-transformation, but slim actors posing as fat are comedic. This often does little to unravel the gender binary or size hierarchies. Thus it makes sense that so many slim, male comedians (such as Robin Wil-liams, Mike Myers, Eddie Murphy, Martin Lawrence, and Tyler Perry) have been so successful in double-drag of slim-to-fat and male-to-female playing fat, older women. The Black older female characters played by Black slim men have been seen as "neo-mammies" (Mason, 2017), continuations of the Black mammy stereotype – loud, poor, fat, caretakers of white people's kids – which bloomed in the golden era of Hollywood from the 1930s to the 1950s.

Fat male bodies as sites of comedy can also be understood in terms of fear of femininity or gender non-conformity. A fat male body is coded as dangerously bordering on femininity, with visible breasts and a protruding belly. The loss of rigid bodily boundaries would mean the loss of rigid, naturalized gender differences – in other words, the fat male body in some ways represents gender instability. However, a fat male actor's fatness does not have to be a central issue in his comedy films or television shows – a privilege that fat women rarely have. Male fatness still tends to support and add to other defining features of the character, most poignantly his "ordinariness" or "realism," especially in television (Mosher, 2001, pp. 167–173).

In comedic images of fat women in mainstream television and film, there has been another recur-ring character since the mid-1990s: the deluded fat woman. This refers to an idea that fat female characters see themselves differently from how others see them. Other people's perspectives are usually presented as the "objective" view, while the woman's own perspective is "deluded," excessive, or too positive. This figure of the deluded fat woman exceeds expectations not only about body size but about properly demure sexual desires, dresses in exuberant style, and/or who speaks too loudly or too much. Typically, this character type thinks she is strikingly gorgeous; perhaps parades in flashy, scanty, or body-accentuating clothing; or acts in a sexually forthcoming way. Examples of the deluded fat woman have included, for instance, the regular supporting character Mimi Bobeck (American actress Kathy Kinney) in the TV sitcom *The Drew Carey Show* (1995–2004) who is a fat white woman who wears glaring, drag-queenish makeup and extravagant costume-like clothes: a woman always-in-excess. Another example is the character Rasputia (played by Eddie Murphy) in *Norbit* (2007) – a super-sized Black fat woman who is voraciously sexual and not shy about showing her body at all.

Even if these female characters are deemed "delusional" and laughable, they can nevertheless also suggest a sort of a coming out as fat (Moon & Sedgwick, [1991] 2001) where fat people refuse to see or hear the potential disapproval around them, and focus on flaunting their bodies and selves without shame or fear. That might be mediated fantasy, but it is a very attractive one.

Sexy fat: pornography and gender

Until the late 2000s, before the rise of social media, there was only scarce material in the media representing fatness in an explicitly "positive" light. Several scholars of television, film, and printed press have noted that the little that there was focused almost exclusively on fat femininity as beautiful or sexy, to a degree where positivity was often collapsed with sexual desirability to others (Feuer, 1999; Hole, 2003; Kyrölä, 2014, pp. 158–165; LeBesco, 2004, pp. 50–52; Murray, 2008). I find the way in which "positivity" and "sexiness" tend to be equated, when it comes to fat in the media, symptomatic of at least three things. First, the rejection from the realm of attractiveness and sexuality has had devastating effects on many fat women and men's images of themselves, and entry into that realm seems all the more attractive due to this denial. As Jane Feuer (1999) has pointed out, it is hard to struggle against sexual objectification without ever having been a sexual object. Second, becoming the willing object of sexually charged looks is habitually and increasingly portrayed as not only pleasurable but empowering for all women (Heyes, 2007; Gill & Elias, 2014), and this promise of empowerment through sexiness is unsurprisingly applied also to fat women. Finally, feminist criticism of too narrowly defined beauty ideals has become mainstream to a large extent, but with ambiguous results. The demands are directed at the narrowness and uniformity of beauty standards, while their gendered, class-related, and racialized structures are not necessarily perceived problematic as such.

An example of commercial appropriation of feminist critique of beauty ideals is the well-known advertisement series *The Dove Campaign for Real Beauty*. The campaign aimed to broaden the range of bodies understood as beautiful, but utilized models who differed only slightly in terms of size, age, gender expression, shape, or race from contemporary body norms, and did nothing to undermine the equation of beauty with women's worth (for example, Johnston & Taylor, 2008; Murray, 2013). Another example is the existence of beauty pageants for fat women in different parts of the world, such as the American Beauties Plus Pageant, Finnish Miss XL, the Thai Miss Jumbo Queen, and Miss Fat South Africa, which critique thin privilege and beauty standards but ignore feminist critique of the beauty pageant institution (Kyrölä, 2014, pp. 165–173; see also LeBesco, 2004, p. 51; Murray, 2008, pp. 117–120).

Advertisements, fat beauty pageants and other mainstream media images where fat bodies are celebrated as "sexy" and "desirable" often exclude very large or supersize fat bodies. Such bodies tend to appear more often in the contexts of tragedy, sensationalism, and the "obesity epidemic" (see also Gurrieri & Cherrier, 2013). In the current media culture, images of supersize desirability cannot expect acceptance from mainstream audiences, but they do however exist – particularly in the realm of pornography. Once fat is imaged in an explicitly sexual context with the aim of arousal, the images stop seeking mainstream acceptance and fat suddenly becomes a quality catering to fetishists, viewers with "deviant" desires. Fat porn appears in the fetish section of pornography websites, while fat activists tend to see the fetish status as insulting, preferring the normalization of sexual desire towards and by fat people. At the same time, it is the very denial and rejection of fat by the mainstream media that easily lends fat a pornographic significance and arouses (Kipnis, 1999, pp. 94–96). As Jerry Mosher (2001, pp. 171, 187) notes, the simultaneous impulse to play up the over-visibility of fat embodiment and hide its sexual connotations easily contributes to seeing fat as pornographic, even if it is not presented in a pornographic context.

Fat pornography, especially in LGBTQ contexts, has been seen subversive by many scholars in redefining fat corporeality as a site of shameless, open pleasure, and pointing to ways of re-imagining non-heteronormative sexualities (Kent, 2001, pp. 142–145; Kipnis, 1999, pp. 114–115; Kulick, 2005, pp. 91–92; LeBesco, 2004, pp. 48–49). Some scholars argue that fat is, in fact, necessarily queer, since fat sexuality is culturally understood as deviant (LeBesco, 2004, pp. 88–89). Don Kulick (2005, pp. 89–92) suggests fat pornography can be seen to challenge both the socially sanctioned forms of pleasurable body zones and the expected temporality of sex, especially when the porn involves practices of feeding, being fed, and gaining weight over time (see also Kyrölä, 2014, pp. 178–189).

In mainstream media culture, fat women tend to be either desexualized or hypersexualized, portrayed as pseudomasculine or ultrafeminine, or both at the same time (see Gailey, 2014). Therefore the strategy of normalizing desire towards fat bodies, and fat people as desiring subjects, is an important one. However, in pornography the denial and pathologization of fat desire and sexuality is not downplayed but emphasized as the very engine of "forbidden" arousal – with controversial results.

Virtual fat: fat activism and online communities

Today, blogs, discussion groups and social media sites abound online, exploring alternative ideas about what kind of bodies are valuable, capable and attractive. A key area of this online world has been called the "fatosphere" which focuses on content by and for self-identified fat people and fat activists (Lupton, 2017; Pausé, 2016). The legacy of the fatosphere can be traced back to the mid-1990s, and American discussion groups such as *FD*, a discussion group for pro-fats, and *FAS*, a bulletin list for fat lesbians specifically. In both groups, discussions varied from where to find right clothes sizes to how to relate to sex as a fat individual, and to struggles against sizeism (LeBesco, 2004, pp. 99–101). The fatosphere is still rather compartmentalized into the more heterosexually oriented and the queer subsections.

The emphasis on straight or queer fat femininity describes the vast majority of the fatosphere (Taylor, 2018). Blogs or communities that focus on fat masculinity or queer fat masculinity center on the gay bear subculture – men attracted to and/or identifying as fat or chubby men. These online communities revolve mostly around sex and dating rather than activism – although they can also be seen as political (e.g. Monaghan, 2005). Most current fatosphere content is created by and focused on white bodies, even though there is an increasing Black and people of color multi-platform activist presence and following (compare to Murray, 2008, p. 118).

Fat activist and "body positive" online spheres have attracted ample attention from feminist media scholars during the 2010s (for example, Afful & Ricciardelli, 2015; Gill & Elias, 2014; Gurrieri & Cherrier, 2013; Hynnä & Kyrölä, 2019; Murray, 2013; Sastre, 2014). While the "body positive" movement has its roots in fat activism, many fat activists see its contemporary forms as depoliticized, since "body positivity" tends to center normative or only slightly larger than the norm bodies, while fat activism stands up for fat, non-white, disabled, and otherwise marginalized bodies (for example Dionne, 2017). One critique, however, that is relevant to both "body positivity" and some forms of fat activism, concerns the way in which discourses of pride and self-love can transfer the cultural demand to change one's body into a demand to change one's affective relationship to one's body (Johnston & Taylor, 2008). Has the imperative to have the right body become an imperative to feel right about one's body? What if in addition to failing to attain a normative-sized body, you might also fail to feel positive about your non-normative body?

While taking these important critiques into consideration, it is nevertheless also important to think about why "body positivity" and the fatosphere have gained such widespread popularity online, how people engage with them, and how they make people feel (Hynnä & Kyrölä, 2019). Online communities and sites which focus on fat activism or body positivity should not be dismissed too quickly as a new form of consumerism, or forced "positivity". In actual practice, many blogs, social media accounts and groups offer opportunities to support, community and practical solutions to issues such as dealing with discrimination and body anxiety, finding stylish clothes as well as romantic partners, and navigating through various everyday activities in a world that often excludes fat people.

The fatosphere changes shape continuously, as media technologies and preferred platforms develop and vary. For example, in the late 2000s, it was still easier for individual fat activists to stand out and make a name for themselves through active blogging only. By the late 2010s, fact activist blogging has lost much of its popularity and status to other social media forms, such as posting on Instagram and vlogging on YouTube. New exciting work is constantly emerging around this cultural arena.

Conclusion

In this chapter, I have outlined some key analytical frameworks for fat in various genres of media, from news to reality TV, from comedy to pornography and social media. The rise of social media, where content is not only created from top down but essentially by followers, commentators, and community members, highlights how there is in fact no media representation that would unequivocally carry only one meaning, or feeling. When it comes to fat in the media, more research is needed on how audience members, as well as content co-creators, actually relate to and engage with images of fatness. Comparisons between fat experience and fat media representation are still rather sparse, although studies imply that there are important connections. For example, the ways in which fat women often experience their bodies as "liminal," or stuck-in-waiting, and the ways in which fat in the media is habitually depicted as matter-on-its-way-to-disappear, yet persistently there (see Kyrölä & Harjunen, 2017). The very existence and popularity of the fatosphere and the body positive movement online imply that at least large portions of the contemporary audiences, fat or not, are getting tired of how humiliation-based reality TV, "obesity epidemic" rhetoric, and fat suit comedies make them feel about their bodies as well as bodies of others. They are looking for something more joyful and unapologetic, and welcoming a broader range of bodies into the mainstream in a broader range of roles.

By looking at fat in the media, we can see how the broader cultural boundaries of "normalcy" and acceptability have shifted within the last few decades not only in terms of body size, but also in terms of gender expression, race, and sexuality. Cultural and mediated anxieties around and calls to manage fat may often function as a (thin) veil for managing something else, such as "normal" sexuality, or class and race antagonisms. Today, we also see bodies in mainstream media that were almost unthinkable to see – and thus to consider existing and valid subjects – twenty or thirty years ago. Supersize bodies exist in contemporary media, whereas there were only a handful of scattered examples up until the 2000s. Until Gabourey Sidibe played Claireece "Precious" Jones in *Precious: Based on the Novel Push by Sapphire* (2009, USA), there were virtually no Black, fat teenage girls in lead roles in western media.

As I underlined in the beginning of this chapter, however, visibility does not necessarily equal power. Increased visibility can also entail ever more complex and insidious forms of marginalization and management, such as how successful Black women can have some access to white middle class privilege through dieting (Thompson, 2015), and how body positivity can take forms that are stripped of its radical fat activist past and address and feature mainly normative-sized people (Johnston & Taylor, 2008. Fat in the media is never only about fat, but about how contemporary culture deals more broadly with bodily vulnerability and transformability. Through the construction of fatness as a somehow "exceptional" and dangerous bodily quality, when it is in fact a very common way of inhabiting one's body, bodies deemed "normal" can perhaps hold on to the illusion of safety a little bit longer, as if all our bodies were not vulnerable and in constant change. Media images of fat bodies make audiences confront that vulnerability, for better or for worse.

References

Afful, A. A., & Ricciardelli, R. (2015). Shaping the online fat acceptance movement: Talking about body image and beauty standards. *Journal of Gender Studies*, 24(4), 453–472.

Bernstein, B., & St. John, M. (2009). The Roseanne Benedict Arnolds: How fat women are betrayed by their celebrity icons. In E. Rothblum, & S. Solovay (Eds.), *The fat studies reader* (pp. 263–270). New York and London: New York University Press.

Bordo, S. (1993). *Unbearable weight. Feminism, western culture, and the body*. Berkeley: University of California Press.

Braziel, J. E. (2001). Sex and fat chics: Deterritorializing the fat female body. In J. E. Braziel & K. LeBesco (Eds.), *Bodies out of bounds: Fatness and transgression* (pp. 231–254). Berkeley: University of California Press.

Coleman, R. (2012). *Transforming images: Screens, affect, futures*. London and New York: Routledge.

Cooper, C. (1998). *Fat and proud. The politics of size*. London: Women's Press.

Cooper, C. (2007). Headless fatties. *Charlotte Cooper*. http://charlottecooper.net/fat/fat-writing/headless-fatties-01-07/

Dionne, E. (2017). Fat activists say body positivity is becoming meaningless. *The Revelist, 24,* Jan 2017. https://www.revelist.com/ideas/fat-acceptance-body-positivity/6632/as-toal-argues-using-body-positivity-as-an-umbrella-to-include-bodies-that-are-already-deemed-conventionally-attractive-defeats-the-purpose/8

Elkins, K. (2018). Melissa McCarthy is Hollywood's 3rd highest paid actress – here's how she negotiated her way to the top. *CNBC,* Apr 25. https://www.cnbc.com/2018/04/25/melissa-mccarthy-the-3rd-highest-paid-actress-negotiated-her-way-up.html.

Farrell, A. E. (2011). *Fat shame: Stigma and the fat body in American culture.* New York: New York University Press.

Feuer, J. (1999). Averting the male gaze: Visual pleasure and images of fat women. In M. B. Haralovich, & L. Rabinowitz (Eds.), *Television, history, and American culture* (pp. 181–200). Durham and London: Duke University Press.

Gailey, J. E. (2014). *The Hyper(in)visible fat woman. Weight and gender discourse in contemporary society.* Basingstoke: Palgrave Macmillan.

Gill, R., & Elias, A. S. (2014). "Awaken your incredible": Love your body discourses and postfeminist contradictions. *International Journal of Media and Cultural Politics, 10*(2), 179–188.

Gurrieri, L., & Cherrier, H. (2013). Queering beauty: Fatshionistas in the fatosphere. *Qualitative Market Research: An International Journal, 16*(3), 276–295.

Hass, M. (2017). After the after: *The Biggest Loser* and post-makeover narrative trajectories in digital media. *Fat Studies, 6*(2), 135–151.

Herndon, A. (2005). Collateral damage from friendly fire? Race, nation, class and the "war against obesity." *Social Semiotics, 15*(2), 127–141.

Heyes, C. J. (2007). Cosmetic surgery and the televisual makeover. *Feminist Media Studies, 7*(1), 17–32.

Hole, A. (2003). Performing identity: Dawn French and the funny fat female body. *Feminist Media Studies, 3*(3), 315–328.

Holland, K., Blood, R. W., Thomas, S., Karunaratne, A., & Lewis, S. (2010). "That's not reality for me": Australian audiences respond to *The Biggest Loser. Annual International Communications Association Conference,* 1–26.

Hynnä, K. & Kyrölä, K. (2019) "Feel in your body". Fat activist affects in blogs. *Social Media + Society, 5*(4), 1–11.

Jester, J. (2009). Placing fat women on center stage. In E. Rothblum, & S. Solovay (Eds.), *The fat studies reader* (pp. 249–255). New York: New York University Press.

Johnston, J., & Taylor. J. (2008). Feminist consumerism and fat activists: A comparative study of grassroots activism and the Dove Real Beauty campaign. *Signs: Journal of Women in Culture and Society, 33,* 941–966.

Kent, L. (2001). Fighting abjection. Representing fat women. In J. E. Braziel, & K. LeBesco (Eds.), *Bodies out of bounds: Fatness and transgression* (pp. 130–150). Berkeley: University of California Press.

Kipnis, L. (1999). *Bound and gagged. Pornography and the politics of fantasy in America.* Durham, NC: Duke University Press.

Kulick, D. (2005). Porn. In D. Kulick, & A. Meneley (Eds.), *Fat. The anthropology of an obsession* (pp. 77–92). New York: Jeremy P. Tarcher/Penguin.

Kyrölä, K. (2014) *The weight of images. Affect, body image and fat in the media.* London: Routledge.

Kyrölä, K., & Harjunen, H. (2017) Phantom/liminal fat and feminist theories of the body. *Feminist Theory, 18*(2), 99–117.

LeBesco, K. (2004). *Revolting bodies? The struggle to redefine fat identity.* Boston: University of Massachusetts Press.

Lupton, D. (2017). Digital media and body weight, shape, and size: An introduction and review. *Fat Studies, 6*(2), 119–134.

Mason, C. (2017). Queering the Mammy: New queer cinema's version of an American institution in Cheryl Dunye's *The Watermelon Woman. Black Camera, 8*(2), 50–74.

Meeuf, R. (2016). Class, corpulence, and neoliberal citizenship: Melissa McCarthy on *Saturday Night Live. Celebrity Studies, 7*(2), 137–153.

Mendoza, K. R. (2009). Seeing through the layers. Fat suits and thin bodies in *The Nutty Professor* and *Shallow Hal.* In E. Rothblum, & S. Solovay (Eds.), *The Fat Studies reader* (pp. 280–288). New York: New York University Press.

Monaghan, L. F. (2005). Big Handsome Men, bears and others: Virtual constructions of "fat male embodiment." *Body & Society, 11*(2), 81–111.

Moon, M., & Sedgwick, E. K. ([1991] 2001). Divinity. A dossier, a performance piece, a little understood emotion. In J. E. Braziel, & K. LeBesco (Eds.), *Bodies out of bounds: Fatness and transgression* (pp. 292–328). Berkeley: University of California Press.

Mosher, J. (2001). Setting free the bears. Refiguring fat men on television. In J. E. Braziel, & K. LeBesco (Eds.), *Bodies out of bounds: Fatness and transgression* (pp. 166–193). Berkeley: University of California Press.

Murray, D. P. (2013). Branding "real" social change in Dove's Campaign for Real Beauty. *Feminist Media Studies, 13*(1), 83–101.

Murray, S. (2008). *The 'fat' female body*. Basingstoke: Palgrave MacMillan.

Pausé, C. (2016). Causing a commotion: Queering fat in cyberspace. In C. Pausé, J. Wykes, & S. Murray (Eds.), *Queering fat embodiment* (pp. 75–87). London: Routledge.

Raisborough, J. (2014). Why we should be watching more trash TV: Exploring the value of an analysis of the makeover show to Fat Studies scholars. *Fat Studies, 3*(2), 155–165.

Raisborough, J. (2016). *Fat bodies, health, and the media*. London: Palgrave Macmillan.

Rowe, K. (1995). *The unruly woman: Gender and the genres of laughter*. Austin: University of Texas Press.

Saguy, A. C., & Riley, K. W. (2005). Weighing both sides: Morality, mortality, and framing over obesity. *Journal of Health Politics, Policy, and Law, 30*(5), 869–921.

Sandberg, H. (2004). *Medier & fetma: En analys av vikt.* (Media & fatness. An analysis of weight.) Lund: Lund Studies in Media and Communication.

Sastre, A. (2014). Towards a radical body positive. Reading the online "body positive movement". *Feminist Media Studies, 14*(6), 929–943.

Shohat, E., & Stam, R. (1994). *Unthinking Eurocentrism. Multiculturalism and the media*. London and New York: Routledge.

Snider, S. (2009). Fat girls and size queens: Alternative publications and the visualizing of fat and queer eroto-politics in contemporary American culture. In E. Rothblum, & S. Solovay (Eds.), *The fat studies reader* (pp. 223–230). New York: New York University Press.

Stukator, A. (2001). "It's not over until the fat lady sings." Comedy, the carnivalesque, and body politics. In J. E. Braziel, & K. LeBesco (Eds.), *Bodies out of bounds. Fatness and transgression* (pp. 197–213). Berkeley: University of California Press.

Taylor, A. (2018). "Fabulously" femme: Queer fat femme women's identities and experiences. *Journal of Lesbian Studies, 22*(4), 459–481.

Thompson, C. (2015). Neoliberalism, soul food, and the weight of Black women. *Feminist Media Studies, 15*(5), 794–812.

Ulaby, N. (2001). Roscoe Arbuckle and the scandal of fatness. In J. E. Braziel, & K. LeBesco (Eds.), *Bodies out of bounds: Fatness and transgression* (pp. 153–165). Berkeley: University of California Press.

Wolf, N. (1991). *The Beauty myth: How images of beauty are used against women*. London: Vintage.

Wykes, J. (2012). "I saw a knock-out": Fatness, (in)visibility and desire in Shallow Hal. *Somatechnics, 2*(1), 60–79.

13

BEING FAT IN A THIN WORLD

The politics of fashion

Amena Azeez

Have you ever loved something with all your heart that has not only not loved you back but has also ignored your existence? That is my relationship with fashion. Since I can remember I have loved all things fashion. However, as a "chubby" kid my earliest encounter of (indirect) rejection from the fashion world came when I was cruelly reminded by my class teacher that I could not become a Miss India. To be a Miss India I needed to be slim and I was (and am) the exact opposite of it.

Since the longest time fat women have been categorically kept out of mainstream fashion narratives. From denying us access to quality clothes to offering fair representation, fat women have been ignored on all fronts. For years the industry has demonised fat bodies and categorically sent us a message: Fashion is not for fatties! We can admire fashion from afar but never have a seat at the fashion table. At every possible opportunity, the fashion industry makes it a point to tell fat women, "You don't belong here". I grew up believing it until I decided there had to be a way for me to "fit in".

Growing up as a fat girl in India, I had no fat role models to look up to. Even when I started blogging there was no Tess Holliday or Ashley Graham or Gabi Gregg in India to seek inspiration from. I had to become my own role model. From understanding why the industry is so resistant towards the inclusion of fat bodies, to figuring out a way to create a new narrative that did not see fat bodies as the ugly other whose sole purpose was to function as a contrast to aspirational thin bodies. As a fat woman I was done with being a joke, a health warning, a before picture. I am my own person and I have as much right to be seen, heard and celebrated as thin women are. After spending my teens and mid-20s denying myself the joy of fashion, I put my foot down to all the self-censoring and self-hate I had towards my body and decided that I too am worthy of fashion. My weight by no means is an indication of my talent, my knowledge and my love for fashion. And I should be allowed to revel in it as much as any thin person. And while the Indian fashion industry still sees the thin body as the ideal, it is at least now aware of my existence. I can no longer be ignored. Fat women like me can no more be kept out of fashion. We matter − whether you like it or not.

My pursuit for acceptance introduced me to plus size fashion blogging and fat activism. Back in 2011 when I started fashion blogging, like most of India, I too was unaware of all the marvellous changes the fat activism and body positive movement was bringing about. Here in India the term "plus size" was an unheard one and most people in the Indian fashion industry could not believe a woman who looked like me could be a fashion blogger. I have heard everything from, "You don't look like a blogger!" to "We don't have your size" to "Fashion blogging is not for you. Try food blogging instead!" The very idea that a fat woman, who did not fit into straight and sample size and by no means was anyone's "body goals", could consider herself as the face of fashion was an alien concept to most. As one of India's first plus size fashion bloggers and body positive influencers, I have closely seen the Indian fashion industry go from size exclusive to marginally inclusive and accepting of non-thin bodies. Even before I started fashion blogging, I had first-hand knowledge that the fashion space is not for women who look like me. We can be a part of it, but never the face of it. After knowing how explicitly fatphobic the fashion industry is, I still chose to put myself out there in the hope of bringing about a change in the Indian fashion industry.

On one hand, the fashion industry has been an inclusive safe space for some marginalised groups, and on the other, it has been highly oppressive towards others. While the LGBTQ community has found a way to thrive, grow and shape the fashion industry, fat women have been intentionally kept out to the point that our very existence is denied and erased at every level. How can an industry that has been an ally to one group of marginalised people be intolerant towards another group of marginalised people? Inclusive for some and excluding of others? This is when it finally dawned on me – fashion is political and fat woman taking up space in the fashion world is an act of rebellion and resistance.

Fashion has never been only about clothes. It has always been a form of self-expression. Since fat women do not conform to the industry's rules, clothes are used as a weapon against fat women to keep us out. Not anymore. Fat activists and plus size fashion bloggers are making it loud and clear to the industry that we exist and we deserve to be seen and celebrated. Fat activism and plus size fashion blogging gave fat people an opportunity to create their own new fashion narrative and put them in charge of it. For the first time fat women are in a position of power. Since clothes are the entry point to the fashion world, fat women started making and modelling their own clothes instead of hoping and waiting that fatphobic brands and designers would change their outlook. Step by step they started shaking the fashion industry that had for years ignored them. Not only did the industry take note of the growing popularity and demand of plus size and "fatshion" but it also realised the significant impact of the body positive movement and size inclusive representation. The industry that once denied entry to plus size and fat women, was now rolling out the carpet for them. While the fashion industry has a long way to go to become 100 percent inclusive of plus size and fat bodies, it is now aware of our power, presence and importance. We exist and can no longer be ignored.

Being an active and vocal member of the body positive and fat acceptance movement for years, I somehow still felt my voice wasn't being heard. It is one thing when those who are not aware of my existence ignore me and another for those who themselves have been marginalised to ignore those voices who don't have the same support as them. As a plus size fashion blogger and body positive influencer from India – a non-western developing country – my voice and work are conspicuously ignored by the global body positive and fat activism space. Brands, magazines, organisers, choose to only take into account the needs of plus size and fat women living in US and Europe and other developed nations and ignore those of us living in South Asia. We are treated as cheerleaders, often invisible, for those in a position of power. We are not considered to be narrative creators and changers. We function only to support those at the top but receive no solidarity and support in return from them. The entire body positive and fat acceptance space is strongly dominated by women from western and developed countries. Not only are we ignored by the mainstream narrative of our own country, we are also ignored by a movement that advocates inclusiveness for all. If we truly want the whole world to become size inclusive, it needs to start with making the very movement that promotes it more welcoming of others who do not have the same access and privilege as those on top.

My journey navigating the fashion space as a fat woman has taught me one very life-changing lesson: Existing as a plus size, visibly fat woman in an industry that has been opposed to the very idea of me and has built itself by keeping women like me out of it, is not only an act of rebellion but also an act of political resistance. For some, fashion is a privilege, for me, it is political.

14

FATTENING EDUCATION

An invitation to the nascent field of fat pedagogy

Erin Cameron and Constance Russell

As a dying wish, Ellen Maud Bennett (2018) called upon other "women of size" to reject fatness as the primary determinant of health and to advocate for themselves in the face of weight bias and discrimination. Her obituary, which shared her personal experience of medical fat shaming and resultant lack of treatment, was retweeted and hashtagged around the world. Her message was simple and powerful, and it struck a chord. As she had hoped, Bennett's obituary became a pedagogical tool, highlighting the urgency of addressing fat oppression.

The existence of fat oppression will not come as a surprise to readers of this book. We are marinated in fatphobia. Discussions about health often focus on weight. Thin bodies drape across the covers of fitness and fashion magazines that run headlines like "lose fat and win." Casual "fat talk" about food choices, exercise, and fit of clothing is ubiquitous. We hear constant cries about the "obesity epidemic" in the media. This dominant obesity discourse moralizes body size, teaching us to abhor fat.

Fatness once symbolized wealth, status, and beauty but now is seen as evidence of laziness, gluttony, stupidity, and lack of control (Farrell, 2011). War was declared on "obesity" in the late 1990s when it was deemed a global crisis akin to climate change and weapons of mass destruction (Russell et al., 2013). There have been many casualties in this war. Many have gone to great lengths to "achieve" an "ideal" body and have the physical and emotional scars to prove it (Wann, 2009). The effects of fat hatred are felt most by fat people who endure judgment, bias, discrimination, and assault in health care, the workplace, the legal system, interpersonal relationships, and all levels of formal education (Nutter et al., 2018). These are heightened when fat intersects with other forms of oppression like ableism, sexism, heterosexism, classism, racism, and colonialism (Prohaska & Gailey, 2019; Van Amsterdam, 2013).

What is particularly galling is that the "evidence" on which fatphobic assumptions is built is shaky at best. The idea that weight is a product of calories "in" and activity "out" is increasingly seen as simplistic given genetics, gut microbiome, stress, and other social and environmental factors can also be at play (Rothblum, 2018). Further, the neoliberal framing of weight as solely an individual's responsibility to monitor and manage has been recognized as highly problematic (Rail et al., 2010).

Dominant obesity discourse that perpetuates simplistic and harmful ideas about body weight abounds in many realms, including in formal and informal sites of learning. As we will discuss below, there is far more evidence of ways education feeds fat oppression than disrupts it. While that is certainly discouraging, it is important to remember that education not only has the power to reproduce the status quo but also has transformative potential (Apple, 2013). Fat pedagogy thus focuses not only on critique but also on developing approaches that tackle fat oppression head on and transform learning spaces so that every body can flourish.

In this chapter, we provide an overview of the fat pedagogy literature, offering a brief history of the field and describing key research foci that have emerged thus far.[1] We then look to the future by reflecting upon the "Fat Pedagogy Manifesto" – nine declarations that emerged through synthesizing insights from *The fat pedagogy reader* (Russell & Cameron, 2016). We hope that the narrative approach taken in the latter half of this chapter models the critical reflexivity that we think will be vital to the further development of this nascent field.

The nascent field of fat pedagogy

The first time the moniker "fat pedagogy" appeared in the scholarly literature was in 2013 (Russell et al., 2013) and the field began to coalesce with the publication of *The fat pedagogy reader* (Cameron & Russell, 2016) and a special issue of the journal, *Fat Studies* devoted to fat pedagogy (Cameron & Watkins, 2018). That said, discussions of fat oppression and education have been going on for at least 30 years now, with fat studies scholars leading the way in illuminating the "perpetual pedagogy" (Bordo, 1993, p. xvii) of living in a fatphobic culture. They observed how we quickly learn that thin and able bodies are the most highly valued and internalize the compunction to adhere to this narrow ideal, describing this process as "biopedagogy" (Cameron et al., 2014; Harwood, 2009; Rail & Jette, 2015) and "body-becoming" (McPhail et al., 2017; Rice, 2015).

There is a growing body of literature examining fatness and education. In formal education, researchers have examined curricula, courses, and programs (e.g., Azzarito, 2009; Cameron, 2015a; Watkins et al., 2012), school policies and cultures (e.g., Petherick & Beausoleil, 2015, 2016; Vander Schee & Gard, 2014), physical settings (e.g., Brown, 2018; Hetrick & Attig, 2009), and teaching approaches (e.g., Cameron 2015a, 2016a, 2016b; McPhail et al., 2017). The social exclusion and bullying of fat elementary and secondary students by peers and by teachers has been documented (e.g., McNinch, 2016; Sykes, 2011; Weinstock & Krehbiel, 2009) as has teachers' perceptions of fat students as incapable academically, physically, and socially (e.g., Kenney et al., 2015; Pringle & Powell, 2016). In post-secondary settings, fat people are less likely to be admitted in the first place (Burford, 2015; Burmeister et al., 2013); if they are, they can face discrimination in assessment, peer exclusion, and harassment, lessening the likelihood of graduating (Brown, 2018; Royce, 2016).

Popular culture is also recognized as a powerful form of "public pedagogy" that teaches normative body ideals and (re)produces fat oppression. Increasing attention is thus being paid to informal learning environments. For example, research has been conducted on the educational implications of media, public health campaigns, theatre, performance art, and fashion (e.g., Christel, 2018; Dark, 2019; Lupton, 2015; Monaghan et al., 2019; Rich, 2016) as well as participation in health and fitness activities (e.g., Dark, 2016; Ward et al., 2018).

The affective dimension of teaching and learning about fatness has also been an important research focus. For example, fat pedagogy scholars have criticized pedagogies of shame, guilt, and disgust (e.g., Leahy, 2009, 2014; Lupton, 2015; Rice, 2015; Russell & Semenko, 2016) and others have written about the potential of pedagogies of discomfort (e.g., Cameron, 2016a; McPhail et al., 2017). As well, scholars of various body sizes have shared frank accounts of their own teaching experiences, modeling the value of critical self-reflection (e.g., Bacon et al., 2016; McPhail et al., 2017).

Because fat pedagogy is still relatively new, it is not a surprise that there are many gaps in the field. For example, we observed that contributors to *The fat pedagogy reader* were mostly white, female, and worked in universities in Australia, Canada, New Zealand, the United Kingdom, and the United States. This echoes the larger field of fat studies that has roots in feminism (Farrell, 2011) and has been critiqued as "a bastion of whiteness" (Pausé, 2020, p. 181). Some disciplines are more represented in fat pedagogy than others (e.g., education, sociology, gender studies, health fields) and most empirical research takes a qualitative approach and tends to be small in scale. As well, there have been requests for more practical resources for educators, which makes sense given the absence of fat pedagogy in teacher education (McNinch, 2016; Pringle & Powell, 2016) and existing resource lists have been pitched primarily to post-secondary educators (e.g., Cameron, 2015b; Watkins et al., 2012).

Revisiting the "Fat Pedagogy Manifesto"

The two of us want this chapter to serve as an invitation to readers to join us in fattening educational ideas and practices. It is also a personal reminder that the two of us still have much to learn and unlearn. Since the publication of *The fat pedagogy reader* in 2016, the field has expanded substantially. Thus, in this section, we revisit the "Fat Pedagogy Manifesto" we wrote for the concluding chapter of the book. We examine each of the nine points as a way of deepening our review and identifying future needs in the field.

> 1. We are marinated in a culture rife with weight-based oppression. Fat or thin or somewhere in between, all of us are impacted by it in one way or another. Some of us feel the effects more keenly, however, and intersectional analyses can help clarify how various oppressions interact in complex ways. Fat pedagogy can and ought to help make weight bias, fat phobia, and fat hatred, in all their complexity, more visible. And fat pedagogy must, in the end, make a positive difference to fat people's lives.
>
> *(Russell & Cameron, 2016, p. 254)*

In hindsight, we see that we packed a lot into that first point; the ideas could have been separated out for clarity. We also note we used "weight-based oppression" rather than "fat oppression." While we were trying to be inclusive in our language, it is less hard-hitting. Fat Studies scholars and activists have made it abundantly clear that most of us around the world now live in fatphobic cultures. And it is true that it impacts everyone, albeit in different ways, which is why intersectional analyses are so important. We wish, however, that we had been clearer that fat people are the most impacted.

One of us (Constance) is a fat woman who has had a lifetime of experiences of fat oppression that have impacted her both personally and professionally. As just one example, prior to her awareness of fat studies, she acquiesced to societal and medical pressure to have weight loss surgery, which did not lead to permanent weight loss and had lasting negative health consequences. In contrast, one of us (Erin) has thin privilege that insulates her from fat oppression. Nonetheless, in some of her early writings she discussed her experience of fat shaming as an elite athlete. While that illuminated one of the ways bodies are policed, she now realizes that she diluted her intended message, akin to what is currently happening with body positivity. Despite its political roots in the fat acceptance movement, body positivity now has become a trendy space for apolitical "self-love" and #AllBodiesMatter statements (Yeboah, 2019). Borrowing from the field of anti-racism and the concept of white fragility (DiAngelo, 2018), Erin identifies her initial positioning as an example of "thin fragility" wherein she sought to defensively include her own experiences of fat shaming. While thin allies can and do play a role in fat pedagogy, she now thinks that others like her need to do more to unlearn thin privilege, challenge co-option, and centre fat people's experiences in all their diversity. As two white, able-bodied, straight cis women, we cannot fully understand how racism, heterosexism, and ableism compound the experience of fatness. We agree with Nash and Warin (2017) who argue that we need more "complex, multi-dimensional framing of fat, fat politics and privilege in order … to more productively grapple with the ambiguity of embodied subjectivity" (p. 71).

> 2. Fat pedagogy needs to be grounded in research and scholarship on weight-based oppression. Since different disciplines offer useful insights that become even more powerful when brought together, fat pedagogy is, and must be, an interdisciplinary, multidisciplinary, and transdisciplinary endeavor. Therefore engaging each other generously, attempting to communicate across our different discourse communities, and collaborating with one another can only serve to benefit this emerging field.
>
> *(Russell & Cameron, 2016, p. 254)*

We continue to support this statement and reiterate that fat pedagogy scholarship must maintain a commitment to addressing fat oppression. There is a tension in the field about the role of "obesity" science in fat pedagogy, which can be tricky to handle, especially in the health care fields where "obesity" continues to be framed only as a problem to be solved. Gard (2016) argues that we are doing a disservice to learners if we do not address this challenge head on. We agree, and argue one of the gifts of multidisciplinary, interdisciplinary, and transdisciplinary learning is that it affords new possibilities as ideas to comingle. Not that it is a straightforward process, which is why we mentioned the importance of striving to communicate across disciplinary and discourse divides. Discussing challenges related to working across and with methodological, ontological, and epistemological difference, Russell (2006) critiques adversarial discourse typical of the academy and advocates instead that we "engage in ways that not merely allow for, but also encourage critical *and* generous, and difficult *and* respectful conversations that have the possibility of continuing" (p. 407).

We also want to reiterate that fat pedagogy is grounded not only in research and scholarship, but also in insights generated through fat activism and the experiences of fat people. As Pausé (2020) states, it is vital that the fat community is involved in all aspects of research. In particular, she asserts that "researchers from outside fat communities must collaborate with fat studies scholars with methodological or content matter expertise to ensure the violence against fat bodies is not (re)produced" (p. 183).

> 3. Fat pedagogy scholars and practitioners need to seek one another out. This is a two-way street; scholars sharing findings in accessible ways and practitioners keeping abreast of research and scholarship in the field are both key.
>
> *(Russell & Cameron, 2016, p. 254)*

Fat pedagogy as a field needs to continue to deepen its understanding of praxis and articulate this intent more explicitly. In education, praxis refers to the dialectical relationship of theory and practice, with each informing and honing the other (Freire, 1970). Given its roots in fat studies, fat pedagogy can be understood as a mix of theory, educational practice, and activism. It may be more productive, then, to think of fat pedagogy not as a "two-way street" but as an intersection where multiple roads crisscross. Thus, not only are accessible research and evidence-informed practice important aspects of fat pedagogy, so too is learning about, from, and through fat activism, which we will discuss further below.

4. Fat pedagogy needs to build on the lived experiences of those who have experienced weight-based oppression and of those who have grappled seriously with their thin privilege … It applies to the research we conduct, the teaching materials and resources we share, and who we invite to lead or participate in our pedagogical activities.

(Russell & Cameron, 2016, p. 254)

As with the first point, we wished we had been clearer about the importance of foregrounding fat folks' experiences, which resonates with recent work on standpoint theory in fat studies (e.g., Cooper Stoll & Thoune, 2019; Pausé, 2020). Cooper Stoll and Thoune (2019) make the compelling point that, "Unfortunately, when it comes to much of the research on fat people, the voices of fat people, including fat researchers and activists, are either marginalized or absent" (p. 1). They suggest that standpoint theory that recognizes "the epistemic advantage" (p. 1) of fat people's situated knowledges could be a useful tool in elevating these voices and a way to collectively develop a "shared angle of vision" (p. 3).

In fat pedagogy research, there is increasing attention to hearing directly from fat people. For example, some researchers have sought fat students' perspectives (e.g., Brown, 2018; McNinch, 2016; Rice, 2007; Sykes, 2011) while others have shared those of fat educators (e.g., Cameron, 2015a, 2016b; McPhail et al., 2017). Already, it is clear that these perspectives are far from uniform – fat post-secondary educators, for example, do not agree on how to address their own fat embodiment when teaching – which demonstrates why hearing diverse fat voices is vital.

What role might thin allies play in fat pedagogy? Like in other social movements, we believe that allies can spend their privilege by speaking up about fat oppression when they witness it, especially given fat people discussing fat oppression are seen as biased and self-interested (Cooper Stoll & Thoune, 2019). Allies also can work with other non-fat folks keen to unpack and address their own privilege as part of the task of dismantling the structures that keep fat oppression in place (Bacon et al., 2016). Nash and Warin (2017) assert, "If fat activism is only tied to particular identities, then fat bodies are the only site through which political action can take place" (p. 74). They thus see power in intersectional collaboration while also recognizing that those with privilege need to avoid taking up space when a "group has the tools to articulate its own demands" (p. 78). Pausé (2020) agrees and further asserts:

All of us have a responsibility to ensure that we are checking our privilege along the way and lifting the voices of those who may not be heard. Highlighting voices of fat people of color, voices of fat working poor, voices of super fats; these are the responsibility of those who hold power by standing outside of those identities. Being honest about where we stand, and the privileges that we bring into our spaces, is key to ensuring that knowledge around fatness does not further oppress fat people.

(p. 184)

5. There is no "one size fits all" approach to fat pedagogy; the efficacy of different approaches will vary by geographical, cultural, linguistic, and sociopolitical contexts.

(Russell & Cameron, 2016, p. 254)

Beyond starting where individual learners are, which we will discuss in the next point, it is vital that we pay attention to the contexts within which we, and the learners with whom we work, are embedded. That includes the type of learning context (e.g., elementary, secondary, post-secondary, informal) and physical setting (e.g., classroom, nature, public space). It also means expanding the geographical, cultural, linguistic, and sociopolitical contexts where fat pedagogy is practiced, which we believe demands that fat pedagogy itself diversifies. As noted above, limited voices have been heard in fat studies generally and fat pedagogy in particular, and that undoubtedly impacts the efficacy of our work. Intersectional approaches also could help fat pedagogy address a range of interconnected problems like white supremacy, colonialism, ableism, classism, sexism, heterosexism, and speciesism, as could engaging with other fields like critical disability studies, critical race theory, critical animal studies, feminist food studies, feminist new materialisms, freak studies, and queer theory (Russell & Cameron, 2016). Broadening our scope theoretically and methodologically may offer us more and better ideas and tools to help us ethically and effectively work in a variety of contexts.

> 6. Regardless of learning context, it is vital that we start where learners are and not work from a deficit position that assumes learners, particularly those expressing fat phobia and demonstrating weight bias, are simply foolish and hateful.
>
> *(Russell & Cameron, 2016, p. 255)*

The two of us come to fat pedagogy with an academic grounding in education so are familiar with constructivist and critical approaches to teaching that acknowledge learners are not "blank slates" and that building on learners' existing knowledge and interests is more engaging and effective (Shor, 1992). Critical and anti-oppressive pedagogies also recognize that all education is political, whether going against the grain or (re)producing the status quo (Kincheloe, 2008). As Kumashiro (2015) illuminates so well, educating "against common sense" is hard work for both teachers and learners, and resistance is to be expected. We have noticed that these ideas are novel to some of our colleagues whose homes are in other disciplines, and they often express disappointment when their students do not respond positively to their efforts. We must recognize that learners, like all of us, are marinated in fatphobic cultures. Resistance, then, does not need to be interpreted as a problem, but as an integral part of a learning and unlearning process that can take years to unfold. Indeed, both of us have taught seemingly resistant students who reach out, sometimes well after a course has ended, to report that they now "get it."

Starting where learners are does not mean that fat pedagogy involves tolerating fat hatred, however, and this is where the process gets especially tricky. On one hand, we want to help folks unlearn fatphobia, and harshly or incessantly criticizing problematic statements can be counterproductive if it leads learners to shut down or depart altogether. On the other hand, allowing fat hatred to circulate in learning environments harms fat leaners, and the reproduction of oppression can be amplified for racialized learners who may already find themselves "tone policed" by educators and peers who unreasonably expect them to quietly listen to hateful statements made under the guise of ignorance. Marginalized learners may find they have little recourse in such situations, so it is incumbent on educators to navigate this tension with care. For us, an intersectional approach that maintains a laser focus on the interlocking systemic forces at play is essential. Farrell (2016) also suggests that deep listening, compassion, and empathy can be helpful and such a "relational ontology" (Wildman, 2006) may enable fat pedagogy to attend more fully to the affective domain, although we would argue only if combined with the analytical tools that critical, anti-oppressive, and intersectional pedagogies afford.

> 7. Fat pedagogy must raise awareness and encourage critical thinking. Learners may have heard little about weight bias and not know that counterhegemonic movements

like fat activism and Health At Every Size even exist ... Helping learners build skills so
that they can critically assess dominant obesity discourse ... is important.

(Russell & Cameron, 2016, p. 255)

While we agree that raising awareness of dominant obesity discourse remains important, then
what? Awareness is somewhere to start but is insufficient on its own. What sorts of skills and
competencies do students and educators need to tackle fat oppression? These questions could be
fruitful for fat pedagogy to consider. For example, in the world of medical education that one
of us works in, there is growing use of simulation activities like having students wear fat suits to
spark reflection and encourage empathy for fat patients (e.g., Hunter et al., 2018). Meadows et
al. (2017) have raised ethical concerns about that practice, which we share. We do not doubt the
good intentions of those medical educators but assert that the hidden curriculum of that simulation needs further consideration. This example highlights that the skills and competencies that
need to be fostered will differ by context and audience. Unpacking dominant obesity discourse
and unlearning weight bias will be more challenging for some.

Learning about and from counterhegemonic fat activism remains a promising pedagogical avenue, and may be particularly so for fat people; Pausé (2020), in writing about fat agency, sees hope
in "[c]rafting positive fat identities, creating fat positive spaces, embodying our fat bodies in the
ways we want" (p. 182). As those working in diverse critical pedagogies have argued, activism *is*
pedagogy (e.g., Lowan-Trudeau, 2017; Marshall & Anderson, 2008). We recognize that those less
familiar with work on the relationship between social movements and education, and the tension
between advocacy and education, may be understandably nervous, especially when working in
conservative contexts. We remind readers, however, that counterhegemonic education can range
from learning *about* social movements and other people's activism to learning *through* participating
in activism. We would like to see more work done on the role of activism in fat pedagogy.

> 8. Emotions can run high in fat pedagogy ... The "affective turn" that is occurring in
> many disciplines, including education, makes it increasingly clear that knowledge alone
> is insufficient in making change.
>
> *(Russell & Cameron, 2016, p. 255)*

In the conclusion to *The fat pedagogy reader*, we noted how the chapters were "peppered with
stories of frustration, discomfort, anger, denial, guilt, curiosity, excitement, love, and hope" (p.
255). Other social movement educations, like anti-racist, feminist, and climate change education, have long advocated attending to the affective dimensions of learning (e.g., Boler, 1999;
Russell et al., 2013). As noted above, fat pedagogy scholars have examined pedagogies of shame,
guilt, disgust, and discomfort. More work of this sort would be welcome, as would attention to
the power of pedagogies of care, love, and hope.

> 9. Given the fat-phobic contexts within which most of us operate, unlearning weight
> bias is an ongoing process even for those who have been doing this work for years. It
> behooves all of us engaged in fat pedagogy, then, to continue to push at the edges of
> our own knowledge and continually engage in thoughtful self-reflection.
>
> *(Russell & Cameron, 2016, p. 255)*

Unlearning our cultures' taken-for-granted assumptions is hard work (Kumashiro, 2015). For
example, the two of us regularly have to grapple with our internalized fatphobia. While we
sometimes find those moments embarrassing, they also help us have more compassion for the

students we teach. We also have found sharing our own stories of unlearning opens space for students to be honest, vulnerable, and more willing to journey with us. Because of the intersectional approach we take, we also discuss our ongoing efforts to unlearn racism, white supremacy, sexism, heterosexism, classism, ableism, and speciesism. In doing so, we seek to model that unlearning need not be a guilt-ridden and discouraging process but can be empowering and exciting. It also keeps us curious about and open to other's experiences, which we see as part of our ongoing commitment to social justice. Autoethnographic work and self-study can be particularly useful self-reflection and pedagogical tools as a number of fat pedagogy scholars have demonstrated. As one example, Pausé (2020) models unlearning in her autoethnographic writing on addressing white supremacy and colonialism and how that has impacted her work in fat studies and activism.

A Fat Pedagogy Manifesto: Take two

By sharing this critical reflection on our first attempt at a Fat Pedagogy Manifesto, we hope that we have illustrated that there remains much to learn about the complex relationship between fat and education. We thus offer this second iteration of the Manifesto not as a definitive statement, but rather hope that it might be generative for others and lead to variations informed by diverse perspectives.

1 Fat pedagogy recognizes that we are marinated in a culture rife with fat oppression and makes fat oppression visible in all its complexity.
2 Fat pedagogy makes a material difference in fat people's lives.
3 Fat pedagogy centres the lived experiences of those who have experienced fat oppression.
4 Fat pedagogy, while grounded in fat studies and critical pedagogies, engages with diverse theories, practices, and social movements in a generous yet critical way.
5 Fat pedagogy is built on praxis grounded in collaborative efforts of scholars, practitioners, and activists.
6 Fat pedagogy must be contextually situated; there is no "one size fits all" approach.
7 Fat pedagogy starts where learners are, attends to the affective dimensions of learning and unlearning, and makes use of intersectional analyses.
8 Fat pedagogy raises awareness of fat activism and encourages learners to contribute to this counterhegemonic movement.
9 Fat pedagogy helps educators and learners build skills and competencies needed to recognize dominant obesity discourse and to develop and maintain alternative discourses and practices that enable all bodies to flourish.
10 Fat pedagogy recognizes unlearning and tackling fat oppression is an ongoing process.

Looking to the future

Fat pedagogy has long been an important element of fat studies and will continue to be so, given the constitutive role education plays in (re)producing fat oppression and its transformative potential. As fat pedagogy develops into a field unto itself, there remains much work to do. Educators keen to incorporate fat pedagogy into their practice have requested more support and resources; thus far, most of what has been developed has been geared to post-secondary settings, although we are starting to see more books for children and youth as well as other materials circulating that could be useful to elementary and secondary teachers. As pedagogical approaches, activities, programs, and professional development opportunities are developed, research that investigates their efficacy would be warranted, including studies that are larger in scale and that follow learners over a longer time period. We also need research to be conducted in a greater variety of formal and informal learning sites and to diversify methodological approaches taken. Further, fat pedagogy has been dominated by English-speaking scholars and, like fat studies, been a bastion of whiteness; expanding the geographical, cultural, linguistic, and sociopolitical contexts in which fat pedagogy is practiced will not only help complexify the field but ensure that our work makes a material difference to more fat people. As intersectional analyses make clear, there is no singular fat voice and we need to ensure that many fat perspectives are sought and heard in fat pedagogy. Theoretically, then, we would like to see more attention paid to intersectionality, decolonization, and standpoint theory, and more work grounded in critical race theory, critical disability studies, critical animal studies, Indigenous theories and practices, feminist food studies, feminist new materialisms, freak studies, and queer theory.

There also are a number of questions that we think warrant attention in fat pedagogy. For example, what are the skills and competencies educators and learners need to tackle fat oppression? What can be learned from critical, anti-oppressive, anti-racist, Indigenous, queer, and feminist pedagogies to help us more productively deal with thin fragility and learner resistance to facilitate the unlearning so vital to fat pedagogy? How might we disrupt pedagogies of shame and disgust, delve deeper into pedagogies of discomfort, and develop pedagogies of care, love, and hope? What is the role of advocacy and activism in fat pedagogy, and how might scholars, teachers, and activists work more productively and playfully together?

These are but a few possible ideas for directions in which fat pedagogy might go. The field needs more scholars who bring other ways of thinking, researching, and practicing, to envision other possibilities. We thus invite you to join us in further developing the praxis of fat pedagogy. Together, we can continue to build the field of fat pedagogy as one way of tackling fat oppression.

Note

1   See Russell (2020) for a more comprehensive review.

References

Apple, M. (2013). *Can education change society?* New York: Routledge.

Azzarito, L. (2009). The rise of corporate curriculum: Fatness, fitness, and whiteness. In J. Wright & V. Harwood (Eds.), *Biopolitics and the "obesity epidemic": Governing bodies* (pp. 183–198). London, UK: Routledge.

Bacon, L., O'Reilly, C., & Aphramor, L. (2016). Reflections on thin privilege and responsibility. In E. Cameron & C. Russell (Eds.), *The fat pedagogy reader: Challenging weight-based oppression through critical education* (pp. 41–50). New York: Peter Lang.

Bennett, E. M. (2018). Obituary. *Victoria Times Colonist*, July 14–15. https://www.legacy.com/obituaries/timescolonist/obituary.aspx?n=ellen-maud-bennett&pid=189588876

Boler, M. (1999). *Feeling power: Emotions and education.* New York: Routledge.

Bordo, S. (1993). *Unbearable weight: Feminism, Western culture and the body.* Los Angeles, CA: University of California Press.

Brown, H. (2018). "There's always stomach on the table and then I gotta write!": Physical space and learning in fat college women. *Fat Studies, 7*(1), 11–20.

Burford, J. (2015). "Dear obese PhD applicants": Twitter, Tumblr and the contested affective politics of fat doctoral embodiment. *M/C Journal, 18*(3). http://www.journal.media-culture.org.au/index.php/mcjournal/article/view/969

Burmeister, J., Kiefner, A., Carels, R., & Musher-Eizenman, D. (2013). Weight bias in graduate school admissions. *Obesity, 21*(5), 918–920.

Cameron, E. (2015a). Toward a fat pedagogy: A study of pedagogical approaches aimed at challenging obesity discourse in post-secondary education. *Fat Studies*, 4(1), 28–45.

Cameron, E. (2015b). Teaching resources for post-secondary educators who challenge dominant obesity discourse. *Fat Studies*, 4(2), 212–226.

Cameron, E. (2016a). Learning to teach every body: Exploring the emergence of a critical "obesity" pedagogy. In E. Cameron, & C. Russell (Eds.), *The fat pedagogy reader: Challenging weight-based oppression through critical education* (pp. 171–178). New York: Peter Lang.

Cameron, E. (2016b). Challenging "size matters" messages: An exploration of the experiences of critical obesity scholars in higher education. *The Canadian Journal of Higher Education*, 46(2), 111–126.

Cameron, E., & Russell, C. (2016). *The fat pedagogy reader: Challenging weight-based oppression through critical education*. New York: Peter Lang.

Cameron, E., & Watkins, P. (2018). Fat pedagogy: Improving teaching and learning for everyBODY. *Fat Studies*, 7(1), 1–10.

Cameron, E., Oakley, J., Walton, G., Russell, C., Chambers, L., & Socha, T. (2014). Moving beyond the injustices of the schooled healthy body. In I. Bogotch, & C. Shields (Eds.), *International handbook of educational leadership and social (in)justice* (pp. 687–704). New York: Springer.

Christel, D. A. (2018). Fat fashion: Fattening pedagogy in apparel design. *Fat Studies*, 7(1), 44–55.

Cooper Stoll, L., & Thoune, D. (2019). Elevating the voices and research of fat scholars and activists: Standpoint theory in fat studies. *Fat Studies*, 9(3), 1–8.

Dark, K. (2016). Fat pedagogy in the yoga class. In B. Berila, M. Klein, & C. Jackson Roberts (Eds.), *Yoga, the body, and embodied social change: An intersectional feminist analysis* (pp. 193–204). Lanham, MD: Lexington.

Dark, K. (2019). Things I learned from fat people on the plane. *Fat Studies*, 8(3), 299–319.

DiAngelo, R. (2018). *White fragility: Why it's so hard for white people to talk about racism*. Boston, MA: Beacon.

Farrell, A. (2011). *Fat shame: Stigma and the fat body in American culture*. New York: New York University Press.

Farrell, A. (2016). Teaching fat studies in a liberal arts college: The centrality of mindfulness, deep listening, and empathic interpretation as pedagogic methods. In E. Cameron, & C. Russell (Eds.), *The fat pedagogy reader: Challenging weight-based oppression through critical education* (pp. 61–70). New York: Peter Lang.

Freire, P. (1970). *Pedagogy of the oppressed*. New York: Herder & Herder.

Gard, M. (2016). Navigating morality, politics, and reason: Towards scientifically literate and intellectually ethical fat pedagogies. In E. Cameron, & C. Russell (Eds.), *The fat pedagogy reader: Challenging weight-based oppression through critical education* (pp. 241–250). New York: Peter Lang.

Harwood, V. (2009). Theorizing biopedagogies. In J. Wright, & V. Harwood (Eds.), *Biopolitics and the "obesity epidemic": Governing bodies* (pp. 16–30). New York: Routledge.

Hetrick A., & Attig, D. (2009). Sitting pretty: Fat bodies, classroom desks, and academic excess. In E. Rothblum, & S. Solovay (Eds.), *The fat studies reader* (pp. 197–204). New York: New York University Press.

Hunter, J., Rawlings-Anderson, K., Lindsay, T., Bowden, T., & Aitken, L. (2018). Exploring student nurses' attitudes towards those who are obese and whether these attitudes change following a simulated activity. *Nurse Education Today*, 65, 225–231.

Kenney, E., Gortmaker, S., Davison, K., & Bryn Austin, S. (2015). The academic penalty for gaining weight: A longitudinal, change-in-change analysis of BMI and perceived academic ability in middle school students. *International Journal of Obesity*, 39(9), 1408–1413.

Kincheloe, J. (2008). *Critical pedagogy primer* (2nd ed.). New York: Peter Lang.

Kumashiro, K. (2015). *Against common sense: Teaching and learning toward social justice* (3rd ed.). New York: Routledge.

Leahy, D. (2009). Disgusting pedagogies. In J. Wright, & V. Harwood (Eds.), *Biopolitics and the "obesity epidemic": Governing bodies* (pp. 172–182). New York: Routledge.

Leahy, D. (2014). Assembling a health(y) subject: Risky and shameful pedagogies in health education. *Critical Public Health*, 24(2), 171–181.

Lowan-Trudeau, G. (2017). Protest as pedagogy: Exploring teaching and learning in Indigenous environmental movements. *Journal of Environmental Education*, 48(2), 96–108.

Lupton, D. (2015). The pedagogy of disgust: The ethical, moral and political implications of using disgust in public health campaigns. *Critical Public Health*, 25(1), 4–14.

Marshall, C., & Anderson, A. (2008). *Activist educators: Breaking past limits*. New York: Routledge.

McNinch, H. (2016). Fat bullying of girls in elementary and secondary schools: Implications for teacher education. In E. Cameron, & C. Russell (Eds.), *The fat pedagogy reader: Challenging weight-based oppression through critical education* (pp. 113–121). New York: Peter Lang.

McPhail, D., Brady, J., & Gingras, J. (2017). Exposed social flesh: Toward an embodied fat pedagogy. *Fat Studies, 6*(1), 17–37.

Meadows, A., Calogero, R., O'Reilly, C., Rodriguez, A., Heldreth, C., & Tomiyama, A. (2017). Why fat suits do not advance the scientific study of weight stigma. *Obesity, 25*(2), 275.

Monaghan, L., Rich, E., & Bombak, A. (2019). Media, "fat panic" and public pedagogy: Mapping contested terrain. *Sociology Compass, 13*(1), e12651.

Nash, M., & Warin, M. (2017). Squeezed between identity politics and intersectionality: A critique of "thin privilege" in fat studies. *Feminist Theory, 18*(1), 69–87.

Nutter, S., Russell-Mayhew, S., Arthur, N., & Ellard, J. (2018). Weight bias as a social justice issue: A call for dialogue. *Canadian Psychology, 59*(1), 89–99.

Pausé, C. (2020). Ray of light: Standpoint theory, fat studies, and a new fat ethics. *Fat Studies, 9*(2), 178–187.

Petherick, L., & Beausoleil, N. (2015). Female elementary teachers' biopedagogical practices: How health discourse circulates in Newfoundland elementary schools *Canadian Journal of Education, 38*(1), 1–29.

Petherick, L., & Beausoleil, N. (2016). Obesity panic, body surveillance, and pedagogy: Elementary teachers' response to obesity messaging. In J. Ellison, D. McPhail, & W. Mitchinson (Eds.), *Obesity in Canada: Critical perspectives* (pp. 245–270). Toronto, ON: University of Toronto Press.

Pringle, R., & Powell, D. (2016). Critical pedagogical strategies to disrupt weight bias in schools. In E. Cameron, & C. Russell (Eds.), *The fat pedagogy reader: Challenging weight-based oppression through critical education* (pp. 123–131). New York: Peter Lang.

Prohaska, A., & Gailey, J. (2019). Theorizing fat oppression: Intersectional approaches and methodological innovations. *Fat Studies, 8*(1), 1–19.

Rail, G., & Jette, S. (2015). Reflections on biopedagogies and/of public health: On bio-others, rescue missions, and social justice. *Cultural Studies<>Critical Methodologies, 15*(5), 327–336.

Rail, G., Holmes, D., & Murray, S. (2010). The politics of evidence on "domestic terrorists": Obesity discourses and their effects. *Social Theory & Health, 8*, 259–279.

Rice, C. (2007). Becoming "the fat girl": Acquisition of an unfit identity. *Women's Studies International Forum, 30*(2), 158–174.

Rice, C. (2015). Rethinking fat: From bio- to body-becoming pedagogies. *Cultural Studies<>Critical Methodologies, 15*(5), 387–397.

Rich, E. (2016). A public pedagogy approach to fat pedagogy. In E. Cameron, & C. Russell (Eds.), *The fat pedagogy reader: Challenging weight-based oppression through critical education* (pp. 231–240). New York: Peter Lang.

Rothblum, E. (2018). Slim chance for permanent weight loss. *Archives of Scientific Psychology, 6*(1), 63–69.

Royce, T. (2016). Fat invisibility, fat hate: Towards a progressive pedagogy of size. In E. Cameron, & C. Russell (Eds.), *The fat pedagogy reader: Challenging weight-based oppression through critical education* (pp. 21–29) New York: Peter Lang.

Russell, C. (2006). Working across and with methodological difference in environmental education research. *Environmental Education Research, 12*(3/4), 403–412.

Russell, C. (2020). Fat pedagogy and the disruption of weight-based oppression: Toward the flourishing of all bodies. In S. Steinberg, & B. Down (Eds.), *The Sage handbook of critical pedagogies* (pp. 1516–1531). London: Sage.

Russell, C., & Cameron, E. (2016). Conclusion: A Fat Pedagogy Manifesto. In E. Cameron, & C. Russell (Eds.), *The fat pedagogy reader: Challenging weight-based oppression through critical education* (pp. 251–256). New York: Peter Lang.

Russell, C., & Semenko, K. (2016). We take "cow" as a compliment: Fattening humane, environmental, and social justice education. In E. Cameron, & C. Russell (Eds.), *The fat pedagogy reader: Challenging weight-based oppression through critical education* (pp. 211–220). New York: Peter Lang.

Russell, C., Cameron, E., Socha, T., & McNinch, H. (2013). "Fatties cause global warming": Fat pedagogy and environmental education. *Canadian Journal of Environmental Education, 18*, 27–45.

Shor, I. (1992). *Empowering education: Critical teaching for social change*. Chicago, IL: University of Chicago Press.

Sykes, H. (2011). *Queer bodies: Sexualities, genders and fatness in physical education*. New York: Peter Lang.

Van Amsterdam, N. (2013). Big fat inequalities, thin privilege: An intersectional perspective on "body size". *European Journal of Women's Studies, 20*(2), 155–169.

Vander Schee, C., & Gard, M. (2014). Healthy, happy and ready to teach, or why kids can't learn from fat teachers: The discursive politics of school reform and teacher health. *Critical Public Health, 24*, 210–225.

Wann, M. (2009). Foreword: Fat studies: An invitation to revolution. In E. Rothblum, & S. Solovay (Eds.), *The fat studies reader* (pp. ix–xxv). New York: New York University Press.

Ward, P., Sirna, K., Wareham, A., & Cameron, E. (2018). Embodied display: A critical examination of the biopedagogical experience of wearing health. *Fat Studies, 7*(1), 93–104.

Watkins, P., Farrell, A., & Doyle-Hugmeyer, A. (2012). Teaching fat studies: From conception to reception. *Fat Studies, 1*(2), 180–194.

Weinstock, J., & Krehbiel, M. (2009). Fat youth as common targets for bullying. In E. Rothblum, & S. Solovay (Eds.), *The fat studies reader* (pp. 120–126). New York: New York University Press.

Wildman, W. (2006). An introduction to relational ontology. In J. Polkinghorne, & J. Zizioulas (Eds.), *The trinity and an entangled world* (pp. 55–73). Grand Rapids, MI: Eerdmans.

Yeboah, S. (2019). The body positivity movement is not for slim bodies already accepted by society. *Metro News.* https://metro.co.uk/2019/07/01/the-body-positivity-movement-is-not-for-slim-bodies-already-accepted-by-society-10081795/

15

FATNESS, DISCRIMINATION AND LAW

An international perspective

Stephanie von Liebenstein

Weight discrimination – as most fat people will confirm – pervades every area of our lives. It is everywhere and comes from everywhere, as Michel Foucault (2006) would probably put it, and it permeates our daily routines. It accompanies us from dawn to dusk, be it at work, in school, in our circle of friends, in our families, whether we watch TV, are active in social networks or open a newspaper, whether we take a walk in the park or look for a place to sit on the subway, whether we play sports, try to find a partner, need health care, are on a plane or in a fashion store, in a restaurant, a cinema or even on jury duty, before court or in a custody battle. Whether we are traveling in the US or in Europe, Australia, New Zealand, Israel, South Africa, Brazil or Iceland: as soon as any corner of the globe comes into contact with Western ideals of beauty, it will not be long before discrimination of fat people begins to proliferate.[1]

Nevertheless, it remains a matter of culture which social discourses revolve around fat bodies. While in Mauritania, for example, a round body is still the epitome of beauty (Harter, 2004), France is notorious for having zero tolerance for body fat – although 54 percent of French men and 44 percent of women fall within the "overweight/obese" BMI range (Esen, 2017); the so-called "Tyranny of the Silhouette" (Robertson, 2013) has a decisive influence on personal and professional success (Huggins, 2015), and fat job applicants face discrimination as strong as that experienced by immigrants (Peretti-Watel & Moatti, 2009).

The situation is similar in other countries around the world: whether in the UK (Thomas, 2005), Germany (Giel et al., 2012), Iceland, Korea, USA, Sweden, Denmark, Spain, Greece or Portugal (Puhl et al., 2015, p. 693, with further references), fat people are severely penalized in professional life, facing unfair hiring practices, lower wages, denial of promotions, and job termination because of their weight even when better qualified than their thin colleagues.

Thus, it is no wonder that increasing numbers of people discriminated against on the grounds of their weight are going to court hoping to be protected by the law or at least to be compensated for their damages. In the United States, the number of reported cases of weight discrimination has risen dramatically in the last two decades, with a 66 percent increase in numbers between 1996 and 2006 alone (Andreyeva et al., 2008). A similarly dramatic rise in legal actions initiated by employees for workers' compensation, unfair dismissal, and discrimination has been reported in Australia (McArthur, 2016). There are still few cases before court in Europe, but numbers are rising every year.[2] All this shows: discrimination on the grounds of weight is a serious legal problem that needs to be addressed immediately.

Weight discrimination, however, is not just relevant in labor law, but equally so in many other areas of civil and administrative law, for instance when fat people are made to pay for two airline seats, are not being served in restaurant, are excluded from scout camp,[3] sign a prenup declaring that they will not gain any weight (*Dewberry v. George*, 2003), are rejected by a university because of their weight or not allowed to enter civil service,[4] when they are excluded from jury duty (*People v. Wynn*, 2004) or cannot get an extension of their work visa because of their weight (BBC News, 2013b). Questions of health insurance law or child and youth welfare law may be affected if fat people are denied health insurance, forced to accept disadvantageous insurance tariffs or when parents lose custody of their child because of their child's weight. Finally, weight discrimination can also become criminally relevant when fat people are bullied, insulted or assaulted.

Weight as a discrimination category

It is therefore particularly unfortunate that weight discrimination does not belong to a class protected by national anti-discrimination legislation in any country in the world. A general and explicit inclusion of "weight" in anti-discrimination legislation has so far only been implemented in a few cities and one US state, namely Michigan. Michigan – which introduced "weight" as a protected class in its Elliott-Larson Civil Rights Act in 1976 – was also one of the earliest places in the world to provide any kind of antidiscrimination protection for fat people at all. The author of the 1976 amendment, then state representative Thomas Mathieu, told the Associated Press in 2010 that he introduced the bill because "he was 'flabbergasted' by the number of cases of unfairness involving women seeking office jobs who possessed the necessary skills and personality, but were overweight" (Engel, 2010, para 9).

San Francisco, too, protects "height and weight" under its Municipal Code (City and County of San Francisco Human Rights Commission, 2001), prohibiting discrimination against fat people in any aspect of employment including, but not limited to, recruitment, selection, hiring, wages, uniforms, hours and conditions of employment, promotion, training, development or benefits. The Compliance Guidelines by the City and County of San Francisco Human Rights Commission cover a wide range of problems caused by weight discrimination, among these the necessity that "employers shall ensure that common areas such as employee lounges, cafeterias, health units and exercise facilities are accessible to people of all sizes." Similar in wording are the ordinances passed by Santa Cruz, CA, (*Municipal Code*, Chapter 9.83) and Binghampton, NY (*Human Rights Law*, Chapter 45.3).

The Icelandic capital of Reykjavik is the only city outside the US that has an antidiscrimination provision explicitly aimed at fighting weight discrimination. Its Human Rights Policy (revised 2016) reads in section 6: "Persons may not be discriminated against due to their build, appearance or body type. The contribution of each individual, regardless of height, weight or appearance, shall be assessed on its merit."

In some cities and states (Victoria, Australia [*VIC Equal Opportunity Act 2010*]; Madison, WI, USA [*Madison City Code*]; Urbana, Ill, USA [*Urbana Human Rights Ordinance*]; Washington, DC, USA) "weight" is officially (meaning either directly through definitions in the relevant Code or through official guidelines) subsumed under "physical" or "personal appearance"; other cities and states protect against weight discrimination only in some delineated areas like advertisement (Berlin, Germany) or health insurance coverage for "obesity" treatments.[5]

However, oftentimes "weight" is subsumed under "physical appearance" without there being a mention of "weight" in the relevant Code or in any official guidelines accompanying the Code. France and Belgium fall in this group of countries and also e.g. Bolivia. As we will see later, "physical appearance" without further clarification usually provides only limited protection to fat people. So does the subsumption of "weight" under "disability".

Finally, many countries in the world follow an open-list approach to anti-discrimination, using phrasings like "any other ground" (South Africa, Employment Equity Act, 1988, Chpt. II, 6 (1)), "in particular" (Canada, Canadian Constitution Act 1982, Part I, 15 (1)), or "other reason" (European Convention on Human Rights (ECHR), Art. 14) at least in their human rights charters or Labor Codes. Russia, for example, protects "sex, race, color of skin, nationality, language, […] *as well as other factors* not relevant to professional qualities of the employee" in Art. 3 of its Labor Code (2001). Open lists have at least the potential to include weight as an "analogous ground". Unfortunately, so far no case has been known in which a plaintiff discriminated against on the basis his weight has successfully invoked such an analogy. The case of the Russian Aeroflot stewardesses who had filed a lawsuit against an Aeroflot uniform size regulation in 2017 and obtained a ruling in Moscow City Court, for example, was a sex discrimination case (Matsnev, 2017), not one based on "other factors".

So far, then, not much has been done by legislation around the world to protect the growing group of fat people from more than often stifling discrimination. This chapter aims to explore the existing and not-yet-existing possibilities of legal protection for fat people, sheds a light on what exactly we aim to protect when demanding legal remedies against "weight discrimination" and makes suggestions what changes could be made both in legislation and in everyday legal practice.

Fat discrimination and law in Fat Studies literature

Scholars and authors in the field of Fat Studies have bemoaned the unsatisfactory legal situation since the very beginning of research into the field. Esther Rothblum, editor of the Fat Studies reader and the Fat Studies journal, pointed out employment discrimination and employment-related victimization as early as 1990 (Rothblum et al., 1990). Ten years later, Sondra Solovay dedicated a whole book (*Tipping the scales of justice: Fighting weight-based discrimination*) on weight discrimination and the legal system in which she also discussed the question of whether fat people should have legal protection and whether the existing protected class of "disability" is suitable for fat people to rely on. She covered a wide range of areas from the question of whether parents are legally responsible when a child becomes fat to medical malpractice, denial of public access, and discriminating public policy. The book is a very enlightening, easy-to-read introduction into the problem(s) fat people face in the US when confronted with the law and public administration. Also, it points out how serious weight discrimination can be and to what extent it destroys life opportunities.

It was Anna Kirkland who first systematically worked through the legal theory of weight discrimination and who devoted an entire book (2008) on *Fat rights: Dilemmas of difference and personhood*. Her approach is to place weight discrimination in the wider context of the civil rights tradition and to discuss "weight" as another candidate for a class protected under antidiscrimination law, highlighting the differences and similarities between "weight" and traditional discrimination classes like gender, race and disability. Kirkland does not stop at this point, however. Her ultimate goal is to shift the focus from the construction of discrimination categories to the underlying presuppositions leading to the recognition that some differences between persons allow for legal protection whereas others do not. These differences, what they mean and how they are constructed – the "logics of personhood" – are the centre of her study. Kirkland's book is a brilliant and enlightening study on a high theoretical level which not only discusses the logics behind discrimination categories in general, but also dismantles arguments often brought forward by those opposing the inclusion of "weight" in antidiscrimination law.

Yofi Tirosh's (2012) article "The right to be fat" goes a step further and argues not only for protection against discrimination but for the right to be fat as a fundamental right, similar to the right to free speech. She argues that in a country in which a great number of highly personal decisions such as marriage, religion, procreation, and education are domains of rights protected by constitutional laws (like most other Fat Studies scholars, she talks about the US here), the (fat) body should be a domain of rights as well: as part of personal liberty, autonomy and dignity. Tirosh will be discussed in more detail towards the end of this chapter.

Charlotte Cooper (1997, 2009, 2016), April Herndon (2002), Hannele Harjunen (2004) and Anna Mollow (2015) have contributed significantly to the debate on whether fatness should be recognized as a disability. Their work, too, will be discussed in the course of this chapter.

Many insights into the legal side of weight discrimination, however, stem from scholars working in what might be termed "Critical Obesity Studies"; that is, they do valuable research into the workings of weight discrimination but are embedded into an "obesity prevention and counteraction" background. That, though, does not keep them from producing highly relevant results for those from a Fat Studies background interested in improving the legal situation of fat people. Many useful (also international) studies have, for example, been conducted by Rebecca Puhl and her research group (Pomeranz & Puhl, 2013; Puhl & Heuer, 2011; Puhl et al., 2015).

Fitting fat people into law's categories

The problem with any legal category, of course, is the fact that life does not come in categories. It is and always has been a challenge to adapt the law to the changing needs of society and, on the other hand, to force real-life situations into the concepts and definitions of law. Where fatness is concerned, one of those challenges is the fact that fat people are a group as diverse as any other group of real-life persons. It is, for example, by no means the case that most lawsuits for weight discrimination worldwide are filed by people whom we, as readers of *The international handbook of Fat Studies*, would call "fat": in fact, those who file complaints based on weight discrimination are often rather thin or at least nowhere near "obesity" in terms of BMI. Mention should be made, for example, of the cases in which flight attendants filed actions against discriminatory BMI regulations,[6] or of the famous case of Abercrombie & Fitch which demanded their salespeople to conform to model measurements instead of just asking for thinness (BBC News, 2013a).

For the legal assessment of an employment discrimination case, for example, it not only makes a significant difference how fat the plaintiff is exactly, but also whether they are completely healthy or have some physical limitations, for instance in terms of mobility. There are fat plaintiffs who function equally well in a particular job as any similarly qualified thin person; likewise, there are plaintiffs who are physically unable or only partly able to exercise the job from which they were dismissed or for which they were not considered. It makes a difference, for example, whether a fat person is "just" considered unattractive by a (potential) employer or whether they actually cannot fulfill the job with all its requirements; in the latter case, again, it is a different situation whether the fat person just needs some adjustments in their work environment to be just as productive as a comparable thin employee (for example, a wider chair, fitting work clothes or an adjustable car seat), or whether it is in fact impossible for the person to do the job as well as a similarly qualified thin person (for example, because they are not mobile enough to effectively rescue passengers in an emergency).

Last but not least fat people differ not only in terms of their weight and their state of health, but in a plethora of other aspects. As a rule, a fat person is not only fat, but entangled in a complex network of characteristics that overlap, reinforce or weaken one another. A fat person, for example, is not only fat, they also have a gender, a race, an age, a sexual orientation, a class, and other physical characteristics beyond their weight. For a comprehensive legal assessment of weight discrimination, it is not enough to just assign a discriminated person to a marginalized group and to ignore all other aspects of their (group) identity. Ultimately, it would take a comprehensive analysis of the power hierarchies within an identity (for more on intersectional identities see Crenshaw, 1989) to do justice to it.

What does "discrimination on the grounds of weight" mean, then?

Similarly, complex and hitherto not yet sufficiently defined is what it actually means to be "discriminated against on the grounds of one's weight"? Even on the purely conceptual level, there are a number of ambiguities since most victims of weight discrimination are by no means discriminated against because of their weight, but because they are fat; the "problem", then, seems to be not so much a certain number on the scale but visible body fat. So, do we conceptualize the discrimination feature correctly when we call it "weight"? The term "size" faces a similar problem, as it signifies not only the width of clothes, but also their length. Even if we use the notoriously controversial "BMI" we are not on the safe side: first, there are the known problems with regard to its significance in terms of body fat percentage; even more serious in this context is that "BMI" invokes a medicalized discourse that in no way adequately embraces what fatness means for an individual in their very own bodily experience. And finally, it is not at all clear who is included in "weight" as a discrimination category: just fat people or also very thin ones or even those usually labelled "normal weight"?

Further lack of conceptual clarity arises when it comes to the theoretical background of weight as a legal category: as it turns out, the underlying legal theory turns out to be radically different whether weight discrimination is construed as discrimination on the grounds of a disability or chronic illness, as indirect discrimination based on age or as sex-plus discrimination, as discrimination based on physical appearance or as a separate discrimination category. Each of these approaches is based on its own theory and its own inherent logic. What is missing for a proper treatment of the category "weight" so far is a convincing theoretical framework which gives meaning to the question of what "weight discrimination" can and should signify in a legal context.

If we aim to effectively protect fat people from discrimination we also need to understand what inherent logic underlies the discrimination category of "weight" (that is, if we decide to use "weight" and not another term like "size" or "fatness") as opposed to other categories of discrimination. The core of weight discrimination seems to be the very fact that "weight" is commonly used as a signifier for supposed negative character traits of a person such as laziness, greed, or impulsivity, and because people assume that it is a "lifestyle choice" whether someone is fat or thin: that weight is subject to the full control of a person, like a haircut or clothing, and thus a mutable characteristic. Fat people, according to this logic, are to blame for their weight, and this "guilt" justifies the negative social consequences often associated with fatness. When compared to, for example, the discrimination category "race", "weight" reveals a reverse discrimination logic: being X race – according to racist logic – makes you prone to having y moral flaw. But having x moral flaw – according to fattist logic – makes you prone to be Y weight (Wang, 2008, p. 1930). More differences appear when "weight" is compared to other discrimination categories.

Questions around the legal dimensions of weight discrimination are thus remarkably complex, and they become even more complex when we take intersectional aspects into account. Simply demanding for "weight" to be added to antidiscrimination law is not enough.

Fatness as a disability?

When filing an action on the grounds of weight discrimination, one popular approach has so far been to subsume high weight under the discrimination class of "disability" – which is protected in most countries in the world (Degener, 2005). Indeed, most successful legal actions on weight discrimination in employment have so far relied on subsuming fatness under "disability", especially since the term has taken on a slightly different slant in international legal debate recently; a slant that turns out to be advantageous for fat people.

In 2008, the Americans with Disabilities Act Amendments Act (ADAAA) became effective in the US, extending the definition of disability significantly in favour of fat people. Its antecedent was the Americans with Disabilities Act (ADA) (1990) which defined disability as "(A) a physical or mental impairment that substantially limits one or more major life activities of such individual; (B) a record of such an impairment; or (C) being regarded as having such an impairment" (42 USC § 12102(2)). ADAAA, now, extends this definition "in favor of broad coverage of individuals under this Act" (Title 42 U.S. Code § 12102, Sec. 4 (A)) on the one hand regarding the listed "major life activities" (they are now detailed by an open list of examples), on the other hand in other relevant aspects. Certainly, "obesity" had the potential to be protected under the ADA before, as in *Equal Employment Opportunity Commission (EEOC) v. Texas Bus Lines*, 1996 where "perceived disability" was invoked (Kirkland, 2003, p. 32). Nevertheless, the regulations in the ADAAA facilitate disability discrimination claims for fat people significantly.

The Equal Employment Opportunity Commission (EEOC), being the antidiscrimination body responsible for labour law issues in the US, in rare cases files complaints itself to protect the rights of individuals and the interests of the public (U.S. Equal Employment Opportunity Commission (n.d.). During the last few years, it has filed several weight-related suits on the basis of ADAAA and advocates a broad interpretation of the notion of "disability" in favour of fat plaintiffs (DelDuca et al., 2016). In their Compliance Guidelines it says that "severe obesity, which has been defined as body weight more than 100% over the norm [...] is clearly an impairment" (Pomeranz & Puhl, 2013, p. 470). This is good news for fat people who fall into this category; however, these guidelines are by no means authoritative for US courts.

In the US, thus, high weight, at least above a certain level, is now sometimes recognized as disability even when the plaintiff has no further "impairment". Only recently, the state of Washington has recognized "obesity" above BMI 40 as an impairment in and of itself (*Taylor v. Burlington Northern Railroad Holdings Inc.*, 2019) because "it is recognized by the medical community as a 'physiological disorder, or condition'" (p. 2 of the ruling). In addition, occasionally there exist local ordinances, such as in New York and New Jersey (DelDuca et al., 2016), in which a high weight at least above BMI 40 explicitly and without further impairments falls under the protected category of "disability".

In Europe, too, the concept of disability seems to be slowly changing towards the inclusion of fat people, at least for BMIs ≥ 40. In the famous case of a Danish childminder, Karsten Kaltoft, who was dismissed because of his weight, the European Court of Justice (ECJ) ruled in 2014 that directive 2000/78/EC of the Council of the European Union be interpreted as meaning that an employee's "obesity" constitute a "disability" within the meaning of the directive if it entails a "long-term physical, mental, intellectual or sensory impairment which in interaction with various barriers may hinder their full and effective participation in society on an equal basis with others" (Fag og Arbejde (FOA), ECJ, 2014, December 18 – C-354/13 FOA). Here, the ECJ cited the UN Convention on the Rights of Persons with Disabilities (UN-CRPD) which, since 2008, understands disability no longer as a purely medical phenomenon but as an interaction between a disabled person and the social environment that holds them back. Not the disabled person is thus impaired, but society disables them.

The social model of disability is not an invention by the UN-CRPD but goes back to the disability rights movement of the 1970s and 80s (Harjunen, 2004, p. 308). In 1976, the Union of the Physically Impaired Against Segregation (UPIAS), a British disability rights organization, redefined "disability" as referring to the disadvantage and restriction of activity that is socially created and imposed on disabled people, as opposed to "impairment" which refers to the physical body and the lack or a defectiveness of a limb, organ or mechanism of the body (Harjunen, 2004, p. 308). It was British sociologist Michael Oliver who used the term "social model of disability" first (Oliver, 1983), opposing it to the "individual model of disability" of which the medical model is a subset.

While the social model of disability focuses on social instead of individual and medical aspects, it still – and Oliver never intended otherwise – requires at least some mild kind of impairment for someone to be labelled "disabled". This aspect is often overlooked in Fat Studies scholarship. Even though it is certainly appropriate to no longer focus on the medical aspects of a disability alone and to take society's part in the making of a disability into account, the medical part of "disability" is still a prerequisite for the debate whether something is a disability in the first place. Even Charlotte Cooper has to admit that when she labels her own fatness an "impairment" although she admits to feeling awkward doing so (Cooper, 1997).

The ECJ, however, in the Kaltoft case did not categorize his fatness as a disability. "Obesity" alone – the ECJ decided – did not qualify as an impairment. Nevertheless, the ECJ's verdict set the tone for a stronger focus on the social model of disability. Also, the ECJ clearly rejected the stigmatizing question of "blame": classification as disabled does not depend on whether a person is to blame of their weight or how high chances are that a person can reduce their weight in the future (von Liebenstein, 2017, p. 10).[7]

The ECJ's "Kaltoft" judgment sparked a world-wide debate about whether "obesity" should be treated as a disability in a legal context. Based on the ruling, occasional national courts in the EU decided in favour of fat plaintiffs, i.a. The Northern Ireland Industrial Tribunal 2016 of a plaintiff who had been bullied on his job because of his weight. The Tribunal ruled that the man with a BMI of 48.5 had been "harassed for a reason which related to his disability, namely his morbid obesity condition" (*Bickerstaff v. Butcher* – NIIT/92/14) and concluded that the plaintiff's "obesity" count as a separate disability independent of the question which other "impairments" the plaintiff "suffered from".

Courts in individual European countries, however, do not normally accept fatness as a disability of its own right so far. A German gardener, for example, who weighed 200 kg and had been terminated because of his weight, sued for damages before the Labor Court Düsseldorf, Germany, and argued that – contrary to his employer's opinion – he suffered from no physical, mental or psychological impairment and was fully able to perform his work (*ArbG Düsseldorf*, 2015, December 15–7 Ca 4616/15). His claim for compensation under the German General Equal Treatment Act (GETA) was dismissed by the court on the grounds that in order to be protected by GETA, he had to qualify as disabled, and that recognition as a disabled person, in turn, require a physical, mental or psychological impairment; however, the plaintiff had just denied having one, and his weight did not qualify as being an impairment in itself.

Without impairment, then, there is no recognition as a disabled person in many European countries and, in fact, many countries in the world (e.g. Hong Kong, Australia i.a.; von Liebenstein, in press).

A particularly strong focus on the "social" aspects of the social model of disability, however, was set by the Supreme Court of Canada when it ruled in the landmark human rights case *Québec v.*

Boisbriand: "Disability is more than a biomedical condition and can exist outside of functional limitations [...] 'Handicap' may be the result of a physical limitation, an ailment, *a social construct*, a perceived limitation, *or* a combination of all these factors. Indeed, it is the combined effect of all these circumstances that determines whether the individual has a 'handicap'" (Ontario Human Rights Commission, n.d.). Furthermore, the court clarified that in assessing whether or not something is a disability, it does not matter whether the disabled person is "to blame" for their disability and how much influence they can exercise over it (Canadian Obesity Network, 2009). This relatively "strong" social model of disability articulated by the Supreme Court of Canada has been followed in many Canadian appellate court and Human Rights Tribunal of Ontario (HRTO) decisions[8] and has paved the way for lawsuits related to weight discrimination as disability discrimination, including, but not limited to, the case law following the "One Person, One Fare" policy introduced in 2009 by the Canada Transportation Agency (CTA) for Canadian airlines.

However, the "strong" social model of disability seems to be much quicker to gain a foothold in those discrimination cases in which marginalized groups other than fat people are involved, probably due to the fact that weight discrimination is still a largely unknown problem to most courts in the world. The German Federal Labour Court, for example, decided in the case of an employee with an asymptomatic HIV infection that he was to be classified as disabled mainly because of the stigma experienced by him (*BAG, 2013*, December 19–6 AZR 190/12; Pärli & Naguib, 2012). Without doubt, fat people also suffer from massive stigmatization. But obviously our stigma does not (yet) seem to weigh heavily enough.

Should we advocate for fatness to be recognized as a disability of its own right, then? Without doubt, there may be practical advantages to it: for an individual plaintiff the path via "disability" may well be a good choice if there is a realistic chance of qualifying as disabled and of thereby obtaining redress for the discrimination suffered. Another advantage of invoking disability discrimination may be that antidiscrimination provisions for disabled people usually demand employers to reduce barriers at the workplace; for fat plaintiffs that may mean an employer has to provide a sufficiently wide office chair or take precautions enabling them to use other working equipment. In some cases, however, the plaintiff is too thin to be considered disabled[9] and would have relatively small chances of qualifying as disabled, even within the widest interpretation of "disability". In cases like this, it might be hopeless to invoke "disability discrimination". Here, another discrimination category would be urgently needed.

Apart from those practical considerations it is a matter of debate whether we should advocate for fatness generally to be recognized as a disability. Charlotte Cooper answers in the affirmative since, she argues, acknowledging fat people as disabled helps them with their identity formation as an oppressed group and their self respect. Additionally, she points to the ableism fat activism has suffered and still suffers from (Cooper, 2016, p. 184 ff.). Fat activists and disabled rights activists have by no means been natural allies in the past (Cooper, 1997) although both fight for similar goals: to not be subjected to a medicalizing and thereby stigmatizing discourse but to be considered a variation in human identity and discrimination as a human rights issue. Both point to the artificiality of the respective categories "disabled" and "fat" and aim to deconstruct them, analyzing society's interest in their existence.

Herndon (2002) argues that fat people are depoliticized when not recognized as disabled: isolated from society and other disabled people as it is, the focus on individual, discrete impairments constitutes an additional hindrance for them to form a political stance as a group. Mollow (2015) agrees when she demands disability rights activists to join forces with fat activists, pointing out the similarities between disabled rights activists' and fat activists' struggles. Harjunen (2004), in turn, argues that the category of "disability" may be a useful tool to force awareness about the stigma and abuse fat people suffer in western societies.

However, none of them acknowledge the fact that even the social model of disability needs an impairment as a prerequisite to be applicable. And it is this prerequisite that many fat activists and Fat Studies scholars, especially those who do not experience their fat bodies as diseased or impaired in any way, feel uncomfortable with.

Marilyn Wann (2013) and the Health at Every Size (HAES) movement have thus always taken the stance against fatness to be labelled a medical deviation, be it an impairment or a disease. They reject mainstream medicalized discourses around fat bodies and contest society's attribution they belong to a "problem" group in need of therapy. The social construction of "disease" has traditionally always recurred to a dynamic of inclusion and exclusion and valuation/devaluation: the "self" being good and healthy, the "other" sick and evil, a ready foil in front of which the self establishes its identity (Foucault, 2006). Probably most fat activists agree with this intuition to draw back from a medicalized discourse forcedly imposed on their bodily existence. Thus, despite the valid debates around ableism and healthism, there are very good reasons to defy medicalization.

Last but not least, a subsumption of fatness under the category of "disability" would mean that a whole range of discriminations would not be covered by anti-discrimination law, namely those experienced by people with a BMI < 40. Weight discrimination experienced by those relatively thin fat people needs to be covered by anti-discrimination law as well as that experienced by fatter people.

At the moment, international support in the general public for fatness to be considered a disability seems to be relatively sparse anyway. In a large international survey from 2015, the overwhelming majority of the Australian, Canadian, US, and Icelandic populations voted against it (Puhl et al., 2015, p. 706).

Fatness as "physical appearance"?

At first glance, it seems more promising to protect the whole spectrum of fat people by subsuming weight under "physical appearance" or a similar category. "Physical appearance" is a protected category e.g. in France (Code Pénal, Art. 225–1), Belgium (Loi tendant à lutter contre certaines formes de discrimination, Art. 3), Bolivia (Ley 045 Contra el Racismo, chpt. V, title VIII, art. 22), the Australian state of Victoria, and some US cities.

The Australian state of Victoria with its Equal Opportunity Act in the version of 1995 was one of the first places worldwide to include "physical features" in its antidiscrimination legislation. "Physical features", in turn, is officially defined as a "person's height, weight, size or other bodily characteristics" (Victorian Equal Opportunity & Human Rights Commission, n.d.). Although few weight-related lawsuits have been brought to court (most of them were ended by settlement before), there are indeed a few cases in which a fat plaintiff received damages invoking discrimination on the grounds of "physical features", for example *Hill v. Canterbury Road Lodge Pty* in 2004. The 120 kg plaintiff had been bullied at work because of her weight. She won the lawsuit and received $ 2,500 in damages. Although the number of weight-related discrimination complaints is constantly rising in Victoria (McArthur, 2016), only very few succeed in invoking "physical features" as there is an ongoing debate as to whether the protected physical characteristics must necessarily be immutable or whether protection is also granted to characteristics which are subject to individual influence or control.[10]

France and Belgium, having a strong human rights tradition, surpassed the requirements of the relevant European antidiscrimination directive as early as 2001 and adopted a number of additional categories of discrimination, including physical appearance (Fornari, 2015). However, this category has so far mostly been applied to relatively thin people. Fat people have failed with their complaints so far because a high weight allegedly is not an "immutable property" (Fornari, 2015), but subject to the "individual will of a person".

"Physical appearance" in the wording of antidiscrimination law does thus not necessarily ensure protection against discrimination for fat people. More often than not, fat people are denied protection with the argument that "physical appearance" only comprises congenital characteristics or ones that are withdrawn from individual control; at least this is what happens in France and Belgium (Fornari, 2015).

In any case, it is debatable whether it makes sense to conceive weight discrimination as a subset of discrimination on the basis of physical appearance. "Yes", Rhode (2010) argues in *The beauty bias*: "Overweight individuals are the most common targets of appearance discrimination and [...] they are overrepresented among low-income and minority groups" (p. 102). Sablonsky (2006) and Baron (2005), too, construe weight discrimination as a form of appearance discrimination when assuming that fat women face employment discrimination because thinness is a standard of beauty.

Wang (2008, p. 1933) takes an opposing stance: weight discrimination is not a subset of "lookism", she argues, since fat people get blamed because they are deemed lazy and incompetent, not simply because they are considered ugly. When discussing fat as a discrimination factor, we should by no means negate the underlying moral dimension of the debate:

> Weight discrimination requires both: (1) that being fat is considered a negative life outcome, and (2) that fat people are considered responsible for their weight. Appearance discrimination contributes to fatness being a negative life outcome. That alone, however, is not enough for weight discrimination; the victim must also be held personally responsible for her negative life outcome. To put it another way, you could eliminate weight discrimination – by eliminating the element of personal responsibility – without eliminating weight-based appearance discrimination.
>
> *(Wang, 2008, p. 1933)*

Solovay (2000) agrees with this argument when she writes: "Unlike biases against thin people perceived as unattractive, stereotypes of fat people tend to include character shortcomings [...] meaning [that] fat people tend to be viewed not as only 'lacking' but also as 'responsible' for the prejudices held against them" (p. 1459). It is at least debatable, then, whether a protected class labelled "physical characteristics" alone would offer sufficient protection against weight-based discrimination.

Alternative strategies of framing weight discrimination

How else might a suitable category be conceptualized, then? That there *is* in fact a need for legal protection against weight-based discrimination is a notion evoking a lot of international support: in a recent study, 65 percent of US-American men and 81 percent of women voted for anti-discrimination legislation for fat people (Puhl & Heuer, 2011); moreover, consent rates are increasing from year to year (Suh et al., 2014). International approval rates for the protection of "weight" as a discrimination category are similarly high, especially when it comes to employment discrimination. In a recent study on the rate of approval in four countries (USA, Canada, Iceland and Australia), 71–95 percent of the more than 3,000 respondents voted for legal protection against weight discrimination in the work environment (Puhl et al., 2015). This positive international atmosphere for the antidiscrimination of fat people should be put to good use.

It seems indispensable to place the category "weight" or "size", or however we decide to phrase it, directly into the text of the law, since so far neither subsumption under "disability" nor under "physical appearance" has produced satisfactory results. Even less successful has been the strategy of using open lists that use phrases such as "and others" or "characteristics such as": so far there are no known weight-related cases worldwide where the reference to such an open formulation has been successful in court.

Open lists have the additional disadvantage that they leave open to interpretation which group is eligible to protection. Some of the standard arguments against the inclusion of fat people in any kind of anti-discrimination policy are the supposed mutability of weight or the claim that fat people are not a "group". It is therefore urgently necessary to develop binding criteria for what constitutes a legitimate ground of discrimination protection and what does not.

One of the strategies to defend against the "immutability" argument has been to demonstrate over and over again that weight is by no means as mutable as is widely believed or, to use Elizabeth Kristen's (2002) words, to "assume that [...] weight is either immutable or so difficult or dangerous to permanently change as to be practically immutable" (p. 71). This argument has convincingly and repeatedly been brought forward by fat rights activists all over the world for more than three decades, but has so far not yet found its way into mainstream society and everyday legal discourse.

Another strategy would be to put forward that the demand for immutability is unreasonable, produces false results, and is not consistently applied to existing protected classes (for more arguments see Clarke, 2015). For example, it can be argued that religion is a self-chosen assignment; at least, however, so is "marital status" which is protected in many countries and, in times of relatively reliable contraception, to a certain degree also "pregnancy". "Disability", too, is, to some extent, a mutable status, depending on the possibilities of rehabilitation and recovery that exist, or might exist in the future. One of the problems with the concept of immutability is that it has been repeatedly invoked in the past to deny protection to discriminated groups, such as LGBTQs, who for a long time had to face the prejudice that their sexual orientations and identities were a matter of choice (for more details and references Solanke, 2017, p. 54 ff., esp. p. 59 n116).

In the recent past, it was i.a. Iyiola Solanke (2017) and, in part, Yofi Tirosh (2012) who attempted to develop a catalog of criteria for the inclusion of new discrimination categories that could be utilized by fat people. Solanke starts off from a concept of "stigma" and frames discrimination as a public health issue. Among other things, her "anti-stigma principle" determines a characteristic's worthiness of protection based on the following questions: "Is the "mark" arbitrary or does it have some meaning in and of itself?" – "Is the mark used as a social label?" – "Does this label have a long history? How embedded is it in society?" – "Is the label used to stereotype those possessing it?" – "Does the stereotype reduce the humanity of those who are its targets? Does it evoke a punitive response?" – "Do these targets have low social power and low interpersonal status?" etc. Tirosh (2012), in turn, points to the question whether the disputed characteristic is "close to the core of the person" (p. 333) and to what extent it defines the sense of who someone is as a person, both from the "inside out" (for oneself) and from the "outside in" (by society's gaze) (Tirosh, 2012, p. 333). To ask questions like that ensures, according to Tirosh, that "there should not be an automatic leap from the right to be fat to smoke or to skydive" (p. 334).

Another issue often raised in the context of discrimination categories and their legitimacy is the question of fatness as a health risk. The reasoning usually is: "We cannot protect a status that constitutes a health risk not only to individual citizens, but to public health as a whole. On the contrary, it is our duty to protect the population against it." The "right to health" – as laid down in a conglomerate of international treaties from 1948 to 2008 and summarized in a fact sheet by the United Nations Commissioner of Human Rights and the World Health Organization in 2008 (World Health Organization, 2008) – thus seems to clash with the right to be fat.

That the health risks of being fat are exaggerated for economic, political and social interests to the detriment of fat people, however, has been common knowledge for fat activists internationally for as long as fat activism exists. Still, so far it has only very rarely been used for a legal critique of international public health efforts. Tirosh (2012) thus rightly warns that efforts to protect the rights of fat people should not only be based on anti-discrimination legislation, but also on the right to be spared government measures aimed at slimming down the population, such as compulsory weighing of schoolchildren, withdrawal of custody of fat children, and the various government campaigns in the "war against obesity": for example, British prohibitions to sell junk food near school buildings or the initiative of New York's former mayor Michael Bloomberg who promoted a ban on using food stamps to buy sugared soft drinks (Tirosh, 2012, pp. 273–274).

Tirosh thus argues convincingly for a "right to be of any body size as part of the general principle of liberty (and, more specifically, as part of autonomy and dignity)" (p. 267). In particular, she criticizes that in a legal context the body is viewed through a purely mechanistic lens, "as if asking legal subjects to lose weight is no more cumbersome than requiring them to get their car fixed by a mechanic" (p. 296). In contrast to the Cartesian dualism of body and soul, the body should be regarded as a "lived body" (Leder, 1992, p. 25) and a domain of rights (Tirosh, 2012, p. 268). Especially in legal theory, Tirosh thinks, the fat body needs to be understood "through social practices associated with it, and through the individual's personal experience of his or her body" (p. 306).

The way fat people are being treated in court is, according to Tirosh, damaging their self-trust in their body and their sense of self-efficacy as an agent, and impedes their full and equal participation in society (p. 283). Especially in the area of legislation and jurisdiction, a non-medical approach to fatness is imperative so fat people are no longer treated as second-class citizens or as inferior. To "limit the extent of the body", she argues, invoking the right to be fat as a fundamental right, is ultimately "as severe as limiting the scope of speech" (p. 314).

Is law a suitable tool against weight discrimination?

In this context the question often arises whether the law is actually a suitable tool to end weight discrimination. Social prejudice against fat people, some say, will not decrease just because there is a law banning weight discrimination, especially since many antidiscrimination provisions that include fat people remain largely unlitigated or produce mixed results. Since the day of its enactment in 1976, for example, only eight to ten cases of weight-related discrimination referred to Michigan's Elliot-Larson Civil Rights Act (Kristen, 2002).[11] France, too, has seen only very few complaints filed so far on the basis of Art. 225–1 of the French Code Pénal and almost none based on "physical appearance" (Fornari, 2015). Similarly unsuccessful with respect to weight discrimination have been the few laws in other countries: the litigation torrent and business backlash so anxiously anticipated by many critics of antidiscrimination legislation have so far failed to materialize (Rhode, 2010, p. 126; Shinall, 2012, pp. 20–30).

On the one hand, this is due to problems of law enforcement, especially where employment discrimination is concerned: in the US Federal court, for example, employment discrimination plaintiffs fare worse at every step of the adjudication process than all other litigants (Clermont & Schwab, 2004, pp. 429–458). They are more likely to lose pretrial, are less likely to settle their claims, and thus, are more likely to go to trial. At trial, employment discrimination plaintiffs lose disproportionately often, and when appealing an adverse trial outcome, they do far worse than the respective defendants.

On the other hand, experience of advocacy groups shows that plaintiffs do not file claims about their weight-based discrimination (the discrimination files of the German Gesellschaft gegen Gewichtsdiskriminierung e.V.; similarly Tirosh, 2012, p. 332). The main reason for this may be the stigma attached to being fat. Anyone who is prepared to publicly stand up for their fatness and, as is common practice in many countries, to connect their name with a weight discrimination case, has usually already come out as fat (on the "fat closet", Sedgwick, 1990). Unfortunately, these are only a few at the moment. Standing up for one's rights as a fat person in the current hostile social climate, and to publicly appear in court, requires a maximum of emotional effort and self-confidence.

However, it is exactly this hostile and stigmatizing social environment that antidiscrimination legislation can help change. It is precisely in those moments when social and moral norms are counterproductive that legal intervention is particularly conducive to regulating behaviour and shaping future norms. In Germany, for example, the public debate during the legislative procedure of the General Equal Treatment Act (GETA) adopted in 2006 has led to a considerable change of values not only in Germany but throughout Europe (Antidiskriminierungsstelle des Bundes, 2016, p. 16 n17). At present, we can witness a similar effect in the discussion about the introduction of a "third sex" called for by the German Federal Constitutional Court in 2017 for all official procedures; legislature is bound to pass the law until the end of 2018 (*BVerfG*, 2017, October 10–1 BvR 2019/16). The decision has greatly spurred public debate about sex, gender, and trans persons; a debate that was previously marginalized is now being conducted in the midst of society.

The mere inclusion of a protective category in anti-discrimination legislation is, of course, by no means enough in the long run. Nevertheless, it could be a first step, especially with a view to stimulating the invaluable social discourse around the issue of weight discrimination. After all, this discourse is absolutely essential if we aim to protect fat people against discrimination not only on a purely legal level, but also in everyday life. Which, in turn, is prerequisite for them to feel strong enough to assert their claims before court.

Into the future

In sum, there remains a lot to be done not only in daily legal practice and legislation but in research about fatness and law as well. Unfortunately, so far there exists only very limited research about fatness and law in countries in which English is not an official language. To quote Charlotte Cooper, Fat Studies has so far largely been "fat American studies" (Cooper, 2009). Fat phobia and weight discrimination, though, are proliferating in most western countries and, in fact, in quite a number of countries in the global south (Contrera, 2018), so research into legal aspects of fatness in these countries is imperative as well. Also, the main focus of legal research into fatness and discrimination has so far been on antidiscrimination provisions and employment law and not so much on other aspects of fatness and law, e.g. public law, especially fundamental rights, youth welfare law, public health law, social law, education policy and law, just to name a few; also, criminal law has so far only sporadically been touched on by Fat Studies scholars. As a basis for activists challenging state campaigns in the "war against obesity", more research into the structure and workings of government "anti-obesity" measures would be desirable.

Furthermore, there is still a great need for debate regarding the question of how intersectionality can be reflected in and mapped onto law. In a world in which people usually do not belong to only one category of discrimination but often even several at a time, how can this fact be represented in legal code and how can we deal with it in legal practice?

Last but not least we need to bring the protagonists of legal fat activism into the spotlight. Which strategies have they employed to change a detrimental legal situation? Which of those strategies have been successful, which have not and why? What can we learn from other oppressed groups and their struggles for legal protection and representation?

Finally, in all our scholarly endeavors we may not forget that those affected by weight discrimination – those who are not hired because of weight discrimination, those whose child has been taken away by youth welfare organizations because of fat phobia, those who have been unfairly treated in court because of weight bias – cannot wait. Their lives continue to be affected by the biases of legal systems every single day. And it is today that we need to make every possible effort to encourage the governments and jurisdiction of all our various countries to take weight discrimination seriously and act.

Notes

1 Even if in many African countries the fat ideal of beauty still prevails and a thin body is still associated with an HIV infection (Matoti-Mvalo, & Puoane, 2011), this ideal is changing towards the Western ideal of thinness not only in many African countries, but also i.a. on the Fiji Islands (eating disorder expert Silvia Uhle in Wüstenhagen, 2007).

2 Researched at juris, the largest German legal information portal, https://www.juris.de/jportal/index. jsp.

3 As has happened in the US (cp. *Overweight Advocates*, 2013).

4 This was a serious problem in Germany until 2013 when the Supreme Administrative Court (BVerwG) decided to drop the hurdles for civil service candidates (cp. BVerwG, 2013, October 30–2 C 16.12, and BVerwG, 2013, December 13–2 B 37.13).

5 e.g. US states Georgia, Indiana, Maryland, and Virginia (Morbid Obesity Anti-Discrimination Act, Ga. Code Ann. § 33.24.59.7 (2005); Ind. Code § 27–8-14.1–4 (2008); Md. Code Ann., Ins. § 15–839; Va. Code Ann. § 38.2–3418.13 (2007)).

6 The Aeroflot case (Russia's Aeroflot Airline, 2017), and Air India (Strochlic, 2015).

7 The Employment Appeal Tribunal, London, argued similarly in Walker v. Sita Information Networking Computing Ltd UKEAT/0097/12: "The question is whether the individual has the impairment, and whether the impairment may properly be described as physical or mental. The Act does not require a focus upon the cause of that impairment."

8 For references and details see Ontario Human Rights Commission, n.d.

9 For example, the applicant for a position as Managing Director of a Lyme disease Association in Darmstadt, Germany, who had not been hired because of her BMI of 28.7 on the grounds that she was not a suitable role model for members of the association because she was "overweight" (*ArbG Darmstadt, 2014, June 12*–6 CA 22/13).

10 There is an ongoing debate, for example, whether tattoos qualify as "physical features".

11 Wang (2008, p. 1928) states that "most cases brought under the weight clause are dismissed for lack of evidence".

References

Literature

Andreyeva, T., Puhl, R. M., & Brownell, K. D. (2008). Changes in perceived weight discrimination among Americans: 1995–1996 through 2004–2006. *Obesity, 16*(5), 1129–1134.

Antidiskriminierungsstelle des Bundes (2016). *Evaluation des Allgemeinen Gleichbehandlungsgesetzes*. Berlin: Antidiskriminierungsstelle des Bundes.

Baron, S. (2005). (Un)lawfully beautiful: The legal (de)construction of female beauty. *Boston College Law Review, 46*(2.2), 359–389.

BBC News (2013a, Jul 25). Abercrombie & Fitch faces French inquiry over "models". *BBC News*. http://www.bbc.com/news/world-europe-23450486

BBC News (2013b, Jul 27). South African chef "too fat" to live in New Zealand. *BBC News*. http://www.bbc.com/news/world-asia-23475583

BBC News (2017, Apr 20). Russia's Aeroflot airline accused of "sex discrimination". *BBC News*. http://www.bbc.com/news/world-europe-39653381

Canadian Obesity Network (2009). *Obesity as a disability.* http://www.obesitynetwork.ca/Obesity-as-a-Disability-156

City and County of San Francisco Human Rights Commission (2001). *Compliance guidelines to prohibit weight and height discrimination.* https://www.shrm.org/ResourcesAndTools/tools-and-samples/hr-qa/Documents/Height_and_Weight.pdf

Clarke, J. E. (2015). Against immutability. *The Yale Law Journal, 125*(2), 2–102.

Clermont, K. M., & Schwab, S. J. (2004). How employment discrimination plaintiffs fare in federal court. *Journal of Empirical Legal Studies, 1*(2), 429–458.

Contrera, L. (2018). *Fat & the Global South.* Fat Studies MOOO, hosted by C. Pausé. https://friendofmarilyn.com/fat-studies-mooo/.

Cooper, C. (1997). Can a fat woman call herself disabled? *Disability and Society, 12*(1), 31–42.

Cooper, C. (2009). Maybe it should be called Fat American Studies? In E. Rothblum, & S. Solovay (Eds.), *The Fat Studies Reader* (pp. 327–333). New York: New York University Press.

Cooper, C. (2016). *Fat activism. A radical social movement.* Bristol: HammerOn Press.

Crenshaw, K. W. (1989). Demarginalizing the intersection of race and sex: A Black feminist critique of antidiscrimination doctrine, feminist theory and antiracist politics. *University of Chicago Legal Forum, 8*(1), 139–168.

Degener, T. (2005). Antidiskriminierungsrechte für Behinderte: Ein globaler Überblick. *Zeitschrift für ausländisches öffentliches Recht und Völkerrecht, 65*, 887–935.

DelDuca, M. V., Diamond, T. E., & Gobalasingham, K. (2016, Aug 11). Is obesity an ADA disability? *Lexology.* https://www.lexology.com/library/detail.aspx?g=71b72322-cfef-4e4e-91b0-3743e613e7a2

Discrimination (n.d.). Belgium.de, Informations et services officiels, https://www.belgium.be/fr/justice/victime/plaintes_et_declarations/discrimination

Engel, J. (2010, May 26). Rare Michigan law may help waitress win weight discrimination lawsuit against Hooters. *MLive Michigan.* http://www.mlive.com/news/index.ssf/2010/05/rare_michigan_law_may_help_wai.html

Équipe de surveillance et d'épidémiologie nutritionnelle (Esen) (2017). *Étude de santé sur l'environnement, la biosurveillance, l'activité physique et la nutrition (Esteban), 2014–2016.* Saint-Maurice: Santé publique France.

Foucault, M. (2006). *History of madness.* New York: Routledge.

Fornari, C. (2015, June 30). L'apparence physique mise à nu: histoire et actualités d'une discrimination. *Respect Mag.* http://respectmag.com/dossiers/discrimination-physique/2015/06/30/faut-il-legiferer-574/

Giel, K. E., Zipfel, S., Alizadeh, M., Schäffeler, N., Zahn, C., Wessel, D., Hesse, F. W., Thiel, S., & Thiel, A. (2012). Stigmatization of obese individuals by human resource professionals: An experimental study. BMC Public Health, 12, 525.

Harjunen, H. (2004). Exploring obesity through the social model of disability. In T. Rannveig, & K. Kristiansen (Eds.), *Gender and disability research in the Nordic countries* (pp. 305–324). Lund: Studentlitteratur.

Harter, P. (2004, Jan 26). Mauritania's "wife-fattening" farm. *BBC News.* http://news.bbc.co.uk/2/hi/3429903.stm

Herndon, A. (2002). Disparate but disabled fat embodiment and disability studies. *Feminist Formations, 14*(3), 120–137.

Huggins, M. L. (2015). Not "fit" for hire: The United States and France on weight discrimination in employment. *Fordham International Law Journal, 38*(3), 889–951.

Kirkland, A. (2003). Representations of fatness and personhood: Pro-fat advocacy and the limits and uses of law. *Representations, 82*(1), 24–51.

Kirkland, A. (2008). *Fat rights: Dilemmas of difference and personhood.* New York, London: New York University Press.

Kristen, E. (2002). Comment, addressing the problem of weight discrimination in employment. *California Law Review, 90*(1), 57–110.

Leder, D. (1992). A tale of two bodies: The Cartesian corpse and the lived body. In D. Leder (Ed.), *The body in medical thought and practice. Philosophy and medicine* (Vol. 43, pp. 17–35). Dordrecht: Springer.

Lynch, A. (1996). Is obesity a disability – actual or perceived – under the Disability Discrimination Act 1992? *Deakin Law Review, 12*, 161–182.

Matoti-Mvalo, T., & Puoane, T. (2011). Perceptions of body size and its association with HIV/AIDS. *South African Journal of Clinical Nutrition, 24*(1), 40–45.

Matsnev, O. (2017, Sept 6). Aeroflot flight attendants win challenge over clothing sizes. *New York Times.* https://www.nytimes.com/2017/09/06/world/europe/aeroflot-flight-attendants-weight-rule.html

McArthur, G. (2016, Dec 18). Victorians sacked or told to lose weight by employers concerned their size makes them too dangerous to work. *Herald Sun.* www.heraldsun.com.au

Mollow, A. (2015). Disability Studies gets fat. *Hypatia: A Feminist Journal of Philosophy, 30*(1), 199–216.

Ontario Human Rights Commission (n.d.). *What is a Disability?* http://www.ohrc.on.ca/en/policy-ableism-and-discrimination-based-disability/2-what-disability#_edn27

Oliver, M. (1983). *Social work with disabled people.* London: Macmillan.

Pärli, K., & Naguib, T. (2012). *Schutz vor Benachteiligung aufgrund chronischer Krankheit. Die Expertise im Überblick.* Berlin: Antidiskriminierungsstelle des Bundes.

Peretti-Watel, P., & Moatti, J. P. (2009). *Le principe de prévention. Le culte de la santé et ses dérives.* Paris: Éditions du Seuil.

Pomeranz, J., & Puhl, R. M. (2013). New developments in the law for obesity discrimination protection. *Obesity, 21*(3), 469–471.

Puhl, R. M., & Heuer, C. (2011). Public opinion about laws to prohibit weight discrimination in the United States. *Obesity, 19*(1), 74–82.

Puhl, R. M., Latner, J. D., O'Brien, K. S., Luedicke, J., Danielsdorrit, S., & Ramos Salas, X. (2015). Potential policies and laws to prohibit weight discrimination: Public views from 4 countries. *The Milbank Quarterly, 93*(4), 691–731.

Rhode, D. L. (2010). *The beauty bias: The injustice of appearance in life and law.* Oxford: Oxford University Press.

Robertson, J. (2013, Dec 24). The perils of being fat, female and French. *BBC News.* http://www.bbc.com/news/magazine-25215641

Rothblum, E. D., Brand, P. A., Miller, C. T., & Oetjen, H. A. (1990). The relationship between obesity, employment discrimination, and employment-related victimization. *Journal of Vocational Behavior, 37*(3), 251–266.

Sablonsky, K. (2006). Probative "weight": Rethinking evidentiary standards in Title VII sex discrimination cases. *N.Y.U. Review of Law and Social Change, 30*(2), 325–328.

Sedgwick, E. K. (1990). *Epistemology of the closet.* Berkeley, CA: University of California Press.

Shinall, J. H. B. (2012). *Obesity in the labor market: Implications for the legal system* [Doctoral dissertation]. ProQuest Dissertations & Theses Database. Order No. 3538186.

Solanke, I. (2017). *Discrimination as stigma: A theory of anti-discrimination law.* Oxford, Portland, OR: Bloomsbury.

Solovay, S. (2000). *Tipping the scales of justice: Fighting weight-based discrimination* [E-Book]. Amherst, NY: Prometheus Books.

Strochlic, N. (2015, Sept 15). Airline grounds 125 Flight attendants for being "fat". *The Daily Beast.* https://www.thedailybeast.com/airline-grounds-125-flight-attendants-for-being-fat

Suh, Y., Puhl, R., Liu, S., & Felming, M. F. (2014). Support for laws to prohibit weight discrimination in the United States: Public Attitudes from 2011 to 2013. *Obesity, 22*(8), 1872–1879.

Thomas, D. (2005, Oct 25). Obesity research: Fattism is the last bastion of employee discrimination. *Occupational Health & Wellbeing (Personnel Today).* https://www.personneltoday.com/hr/obesity-research-fattism-is-the-last-bastion-of-employee-discrimination/

Tirosh, Y. (2012). The right to be fat. *Yale Journal of Health Policy, Law, and Ethics, 12*(2), 264–335.

United Press International (2013, Jul 19). Overweight advocates decry Boy Scout Jamboree policy. *United Press International.* https://www.upi.com/Odd_News/2013/07/19/Overweight-advocates-decry-Boy-Scout-Jamboree-policy/UPI-88661374259634/?spt=hs&or=on

U.S. Equal Employment Opportunity Commission (n.d.). *About EEOC.* https://www.eeoc.gov/overview

U.S. Equal Employment Opportunity Commission (2020). *What You Should Know: The EEOC and Protections for LGBT Workers.* https://www.eeoc.gov/eeoc/newsroom/wysk/enforcement_protections_lgbt_workers.cfm

Victorian Equal Opportunity & Human Rights Commission (n.d.). *Physical features discrimination.* https://www.humanrightscommission.vic.gov.au/discrimination/discrimination/types-of-discrimination/physical-features von Liebenstein, S. (2017). Gewichtsdiskriminierung. In S. Berghahn, & U. Schultz (Eds.), *Rechtshandbuch für Frauen- und Gleichstellungsbeauftragte* (sec. 2/3.1, pp. 1–22). Hamburg: DasHöfer.

von Liebenstein, S. (in press). Discrimination categories and their potential to cover fatness. An international approach [working title]. *Fat Studies, An Interdisciplinary Journal of Body Weight and Society*.

Wang, L. (2008). Weight discrimination: One size fits all remedy? *The Yale Law Journal, 117*(8), 1900–1945.

Wann, M. (2013). Fat people: #IAmNotADisease. *CNN*. https://edition.cnn.com/2013/06/25/opinion/wann-obesity-disease.

World Health Organization (2008). *The right to health*. Fact Sheet No. 31. Geneva: World Health Organization. https://www.ohchr.org/Documents/Publications/Factsheet31.pdf

Wüstenhagen, C. (2007, Oct 20). Globales Fasten. *ZEIT online*. http://www.zeit.de/2007/43/Fis-Bulimie

Legislation

Allgemeines Gleichbehandlungsgesetz (AGG) (General Equal Treatment Act (GETA)) (2006). http://www.antidiskriminierungsstelle.de/SharedDocs/Downloads/EN/publikationen/agg_in_englischer_Sprache.pdf?__blob=publicationFile

Americans with Disabilities Act (ADA) (1990). https://www.gpo.gov/fdsys/pkg/USCODE-2015-title42/pdf/USCODE-2015-title42-chap126.pdf

Americans with Disabilities Amendments Act (ADAAA) https://www.eeoc.gov/laws/statutes/adaaa.cfm

Binghampton Human Rights Law (2008). http://www.binghamton-ny.gov/ordinance/binghamton-human-rights-law

Canadian Constitution Act (1982). http://laws-lois.justice.gc.ca/eng/const/page-15.html#h-39.

Charter of Fundamental Rights of the European Union (CFR). http://www.europarl.europa.eu/charter/pdf/text_en.pdf

Code Pénal, Art. 225–1 (2001, revised 2016). https://www.legifrance.gouv.fr/affichCodeArticle.do?cidTexte=LEGITEXT000006070719&idArticle=LEGIARTI000006417828

Elliott-Larsen Civil Rights Act (1976). https://www.michigan.gov/documents/act_453_elliott_larsen_8772_7.pdf

Employment Equity Act (1988). http://www.labour.gov.za/DOL/downloads/legislation/acts/employment-equity/eegazette2015.pdf

European Convention on Human Rights (ECHR). http://www.echr.coe.int/Documents/Convention_ENG.pdf

Ley 045 Contra el Racismo y Toda Forma de Discriminación (Law 045 Against Racism and All Forms of Discrimination) (2010). http://www.comunicacion.gob.bo/sites/default/files/dale_vida_a_tus_derechos/archivos/Ley%20045%20Contra%20el%20Racismo%20y%20Toda%20Forma%20de%20Discriminaci%C3%B3n.pdf

Morbid Obesity Anti-Discrimination Act, Georgia Code Ann., § 33.24.59.7 (2005). https://law.justia.com/codes/georgia/2010/title-33/chapter-24/article-1/33-24-59-7/

Indiana Code, § 27–8-14.1–4 (2008). Retrieved via LexisNexis

Maryland Code Ann., § 15–839 (2006). Retrieved via LexisNexis

Virginia Code Ann., § 38.2–3418.13 (2007). https://law.lis.virginia.gov/vacode

Madison City Code (n.d.). https://library.municode.com/wi/madison/codes/code_of_ordinances?nodeId=COORMAWIVOII_CH39DECIRI_39.03EQOPOR

Santa Cruz, CA, Municipal Code (1995). http://www.codepublishing.com/CA/SantaCruz/

The City of Reyjavik's Human Rights Policy (2006, revised i.a. 2016). http://reykjavik.is/en/city-of-reykjaviks-human-rights-policy#6.%20Body%20build%20and%20type

UN Convention on the Rights of People with Disabilities (CRPD) (2008). https://www.un.org/development/desa/disabilities/convention-on-the-rights-of-persons-with-disabilities.html

Urbana Human Rights Ordinance (n.d.). http://www.urbanaillinois.us/sites/default/files/attachments/03-urbana-human-rights-ordinance-urbana-municipal-code-sec-12-1.pdf

Case Law

ArbG Düsseldorf (Labour Court Düsseldorf, Germany), 2015, December 15–7 Ca 4616/15

ArbG Darmstadt (Labour Court Darmstadt, Germany), 2014, June 14–6 CA 22/13

BAG (Federal Labour Court, Germany), 2013, December 19–6 AZR 190/12

Bickerstaff v. Butcher – NIIT/92/14

BVerfG (Federal Constitutional Court, Germany), 2017, October 10–1 BvR 2019/6

BVerwG (Federal Administrative Court, Germany), 2013, October 30–2 C 16.12

BVerwG (Federal Administrative Court, Germany), 2013, December 13–2 B 37.13

Dewberry v. George – 62 P.3d 525, 526 (Wash. 2003)

EEOC v. Texas Bus Lines – 923 F. Supp. 965 (S.D. Tex. 1996)

Fag og Arbejde (FOA), ECJ (European Court of Justice) 2014, December 18 – C-354/13 FOA

Hill v. Canterbury Road Lodge Pty Ltd – [2004] VCAT 1365

People v. Wynn – 2004 WL 417221 (Cal. Ct. App. 2004)

Taylor v. Burlington Northern Railroad Holdings Inc. – 2019 No. 96335–5

Walker v. Sita Information Networking Computing Ltd – UKEAT/0097/12

16

PREGNANCY, PARENTING AND THE CHALLENGE OF FATNESS

May Friedman

Introduction

As this book amply displays, it's hard to be fat. Living in a larger body is hard on one's heart, though not in the ways we are often told. Rather than suggesting that our cardiovascular health is irreparably compromised, I would argue instead that being fat often hurts our feelings, exposes our vulnerabilities, leaves us reeling from insults to our souls. While many of us have fought back toward fat acceptance (and even fat delight!), the penalties of living in a reviled body are steep, and the daily impact of revolutionary living can feel very daunting. The challenges of fat life are exacerbated in their overlaps and their intersections with other areas of tension and oppression. Just a few of these include racism, homophobia, sexism, ableism, sanism and other sites of persecution and grief.

This chapter aims to look at a specific site of vulnerability in exploring the tensions of fat and parenthood, in both biological and sociological contexts. As many Fat Studies scholars have exposed, situating fat within this context is crucial, as parenthood is its own site of surveillance, judgment and impossible expectations (Herndon, 2010; Boero, 2009; McNaughton, 2011; Parker, 2014, among others). Transitions to motherhood, specifically, come with gendered beliefs about women's inherent nurturing potential. Reproductive bodies may be found lacking in both physiological and social respects. This gendered and judgmental context is exacerbated around parenting by fat people, which is viewed with particular suspicion and surveillance, and scorn. The lens is subtly shifted in the context of parents raising fat children. The extent to which children are viewed as linear and uncomplicated products of parental labour is laid bare when fat children are the subject of discussion. The use of Fat Studies scholarship to examine fat parents and fat children thus peels back the deep cultural expectations of both fat people and parents by exploring the overlap between these institutionalized and discursive identities and experiences.

Exploring fat in relation to reproduction exposes key questions that are central to Fat Studies: around fat and health, around autonomy and responsibility, and around both the physical and social aspects of reproduction and reproductive labour. Furthermore, a consideration of fatness and reproduction sits at the core of many intersections around race, poverty, ability, sexuality, madness and beyond. This chapter seeks to examine existing literature from Fat Studies as a field, as well as from adjacent disciplines, around fat and parenthood/motherhood to expose the tensions and opportunities afforded by considering fatness in relation. Beginning with the literal sharing of flesh in the context of fat pregnancy, this chapter will consider the role of epigenetics as well as the increasing surveillance and regulation of pregnant people, suggesting that "fat pregnant bodies are constructed as bio-cultural anxieties, distilling biological and social causes into the one embodied location" (Warin et al., 2012, p. 361). Moving away from physical conjoinment, the chapter will then explore the implications of parenthood for both fat kids and fat parents and the ways that parental responsibility is exposed, surveilled and confronted when larger bodies are at play, especially those which sit at the intersection of multiple oppressions. Finally, this chapter will consider the role of Fat Studies as a discipline and a practice, exploring what a fat positive approach to parenthood might look like, and considering the possibilities for shifting discourses around size oppression through parental labour, societal change and responses from the discipline as a whole.

But first: thinking about words

Any analysis of fat and its overlaps may be immediately derailed by terminological quandaries. In the attempt to attend to both intersections and complexities, language becomes fraught. Fat Studies offers space in which to take up fat as a neutral, if not celebratory descriptor. Within the fervent reclamation of "fat" as the word to describe ample bodies, there are nonetheless divisions and tensions: between the "regular" fatty and the supersized person next to her; in the experiences of a person who navigates the specificities of Black fatness; in the nuances of fatness and medicalization for someone who seeks gender affirming surgeries, or someone who lives with chronic illness or disability. While it becomes difficult to resist the seduction of hierarchizing fat experiences, Fat Studies scholarship suggests that fundamentally all that can be said is that fat experiences, like fat bodies, come in many shapes, sizes and textures.

As a "floating signifier" with a long and complicated history (Wann, 2009; Santolin & Rigo, 2015), the word "fat" is deliberately vague in its terminology, resisting the specificity and pathologization of terms like "overweight" and "obese". This flexibility is the chief asset of the word, yet much of Fat Studies scholarship also explores the terminological tensions. How fat, for instance, does one need to be to truly understand fat oppression? What about the mitigating effects of race, class, gender, sexuality and ability? Can we truly speak of shared trauma or celebration given the diversity of our experiences? The potential of including the size 12 cousin-in-in-law or dieting co-worker in our own personal fat politic can make many of us dubious. However, terminological openness is vastly superior to the limiting terminology – in both medical and identity politics contexts – which it replaces. Furthermore, it is evident that, in the pervasive moral panic of the obesity epidemic (LeBesco, 2010), there are no winners. People who are thin "enough", for instance, are still governed by the fear of fat. Size oppression, while uniquely experienced by different bodies, is indiscriminate in its scope.

In the context of reproduction, these terminological issues may carry a new valance. The physiology of reproduction can result in rapid and potentially overwhelming physical shifts, changing the relationship with size oppression and fat politics. Pregnancy, for most people, results in rapid weight gain, which may predicate a self-consciousness about size and weight no matter the body size of origin (Johnson, 2010; Shloim et al., 2014). Yet not all parenting labour is rooted in pregnancy, and it is important to acknowledge that parenthood is as terminologically fraught as fatness. Families are built in many ways. While many families begin with pregnancy, others are built through adoption and surrogacy. Many people parent in non-traditional arrangements with aunties, othermothers or others taking on parenting labour without biological connection (O'Reilly, 2008). Furthermore, an analysis of parenting must acknowledge the tensions between looking at mothers and looking at parents. Assuming all pregnant people are women excises the experiences of many trans people, as assuming that mothers and fathers are different erases the efforts made toward egalitarianism and revolutionary parenting in many households and communities. At the same time, it is facile to ignore the extent to which parenting within patriarchal cultures strongly reinforces heterosexist and binary models. People who are understood as "mothers" are laden with specific expectations and judgments that are distinct from those pushed on "fathers" or "parents" (O'Reilly, 2008). Furthermore, fat women "are uniquely situated in a culture that not only exhibits a strong body hierarchy mandating thinness, but also a gendered body hierarchy mandating female thinness" (Kwan, 2010, p. 156). In this chapter, I will explore some of the specific tensions that are experienced by mothers, fathers and parents. I will extend the same terminological porousness to these terms that I extend to the word "fat". In so doing, I aim to acknowledge the diversity of parental and reproductive experiences across the gender spectrum while also recognizing the stronghold of the gender binary, especially in reproductive and parenting contexts.

Policing the pregnant body

Both Fat Studies scholars and others consider the limited possibilities and shaming contexts offered to fat pregnant people, or fat people attempting pregnancy. Pregnancy, as an intrinsically conjoined state, sits uneasily with neoliberal and modernist notions of personhood that privilege individualism and free will (though arguably, these ideals have only ever been offered to particular subjects, and seldom to mothers (Chandler, 2007)). Arguably, this makes pregnancy uniquely useful as a space for examination by Fat Studies scholars, as fat bodies themselves likewise threaten notions of individual merit and free will. Parker (2014) suggests that "In the search for the cause of and solution for 'obesity', medical research has become increasingly focused on women's reproductive bodies, and in particular, the 'womb environment' during pregnancy" (p. 107).

Warin et al. (2012) suggest that "the fetus distorts the category of subjectivity, feeding from the mother's body through the placenta" (p. 367). When people become pregnant, all behaviour is open to a heightened degree of surveillance and condescension. In 2016, Henriques and Azevedo stated that, "Pregnancy has been widely referred to as a teachable moment because of mothers' strong motivation to protect the well-being of the foetus and strong social pressure to avoid unhealthy habits" (p. 62). In spite of feminist resistance to the notion of "fetal personhood" (Warin et al, 2012; McNaughton, 2011), the needs of fetuses are often presented as trumping those of their hosts, even where there is limited evidence of changed outcomes contingent on changed behaviours (Drong et al., 2012; McNaughton, 2011). As a result, pregnant people may find that they are rapidly thrust into the full judgment of parenthood with their every choice policed, or at least noted, by family members, strangers, medical workers and beyond. This troubling surveillance extends to assumptions made about who will produce a problematic infant: Fat Studies scholarship chronicles the ways in which fat people trying to get pregnant may be cautioned about diminished fertility or potential "bad outcomes" prior to even achieving pregnancy (Friedman, 2015). This may be especially true for fat people who require reproductive technologies to become pregnant. Despite the fact that there are underlying physiological conditions, such as polycystic ovarian syndrome (PCOS) that correlate with both easy weight gain and also infertility, fat parents-to-be may be denied access to IVF and other reproductive technologies until they reduce their weight (Keenan & Stapleton, 2010). In these contexts, the stigma of fatness is revealed fully. Even when weight is clearly established as outside of a person's "fault", people are not treated with the respect accorded other medical conditions, but are instead expected to change their bodies through personal effort.

Guidelines suggest that fat people, upon becoming pregnant, should gain less weight than thinner pregnant people. This is true despite evidence that limiting caloric intake in pregnancy has a limited impact on weight gain (Shloim et al., 2014). When miscarriages or stillbirths occur, even when no direct cause is found, fat people may be blamed for their weight as a mitigating factor (McNaughton, 2011).

On a social level, body management is uniquely experienced in pregnancy. For thinner people, pregnancy may be a fresh lens into the tensions experienced by larger bodies. This may also result in social discomfort, as bodies, even those of thinner people, rapidly shift and become fair game for open commentary. For fat people, the social experience of pregnancy is variable. For some fatter people, pregnancy may be a moment where a larger body is rationalized and justified in ways that are unavailable in non-reproductive contexts (Johnson, 2010). For others, however, some of the milestones of traditional commodified pregnancy may be erased. For instance, clothing for pregnant people is difficult to find in larger sizes, and larger bodies may conceal pregnancy for longer, inviting fewer of the positive interactions that visible pregnancy may bring (Keenan & Stapleton, 2010). Larger pregnant people may also be susceptible to negative interactions from both lay and medical people, suggesting that "there are only certain, somewhat limited, ways-of-being readily accessible to pregnant women" (Johnson, 2010, p. 253). Finally, visibly fat and pregnant people may be already judged as dysfunctional parents for choosing to reproduce while living in socially "unacceptable" bodies (Herndon, 2010; McNaughton, 2011).

Epigenetics: "protecting" the fetal environment

The recent surge of research into epigenetics has unique impacts on fat pregnant people. "The term *epigenetics* literally means on top of genetics and refers to processes that induce heritable changes in gene expression without altering the gene sequence" (Lillycrop & Burdge, 2011, p. 76), indicating that many physiological conditions may have complicated and unstable origins. Indeed, even articles which indicate epigenetic roots to the obesity "epidemic" suggest that obesity is born in "fetal metabolic programming, the mechanisms of which are not well understood" (Heerwagen et al., 2010, p. 711). Looking through the lens of Fat Studies, Parker argues that "fetal programming theory is in its infancy and scientific claims about the long-term effects of 'maternal obesity' in these studies are currently based on observation, correlation and speculation, rather than any demonstrable causation" (2014, p. 107). In other words, epigenetic theories, which have been used to blame fat pregnant bodies for "a range of population health problems" (Parker, 2014, p. 107) must be explored with extreme caution.

The analysis of epigenetic origins of obesity may initially appear advantageous when applied to fat people who are pregnant and parenting. Notably, it suggests that fat people are not responsible for their own weight, but can instead understand fat as, in part, a product of the fetal environment prior to their own births. Unfortunately and unsurprisingly, epigenetic analyses of obesity, which generally exist outside of Fat Studies scholarship, are seldom used to exonerate fat people in the context of future reproduction. Instead, "core assumptions at the heart of obesity science regarding the scale of the obesity problem, the nature of the risk and where responsibility for health should fall, have been taken up uncritically in medical arenas focused on conception, pregnancy and reproduction" (McNaughton, 2011, p. 180). While fatness is shown to be both multifactorial and intractable (Mann et al., 2007; Friedman, 2004), epigenetic analyses hone in on the possibilities that shifts in the fetal environment may end the "obesity epidemic" (Henriques & Azevedo, 2016; Lillycrop & Burdge, 2011), and in so doing, explicitly takes a gendered tone in blaming mothers:

> The gendered nature of child feeding and pregnancy link women's and children's flesh together and this link is an important element in establishing and preserving maternal responsibility for children. At the same time, women's bodies are problematic entities … women are presented as particularly prone to failures of will resulting in an excess of flesh.
>
> *(Maher et al., 2010, p. 240)*

In other words: instead of assuming that any given fat pregnant person may be fat for a range of complicated reasons, that person is now held accountable for ensuring that the baby they are carrying does not "catch" fat by trying, likely in vain, to change the fetal environment. In so doing, stigma is reproduced by suggesting that the fat pregnant body is so objectionable that it must avoid replicating itself at any cost.

Epigenetic research is deeply troubling in its insistence on eradicating diversity and, like much weight "science", betrays a focus on narrow thresholds of normativity with regard to both bodies and behaviours. Fundamentally, epigenetic research is being used as a form of biopower (McPhail et al., 2016): rather than merely observing the impacts at the intersections of biology and environment, epigenetics is deeply invested in changing perceived "bad" outcomes. As Fat Studies scholar LeBesco (2009) eloquently argues, ongoing attempts to locate a "gay gene" or a similar "cause" for fatness are rooted in the desire for cure, suggesting that fat and/or unhealthy bodies are intrinsically unwelcome and abnormal.

The underlying motivations of epigenetic research are revealed in the ways that this research is largely unconcerned with structural impacts on the fetal environment, ignoring the ways that "a gendered and class analysis of obesity provides a different entry point for examining 'obesogenic environments'" (Warin et al., 2008, p. 108). Rather than considering what an overall healthier environment might do to the fetal context, individual behaviours are zeroed in on, concluding that "maternal obesity may be the most common health risk for the developing fetus" (Heerwagen et al., 2010, p. 718). A Fat Studies approach, by contrast, may ask questions such as: what would the epigenetic outcome look like if stress was mitigated by allowing pregnant people to shift their work lives to accommodate any discomforts? What would a reproductive experience free from weight stigma entail? What would be the outcome of providing access to non-judgmental care, or access to fresh, inexpensive and nourishing food (Kukla, 2008)? An examination of socio-economic status and pregnancy reveals that being poor may be much worse for fetuses than being fat (Warin et al., 2008); and of course, the intersection between poorness and fatness may cause exponential challenges (Wann, 2009), yet the overall effort (in both policy and medical contexts) is focused on individual regulation rather than broad scale environmental and societal change.

Fat Studies scholarship offers further alternatives to epigenetic approaches. Taken in tandem with research that reveals the impossibility of successful weight loss (Mann et al., 2007), Fat Studies approaches indicate that fat pregnant people should instead be treated like any other pregnant people with unique bodies. In this context, fatness becomes just another variation of the human condition, one which might require specific decisions to be made in pregnancy: a state of diversity as innocent as our relationship with height. A very short-waisted pregnant person might require measurements to be taken slightly differently; a very tall pregnant person might want to choose to deliver in specific positions or locations to accommodate their body's needs. Similarly, a supersized pregnant person might require an anaesthetic consult prior to delivery so that their body's specific needs are considered. Specific management or monitoring might be required or suggested for larger bodies, but without judgment or the presumption of a changed body as possible or desirable.

Beyond pregnancy: interdependence and mother blame

The field of epigenetics, rich with complexity, and as yet not thoroughly understood, can complicate analyses of fatness but, in practice, becomes yet another tool for policing pregnancy. This surveillance is predicated on the assumption that, feminist analyses of abortion notwithstanding, the rights of fetuses are of greater worthiness than those of the people housing them. While remaining cognizant of the problematic impact of the "fetal origins hypothesis" or "fetal personhood" (Warin et al., 2012; McNaughton, 2011), it is important to also consider the impact of conjoinment beyond pregnancy. Warin et al. suggest that "Fetuses and children are portrayed as innocent victims in need of protection from irresponsible parents. In some cases, mothers have been prosecuted for neglect and abuse in raising obese children" (2012, p. 366), showing the ways that judgment in pregnancy extends into surveillance of parenthood. Fat Studies scholars have explored the many dimensions of mother and parent blame that fall on fat parents and their fat children.

While parenthood after birth lacks the explicit physical conjoinment of pregnancy, early parenthood is an intrinsically linked state. This is most obvious for parents who breastfeed or chestfeed, where the physiological connection between parent and infant is maintained, but even outside of these arrangements, the early years of a child's life involve near total dependence on the adults around them. Specifically, children must be fed, and for many years of early life, they are utterly dependent on the choices and capabilities of their parents and/or caregivers:

> One must feed one's child over and over again, and there is no discrete moment at which one can prove one's *proper* maternality through feeding. On the other hand, at any moment a mother may prove herself an *improper* mother through an act of feeding. Hence this is a test that one can never pass but is always at risk of failing.
>
> *(Kukla, 2008, p. 79)*

Beyond the realm of food, virtually all decisions made for and about children must be the domain of their parents, suggesting that children are in the unique position of both being constructed as individual subjects and simultaneously the conjoined attachments of their often female-identified caregivers. The sanctity of neo-liberal notions of individualized subjectivity are worthless in examining the dependence of young children (Chandler, 2007). Kukla suggests that "reproduction not only happens in women's bodies, but through women's ongoing, richly textured labour" (2008, p. 69). As a result, judgment of children who are deemed to be living at-risk or unworthy lives is explicitly a judgment of parents, and, in most cases, mothers. Furthermore, this judgment is only increasing in tandem with ongoing hysteria about the "obesity epidemic" (Quirke, 2016).

While judgment is heaped on fat parents, and on parents of fat children, "women in particular are held responsible for the future (fat free) health of their offspring from the womb to the tomb" (McNaughton, 2011, p. 179). The specific positioning of fat mothers, or mothers of fat children, is underpinned by the patriarchal institution of motherhood (O'Reilly, 2008) which suggests that mothers are responsible for parenting outcomes and should subsume their lives to their children. Effectively, girl children are taught that their own autonomous lives should only exist until they reproduce, cutting short the potential for female subjects to achieve any type of independent, empowered or self-oriented existence. In the realm of fat, there is little acknowledgement that "Mothering is fundamentally relational, and at odds with the individualistic approach of current health-promotion messages and directives that address energy in/energy out understandings" (Warin et al., 2008, p. 107).

The history of mother blame around fat is long and varied (Bell, McNaughton, & Salmon). Indeed, "the positioning of women as producing ill health in their children has long been a central element of public health initiatives and biomedicine more broadly" (McNaughton, 2011, p. 182). Maternal blame is taken up in the context of fat and motherhood (Warin et al., 2012; Zivkovic et al., 2010; Herndon, 2010) and "the role of mothers as managers and carers of children emerges as central to the framing of childhood obesity" (Maher et al., 2010, p. 235). Particular attention is given toward maternal labour, with some research suggesting that the introduction of women, typically privileged and white, into the workforce has led to the alleged increase in prevalence of fat children (Herndon, 2010; Bell et al., 2009).

The scapegoating of particular bodies and maternal blame for non-normative subjects are intimately related. Fat people, as quintessential neo-liberal modernist failures, are the obvious sites of panic about diminished self-reliance, independence and failed health. As fat people become increasingly surveilled and punished, it is unsurprising that the approbation offered fat people is exponentially realized on fat mothers and mothers of fat children (McNaughton, 2011; Herndon, 2010).

Beginning at birth, the first information we learn about new babies is their sex and their weight. Both pieces of information enter these new people into systems of significance and performance. Babies who "fail to thrive", who do not easily and quickly grow, are immediately targeted as problems. But increasingly, children who thrive all too well and remain at the top of the arbitrary and nonsensical growth charts are likewise constructed as problematic (Keenan & Stapleton, 2010). In the same way that adults' ill health is popularly understood as visibly marked on the fat body, fat children's bodies are presumed to be marked by their poor parenting. Zivkovic et al. state that "children are thus put forward as potential problems and a solution since they represent … the future generations of obese adults, and bodily sites to prevent such medical and socio-economic disaster" (2010, p. 376). This rhetorical construction presents multiple concerns.

First, as discussed above, the multifactorial nature of obesity means that children may be fat for many different reasons drawing on the complex overlay of genetics and environment, since "the true impact of fatness on health is not known and obesity science is permeated with ambiguity and contradiction" (McNaughton, 2011, p. 187). Poverty may have a huge impact on children's access to food and activity (Mainland et al., 2017; Henriques & Azevedo, 2016). Children with differently abled bodies may move differently or not at all, and likewise children with invisible differences may have a range of capacities. Children who fear racism or homophobia may make different choices about how to participate in public space. Beyond this facile analysis, there is limited acknowledgement in popular culture of children as willful and semi-autonomous creatures. It is exceedingly difficult to feed a baby who does not want to eat, and it is similarly difficult to comfort a child who is hungry without providing nutrition (Zivkovic et al., 2010). Mothers are in the impossible position of being expected to scrutinize their children's every bite and movement, perhaps to an even greater extent than the scrutiny which they are expected to offer their own bodies (Quirke, 2016). Mothers who over manage their children's intake, however, are viewed as "helicoptering", fearsome creatures who do not allow their children freedom, suggesting that,

> mothers thus tread a fine line between permissive parenting and being disciplinarian. They are both dangerous and morally responsible for feeding their children according to appropriate social conventions and, on the other hand, their food choices can have potentially dangerous consequences such as overweight and obesity.
>
> *(Zivkovic et al., 2010, p. 384)*

Fundamentally, the core tenet of mother blame is the notion that children are products, and that the success or happiness of children is predetermined based on maternal effort. Such an acknowledgement fails in the realm of physiology wherein the physical characteristics of any given child, including weight, are drawn from complex origins. Looking beyond the physical realm, children's health, happiness, success, politeness, cleanliness likewise occur or do not occur based on complex and multifaceted criteria. This complexity is consistently overlooked, as instead, "overweight or obese children are presented as visible signs of overconsumption and excess, but it is their mothers' misdirected appetites and desires that are really the targets" (Maher et al., 2010, p. 234). Mothers are blamed for failed children; fat children are visibly and irreparably failing (Herndon, 2010; McNaughton, 2011; Maher et al., 2010).

Obviously, children are not products. Likewise, children who are different in any way, including fatness, are not failures. At the centre of mother blaming arguments is a deep value-laden belief in the notion of worthiness, and of fat people as intrinsically unworthy. At the time of writing this chapter, *Esquire* magazine published an article titled "I don't care what my son becomes ... as long as he's not overweight" (Coren, 2017). While obviously positioned as sensationalist clickbait, this article exposes a deeply held social belief, that a fat body is evidence of a flawed subject, and that parents, specifically mothers, who love their children should save them from this fate. The author of this article suggests that his fat son is the product of his mother's mistakes, and that she should immediately change her approach to eradicate his fatness, a perfect storm of fat shame and mother blame. Perhaps most alarmingly, this article reveals a taken-for-granted "truth": that to be fat somehow results in the worst life imaginable.

Exploring the intersections

Fat and parenting does not occur in isolation of other social locations. Fat Studies scholarship is increasingly attenuated to the nuances of intersectionality, considering the ways that, for example, racism, ableism, sanism and other oppressions may work in relation to one another (Friedman et al., 2019). For example, while all fat kids may experience social sanctions for normative/"healthy" children, their experience of the medical system may be reduced to an annual pediatric checkup. For children with special physical or developmental needs, however, the ongoing scrutiny of the medical establishment may be unavoidable and endless. Importantly, the oversight of the medical system may be pervasive even when weight is not a presenting issue. Children with complex social and physical needs may be subject to weight shame and scrutiny regardless of whether weight plays a role in their diagnosis. Parents of fat children may recognize the damaging effects of this ongoing scrutiny (particularly as intersected with problematic interventions around disability and illness from medical professionals) but may be powerless to avoid these interactions for children with special needs.

A fat adult may choose to avoid an appointment with a specialist out of a need to limit fat shaming experiences. While there may be medical consequences to this decision, the person is nonetheless deemed autonomous. By contrast, the same person, choosing to avoid a specialist appointment for her child, is potentially subject to the scrutiny of child welfare systems and may be deemed to be putting her child at risk of extreme harm. The extreme harm of partaking in an ongoing system of stigma and discrimination is, of course, ignored in this analysis. Notably, "the cases of fat children removed from their homes inevitably involve people of colour and the poor" (Bell et al., 2009, p. 163), suggesting further stigma and discrimination.

Children with complex identities may find themselves accumulating layers of fat stigma. A colleague in the field of trans health care recently shared that one of few doctors to work with trans children in Southern Ontario refuses to prescribe puberty blockers to children who are in the overweight or obese weight categories. This doctor made clear that they would prefer to police weight for all people but are only able to manipulate their influence over this particular population by holding back access to desired and necessary medication as "bait" for weight loss. While this data is purely anecdotal, it speaks to the extent to which children who have any non-standard need to engage with the medical system may be uniquely punished for non-normative weights.

Medicalization is only one area of intersection. Beyond the medical realm, newcomer children may face distinct scrutiny from their second language teachers, agencies who support "integration" or other social service spaces. Racialized newcomers may learn that their skin colour and body size are both deemed antithetical to successful integration: Dame-Griff's analysis, for example, looks at the ways that racialized and newcomer families are scrutinized through rhetoric that ties together migration, race and fatness in deeply negative ways (2016). Thinking through anti-black racism, big Black boys may be characterized as uniquely threatening while big Black girls may be simultaneously sexualized and relegated to the sidelines as the "Precious" or "Mammy" figure (Stoneman, 2012). Indigenous children are demonized for fatness and are framed as the products of deficient parenting in many different contexts with virtually no acknowledgement of the impact of colonialism and sustained violence and disruption toward physical and mental health outcomes (Lavallee & Poole, 2010). Each of these social locations may intersect with poverty, which has its own complex relationship with fatness. Poverty may make thinness even less achievable, but being fat may also lead to poverty through limited employment and promotion opportunities, educational dead ends and other sites of systemic discrimination (Wann, 2009). This snapshot cannot begin to do justice to the complexity of fat identity. The examples are virtually endless: of the unique discrimination aimed at a fat kid with two moms, for example; or the implications of parenting a fat kid with ADHD or other "disruptive" diagnoses; or the ways that being fat alongside any chronic health condition such as asthma or juvenile diabetes may complicate care and amplify stigma.

There are literally as many ways to be fat as there are ways to be. Fatness coincides with every other social location and in every liminal identity between social locations. There is a duality, then, in speaking of fat parenting. There is a synchronicity to the overwhelming negativity associated with being the parent of a fat child; concurrently, there are multiple variables that impact the specific flavour that that negativity may take.

While the experiences of parenting fat children are truly endless in their variety, it is useful to quickly pause and consider the specificity of fat parents raising fat children. Fat adults are already presumed to have flawed decision-making capacity, such that their ability to parent is already suspect. Fat parents raising fat children are thus at the nexus of low expectations and heightened scorn, especially in medicalized contexts (Friedman, 2015). On the one hand, fatness may exist, for many families, as a "vertical" identity, one that is shared within families, such as race. On the other hand, because fatness is not always politicized and fat acceptance may be limited to very specific social environments, fat parents may simply layer on additional shame without having the resources to equip their children to deal with the intricacies of fat stigma. A fat parent who is continuously dieting, as most fat people are, makes clear with every bite and every workout that they reject their child's subjectivity. A fat parent who celebrates their child's fat body may be even more reviled in the public sphere (Friedman, 2014). As a result, the specificities of parenting fat children as a fat parent are endlessly fraught and may stretch the existing tensions and turmoil of parenting and judgment toward their breaking point.

Where do we go from here? Exploring fat positive approaches to parenting

In light of the overwhelming evidence of the challenges associated with fat and reproduction, what possibilities exist to shift discourses of blame and instead move toward more fat positive approaches to parenting? Fat Studies scholars and others have offered a range of different ways to approach this task, spanning from advice in the context of individual families to broader scale social transformation.

At the individual/familial level

Fat must be seen as intrinsic and immutable, neither the fault of the child or the parents, and negative associations with fat must be excised. This latter task is of great importance: as Maher et al. suggest, "When women's bodies, children's bodies and maternal responsibilities are viewed together in the context of obesity, the expectation that women will now be watchful of children's weight as well as their own becomes apparent" (2010, p. 243). Fat positive parenting may require intense personal work to shift toward a size acceptance lens on the part of parents toward their own bodies: it is extremely difficult to tell a child their body is perfect while policing the parental body.

Without minimizing the impact of living in diverse bodies beyond weight, and without erasing the intersections between fat, race, ability, and other social locations, there are spaces emerging that support celebration of diversity that may provide guidance for parents of fat children (Thomas, 2016). For example, fat positive parenting might benefit from engagement with critical parental approaches to neurodiversity that seek to recontextualize stigmatized conditions such as autism spectrum disorders as celebrated variations of human identity (Cascio, 2012). While neurodiverse people, for instance, are still often characterized negatively in public spaces, there exists a script for parenting children with diverse minds in more positive ways. Similarly, gender diverse children were either reviled or excised from mention in Western parenting contexts. More recently, critical approaches to parenting from gender fluid positions have allowed for a more celebratory approach to raising non-binary and gender creative kids (Green & Friedman, 2013; Meadows, 2011). Critical and diversity focused models of parenting are still far from mainstream, but there are blueprints for viewing parenting of non-normative children with positivity. Celebrating a child's diversity cannot erase fat phobia from the broader environment. However, the shift toward supportive parenting would nonetheless have a major impact on the lives of fat children, building on the belief that "parental support is *the* most important determining factor in how children come to feel about themselves and whether or not they succeed in their lives" (Herndon, 2010, p. 346).

For parents, a fat positive approach must also engage with Fat Studies work to acknowledge the deep impact of fat phobia in the broader culture (Wann, 2009). Parenting a fat child requires critical conversations about how to respond to stigma and discrimination, how to interact with the environment in the safest possible way, and how to respond to negativity. These are difficult conversations. Fat parents raising fat kids may have to contend with their own wounds based on their own experiences of fat phobia. Thinner parents may have a hard time understanding the extent of their child's trauma, or, conversely, may be triggered with regard to eating disorders or other thin maintaining behaviours. Once again, however, there are blueprints. In the context of other "vertical" identities such as race or ethnicity, parents and children may need to approach these conversations frankly and constantly as Black parents and children may do in considering the impacts of racism. For thinner parents raising fat kids, looking toward models of other "horizontal" parenting may be useful. For instance, critical approaches to trans-racial adoption, or the experiences of straight/cis people raising queer or gender fluid kids may prove useful in creating a framework for acknowledging trauma that is not directly experienced by the parent. As with many shifts toward critical parenting, there is a need for constant conversation and checking in. Furthermore, such an approach is not without its dangers, given that a refusal to force a child to lose weight may be deemed as neglect, especially for parents who are racialized, poor, queer or otherwise viewed as non-normative. Keeping this risk in mind, "the rush to treatment [of obesity] should not be construed as love for the child any more than not rushing to treatment should be construed as neglect" (Herndon, 2010, p. 344).

A truly fat positive approach to parenting, however, must look outside of the household and instead consider the need for widespread societal change. Approaching fat positive parenting only through shifts in parental behaviour merely replicates the same potential for blame and shame that exists around current models of parenting, suggesting that if fat kids are miserable, it is because their parents are not doing enough to support them. Fat kids don't live in isolation, and while positive shifts from parents are obviously deeply meaningful, they still keep the responsibility for supporting fat children solely with primary caregivers. Left alone, this merely replicates the type of parent-blaming rhetoric that holds mothers accountable for eating disorders or obesity by suggesting that unhappy fat kids are merely insufficiently loved. Fat Studies scholarship lays the groundwork for consideration of how to understand fat within the broader social context.

Changing the social context

The need to shift the dialogue about fat children and their families has never been more important. While size acceptance movements have a long history, there is a curious gap in size acceptance materials for young children. Simultaneously, "the sporadic interest in this issue witnessed in previous periods bears little resemblance to the intense frenzy that childhood obesity and overnutrition have generated over the past decade amongst health professionals, the media and the public" (Bell et al., 2009, p. 159). Importantly, Fat Studies scholarship has increasingly responded to the heightened scrutiny of fat children by documenting the tensions in this realm and positing alternatives (see, for example, Boero & Thomas, 2016). Likewise, social media and popular culture have increasingly amplified the work of fat activist parents who are self-consciously responding to both personal and structural environments with radical alternatives (see, for example, plusmommy.com).

Parents of fat children must acknowledge the trauma of living in larger bodies, but this acknowledgement must move outside of the primary environment. Education, medicine, social services, popular culture, media – all of these spaces must respond to Fat Studies scholarship that aims to acknowledge fat phobia and size acceptance. A fat positive approach to parenting would acknowledge that the "whole village" that is notionally responsible for any given child must shift its lens toward size acceptance. While tiny footholds have been made toward shifting the normativity of slender bodies in the public sphere in terms of plus size models gaining limited currency, or television's rare inclusion or acknowledgment of fat people (Friedman, 2014), this is absent with respect to fat children. Parents and teachers need books that include fat kids, media that shows a range of body sizes. Gym classes need to shift toward celebrating a range of capacities and abilities including activities that are meaningful for larger bodies.

On the level of policy, resources that have been devoted to the eradication of fat bodies in the guise of "anti-obesity" could instead be re-allocated toward funding education, health care and social services. This shift might result in an actual impact to population health in opposition to the ill-considered shaming outcomes of anti-obesity initiatives (Thomas, 2016). Exposing hidden sites of anti-obesity rhetoric (such as Mason, 2016) might likewise shift policy focus toward a deeper commitment to substantive and robust wellness rather than the attempted eradication of fatness.

In short: a fat positive approach to reproduction requires a range of tactics that span from the most personal private interactions between parents and children to the most broad-based activist approaches to altering the fat phobic environment from cradle to grave. Children must be meaningfully involved in this societal shift: in giving talks to young people about size acceptance, I have found that children readily accept the idea that discrimination based on fat is as problematic as other sites of discrimination, and are easily able to identify and speak out about fat phobia. Part of the societal shift, however, requires naming the "elephant in the room" and becoming more confident about talking about fat with children and adults alike. This may be especially urgent due to the ways that the obesity epidemic has constructed only two possible types of parents: "those who are expected to guard against children becoming fat and those who are urged to treat children who are already fat" (Herndon, 2010, p. 333). No children or parents are immune to weight stigma or policing in the current climate of fat hatred.

Growing Fat Studies...

As a discipline, Fat Studies has invested in considering the intersections of fat, reproduction and parenting. As the literature gathered here displays, there has been attention given to the ways that examinations of the nuances of fat and parenting are essential to understanding fatness broadly. Thinking through Fat Studies as a theoretical discipline, however, there is a great deal of merit in examining work on the ideologies and epistemologies of motherhood, parenthood and reproduction alongside considerations of fatness. As Fat Studies continues to explore, for example, nuances of fat temporalities (Tigwell et al., 2018 for example), considerations of normative life cycles are brought into focus. Likewise, there are fruitful congruities in thinking through the impact of normative expectations of family alongside normative expectations of bodies. Fat Studies must thus extend its disciplinary focus beyond the *examination* of fat alongside parenting and reproduction and instead consider the *theoretical extensions* that gender, motherhood, and family scholarships may offer to thinking through fat differently.

Fat Studies scholarship delights in exposing the corporeality of fat bodies, considering the ways that the grotesquerie of fat embodiment may provide a different view of the human condition. Similarly, work in motherhood studies considers the impact of relationality and the ways that the embodied relationality of mothering/parenting may threaten neoliberal notions of individuality. Taken together, these scholarships begin to threaten modernist and essentialist notions of human life in profoundly delicious and exciting ways. Thinking through fat and family allows for meaningful and nuanced extensions of thinking through fat bodies that will allow Fat Studies to grow into interesting and essential directions.

Conclusions

A consideration of Fat Studies and other adjacent work at the intersections of fat, reproduction and parenting comes to the inevitable conclusion that there is a lot of work to be done. Activist projects such as "It Gets Fatter" (It Gets Fatter, n.d.) may unwittingly suggest that the inevitability of a miserable fat childhood can only be interrupted by achieving adulthood, autonomy and agency. Even this sub-optimal forecast, however, minimizes the extent to which fat people may be infantilized, reduced to the same shame and disruption of childhood, when they themselves attempt to add children to their families. As with other politicized and scrutinized identities, the need to protect vulnerable children masquerades as an excuse for hateful attention. Who will think of the fat children if their parents are not policed? How will the children of fat people escape their substandard and indulgent parenting? Beginning in the reproductive sector, maintained in epigenetic analyses of pregnancy as well as the medicalization and pathologization of individual pregnant people, and finally exposed in judgment of the endless minutiae of parenting, fat people, and parents of fat children, are constantly found to be lacking. As the field of Fat Studies amply displays, to be seen as insufficient is an ironic judgment to place on people who have been constantly judged for being too much.

While the outlook for fat parents and fat children looks grim, there is hope, nonetheless. With the help of Fat Studies and fat activism, more children are born into fat-politicized environments, allowing the younger generation to become empowered to speak back to the witch hunt of the "obesity" epidemic. If, as Herndon offers, "in a political climate where parents are prosecuted and children are removed from homes and we are told that we are at war with obesity, the expectation is that all parents and all children be involved in the battle" (2010, p. 346), then neutrality is no longer an option. Instead, families, communities, and societies need to make a determined choice to fight back. In contexts in which diversity is celebrated and politicized, fat people fight, and Fat scholars write, using all of the weight of their experiences of scorn and judgment to push against an establishment intent on their extinction. Fat kids view this struggle and potentially find solace as well as tangible tools for fighting fat-phobia. As with any civil rights struggle, opinions may shift, structures may fall and fat may come to be recognized as just another way of being, another way of parenting, and another valuable addition to the human condition.

A consideration of fat and parenting also has the potential to shift analyses of fat more broadly. Fat Studies needs to be in the family way. While existing Fat Studies scholarship on family, children, reproduction and parenting is meaningful and important, it still largely exists in the realm of descriptive explanations of the challenges facing fat life. An embedded and intersectional engagement with the theoretical scholarship coming out of motherhood studies and other family studies scholarships might contribute a great deal to exciting theoretical breakthroughs for both Fat Studies and other fields. Likewise, it would extend the intrinsic interdisciplinary and intersectional focus of Fat Studies. Taking up fat in relation to family thus offers a renewed view of Fat Studies that is essential, timely and exciting and offers new directions in both practical and theoretical realms.

References

Bell, K., McNaughton, D., & Salmon, A. (2009). Medicine, morality and mothering: Public health discourses on foetal alcohol exposure, smoking around children and childhood overnutrition. *Critical Public Health, 19*(2), 155–170.

Boero, N. (2009). Fat kids, working moms, and the "epidemic of obesity": Race, class, and mother blame. In E. Rothblum, & S. Solovay (Eds.), *The fat studies reader* (pp. 113–119). New York: New York University Press.

Boero, N. & Thomas, P. (Eds.). (2016). Fat kids [Special issue]. *Fat Studies, 5*(2).

Cascio, M. A. (2012). Neurodiversity: Autism pride among mothers of children with autism spectrum disorders. *Intellectual and Developmental Disabilities, 50*(3), 271–283.

Chandler, M. (2007). Emancipated subjectivities and the subjugation of mothering practices. In A. O'Reilly (Ed.), *Maternal Theory: Essential Readings* (pp. 529–541). Toronto: Demeter Press.

Coren, G. (2017, Nov 9). I don't care what my son becomes … as long as he isn't overweight. *Esquire.* http://www.esquire.co.uk/life/a18073/giles-coren-overweight-son/

Dame-Griff, E. C. (2016). "He's not heavy, he's an anchor baby": Fat children, failed futures, and the threat of Latina/o excess. *Fat Studies, 5*(2), 156–171.

Drong, A. W., Lindgren, C. M., & McCarthy, M. I. (2012). The genetic and epigenetic basis of type 2 diabetes and obesity. *Clinical Pharmacology & Therapeutics, 92*(6), 707–715.

Friedman, J. M. (2004). Modern science versus the stigma of obesity. *Nature Medicine, 10*(6), 563–569.

Friedman, M. (2014). Here comes a lot of judgment: *Honey Boo Boo* as a site of reclamation and resistance. *Journal of Popular Television, 2*(1), 77–95.

Friedman, M. (2015). Reproducing fat-phobia: Reproductive technologies and fat women's right to mother. *Journal of the Motherhood Initiative for Research and Community Involvement, 5*(2), 27–41.

Friedman, M., Rice, C., & Rinaldi, J. (2019). *Thickening fat: Fat bodies, intersectionality and social justice.* New York: Routledge.

Green, F. & Friedman, M. (2013). *Chasing Rainbows: Exploring gender fluid parenting practices.* Toronto: Demeter Press.

Heerwagen, M. J. R., Miller, M. R., Barbour, L. A., & Friedman, J. E. (2010). Maternal obesity and fetal metabolic programming: A fertile epigenetic soil. *American Journal of Physiology, 299*(3), R711–R722.

Henriques, A., & Azevedo, A. (2016). A biopsychosocial approach to the interrelation between motherhood and women's excessive weight. *Porto Biomedical Journal, 1*(2), 59–64.

Herndon, A. M. (2010). Mommy made me do it: Mothering fat children in the midst of the obesity epidemic. *Food, Culture & Society, 13*(3), 331–349.

It Gets Fatter. (n.d.) http://itgetsfatter.tumblr.com. Tumblr.

Johnson, S. (2010). Discursive constructions of the pregnant body: Conforming to or resisting body ideals? *Feminism & Psychology, 20*(2), 249–254.

Keenan, J., & Stapleton, H. (2010). Bonny babies? Motherhood and nurturing in the age of obesity. *Health, Risk & Society, 12*(4), 369–383.

Kukla, R. (2008). Measuring mothering. *International Journal of Feminist Approaches to Bioethics, 1*(1), 67–90.

Kwan, S. (2010). Navigating public spaces: Gender, race and privilege in everyday life. *Feminist Formations, 22*(2), 144–166.

Lavallee, L., & Poole, J. (2010). Beyond recovery: Colonization, health and healing for Indigenous people in Canada. *International Journal of Mental Health and Addiction, 8*(2), 271–281.

LeBesco, K. (2009). Quest for a cause: The fat gene, the gay gene and the new eugenics. In E. Rothblum, & S. Solovay (Eds.), *The fat studies reader* (pp. 65–74). New York: New York University Press.

LeBesco, K. (2010). Fat panic and the New Morality. In J. Metzl, & A. Kirkland (Eds.), *Against health: How health became the new morality* (pp. 72–81). New York: New York University Press.

Lillycrop, K. A., & Burdge, G. C. (2011). Epigenetic changes in early life and future risk of obesity. *International Journal of Obesity, 35*, 72–83.

Maher, J., Fraser, S., & Wright, J. (2010). Framing the mother: Childhood obesity, maternal responsibility and care. *Journal of Gender Studies, 19*(3), 233–247.

Mainland, M., Shaw, S. M., & Prier, A. (2017). Parenting in an era of risk: Responding to the obesity crisis. *Journal of Family Studies, 23*(1), 86–97.

Mann, T., Tomiyama A. J., Westling, E., Lew, A., Samuels, B., & Chatman, J. (2007). Medicare's search for effective obesity treatments: Diets are not the answer. *American Psychologist, 62*(3), 220–233.

Mason, K. (2016). Women, infants, and (fat) children: Hidden "obesity epidemic" discourse and the practical politics of health promotion at WIC. *Fat Studies, 5*(2), 116–136.

McNaughton, D. (2011). From the womb to the tomb: Obesity and maternal responsibility. *Critical Public Health, 21*(2), 179–190.

McPhail, D., Bombak, A., Ward, P., & Allison, J. (2016). Wombs at risk, wombs as risk: Fat women's experiences of reproductive care. *Fat Studies, 5*(2), 98–115.

Meadows, T. (2011). Deep down where the music plays: How parents account for childhood gender variance. *Sexualities, 14*(6), 725–747.

O'Reilly, A. (2008). *Feminist mothering.* Albany: SUNY Press.

Parker, G. (2014). Mothers at large: Responsibilizing the pregnant self for the "obesity epidemic". *Fat Studies, 3*(2), 101–118.

Quirke, L. (2016). "Fat-proof your child": Parenting advice and "child obesity". *Fat Studies, 5*(2), 137–155.

Santolin, C. B. & Rigo, L. C. (2015). The birth of pathologizing discourse of obesity. *Movimento: Revista da escolar de Educacao fisica da URFGS, 21*(1), 77–90.

Shloim, N., Rudolf, M., Feltbower, R., & Hetherington, M. (2014). Adjusting to motherhood: The importance of BMI in predicting maternal well-being, eating behaviour and feeding practice within a cross cultural setting. *Appetite, 81*, 261–268.

Stoneman, S. (2012). Ending fat stigma: Precious, visual culture and anti-obesity in the "fat moment". *Review of Education, Pedagogy, and Cultural Studies, 34*(3–4), 197–207.

Thomas, P. (2016). Doing it for the children. *Fat Studies, 5*(2), 203–209.

Tigwell, T., Friedman, M., Rinaldi, J., Kotow, C., & Lind, E. R. M. (Eds.) (2018). Fatness and temporality [Special issue]. *Fat Studies*, 7(2).

Wann, M. (2009). Foreword: Fat studies: An invitation to revolution. In E. Rothblum, & S. Solovay (Eds.), *The fat studies reader* (pp. ix–xxv). New York: New York University Press.

Warin, M., Turner, K., Moore, V., & Davies, M. (2008). Bodies, mothers and identities: Rethinking obesity and the BMI. *Sociology of Health & Illness*, *30*(1), 97–111.

Warin, M., Zivkovic, T., Moore, V., & Davies, M. (2012). Mothers as smoking guns: Fetal overnutrition and the reproduction of obesity. *Feminist & Psychology*, *22*(3), 360–375.

Zivkovic, T., Warin, M., Davies, M. & Moore, V. (2010). In the name of the child: The gendered politics of childhood obesity. *Journal of Sociology*, *46*(4), 375–392.

17

FAT STUDIES AND PUBLIC HEALTH

Natalie Ingraham

Introduction

Public health and such fat politics as Fat Studies and fat activism often have fundamentally different approaches to large body size. Public health framing of large body size is generally understood in medical terminology of "overweight" and "obesity",[1] while fat politics focus on the lived experience of fatness in society. The following essay describes fat politics perspectives on fatness, public health perspectives on fatness, and conflicts between the two. Additionally, the work of professional movements such as Health at Every Size is described in their attempts to bridge the gap between the two. Finally, this essay covers how public health has taken up fat activism critiques to address issues such as weight stigma or weight bias.

Fat politics perspectives on fatness

I use the term *fat politics* to describe both fat activism as a civil rights-focused social movement and Fat Studies as an interdisciplinary, academic field. However, these are not mutually exclusive categories, and many professionals researching and writing in Fat Studies also consider themselves fat activists. Broadly, fat politics frames "obesity" as fatness or large body size that is a natural variation in bodies, much like height or eye color. However, the actions taken on how and where this framing occurs differs between activism-based social movement work and more academic-focused activities. Both fat activism and Fat Studies often address health as a central issue of their work, because it is the most commonly voiced "concern" about the impact of fatness – *what about their health?* However, fat politics is just as inclined to ask "why does health matter?" or "is health our only measure of worth as people?", as they are to address health concerns directly in their academic or activist work. Importantly, fat politics does not center health as a primary concern related to fatness. Rather, it addresses a full spectrum of the lived experience of fatness as well as producing and examining fatness in art, media, and online representations.

Fat activism

Cooper's (2016) compendium on the history of fat activism argues that it centers civil rights and fights against discrimination or mistreatment of fat people. Fat activists fight against fatphobia or fear of fatness that they say often fuels mistreatment of fat people across all aspects of society, from structural discrimination in employment and medical settings to interpersonal mistreatment by family, friends, or strangers based on their body size. Previous scholars like Saguy (2013) have also categorized fat activism as a civil rights-based social movement. Cooper (2016) argues that some fat activist-associated movements like Health at Every Size do not fit into this framework because they center on health and well-being instead of civil rights and discrimination. Fat activists work to disrupt the connection between fatness and health by asserting, among other things, that fatness does not equal ill health or health problems or that good health is not an obligation to be a worthy human being. In this way, fat activism is closely connected to other embodied rights-based movements such as the disability rights movements.

Fat Studies

The academic field of Fat Studies is often grounded in fat activism and has expanded rapidly in the last two decades, including the publication of several Fat Studies readers and the launch of the *Fat Studies* journal in 2012. Scholars in the field come from a wide range of academic disciplines, though most are concentrated in social sciences like psychology and sociology or in cultural or media studies fields. As part of fat politics, Fat Studies examines a wide range of topics including intersectional oppressions (class, race, body size, disability), dating and sexuality, media representations of fatness, policy impacts, employment and education. It also often includes critical approaches to the connection between fatness and health. Fat Studies, like critical obesity studies (detailed in the last section of this chapter), takes a critical approach to medical understandings of large body size – based on BMI category (Aphramor, 2005; Gard & Wright, 2005). Fat Studies observes and describes mistreatment of fat people in society, including scholarship on the ways *fat stigma*, the socially negative views of those with fat bodies, has more direct links to negative physical and mental health than fatness itself. Fat Studies also occasionally includes some intervention studies that test ways to reduce fat stigma or tests therapeutic techniques to help fat people cope with mistreatment based on their body size. However, most of the work on health within Fat Studies is observational, analyzing media portrayals of fatness, interviewing fat people, or critiquing fat people's experiences with medical providers.

Public health perspectives on fatness

Medical understandings of fatness

Public health builds on current medical knowledge to improve the health of individuals and society in most countries and across many professions. "Obesity" has become a large, sustained focus for most industrialized nations in the last 30 years. This is especially true around "childhood obesity" and "obesity"-associated conditions such as heart disease and type II diabetes (Colosia et al., 2013). Public health relies mainly on medical definitions of large body size as defined by Body Mass Index (BMI) categories of underweight, "normal" weight, overweight, obese, and morbid obesity. Social science studies of the rise of the "obesity epidemic" show how popular media has reflected increasing alarm at obesity since the late 1980s (Boero, 2007) with language such as "time bomb" and "war" being used to describe the fight against large body size (Meleo-Erwin, 2011; Saguy & Riley, 2005). Thus, the belief that high weights are an immediate social threat and health hazard persists (Chrisler & Barney, 2017). To address this hazard, billions of dollars of public and private funding have gone into finding a "cure" or at least stopgap treatments for obesity, as well as investigating obesity causality.

Public health research on obesity focuses on two main areas: finding "causes" for overweight and obesity (Allen & Safranek, 2011; Hamin, 1999) and designing interventions to "treat" obesity, generally through calorie reduction and/or increased exercise (Samuel-Hodge et al., 2009; Teixeira et al., 2015). Public health has also pursued more systemic or environmental interventions in the last ten years, such as soda tax policies or policy shifting land use practices, such as creating housing, shopping, and recreational areas that are within walking distance to encourage more physical activity (Eisenberg, 2015). In particular, "childhood obesity" has been a rising public health concern (Ward et al., 2017) and the rationale behind several prominent public health programs such as Michelle Obama's Let's Move! campaign (Lupton, 2014).

Public health interventions for adults with obesity also include extreme medical interventions like weight loss surgery or inpatient weight loss treatment programs. Most public health interventions focus on individual behavior change for weight loss and movement out of overweight or obesity. Common interventions include keeping detailed food and calorie logs (Lieffers & Hanning, 2012) or tracking physical activity through technology such as pedometers or more modern fitness trackers (Acharya et al., 2011). Some public health efforts to "fight against the obesity epidemic" also target genetic components or environmental impacts, though these are less common.

"Obesity" as a disease

The American Medical Association (AMA) classified obesity as a disease in 2013 as defined by a BMI over 30, despite objections from its own Public Health and Science Committee (Stoner & Cornwall, 2014). This decision reflects research with medical professionals indicating that obesity is a disease in need of treatment by physicians (Davis, 2008). However, the decision to categorize obesity as a disease was controversial, sparking discussion and disagreement from medical providers as well as fat activist communities. The act of classifying obesity as a disease has worldwide implications for healthcare and insurance coverage. While some argue that labelling obesity as a disease may help distance individuals from a personal responsibility for the "illness", others argue that obesity is better treated as a risk factor. It is further asserted that labelling it a disease would not reduce associated discrimination or stigmatization, but rather increase it, as these bodies would then be labelled as diseased or deviant (Vallgårda et al., 2017). This shift in particular, generated intense pushback from activists and researchers in fat politics, particularly Fat Studies.

Conflicts between public health and fat politics

Many of the critiques aimed at public health by fat politic academics and activists focus on the missing lived experiences of fat individuals. These critiques tend to focus on a few key areas: language choices in describing large bodies, critiques of measurement of bodies in public health, and critique of public health education campaigns. Critiques also emerge on the so-called "war on obesity" that joins similar "wars" on poverty and immigration that tend to converge on one body – that of the fat, poor, generally non-White immigrant (Herndon, 2005, p. 139). Herndon further argues that while there may be public backlash against critiquing the poor or immigrants, there is often very little backlash when attacking fat bodies, and that this is a pathway for discrimination for people who live at the intersections of these categories.

Social scientists have examined many of the conflicts between fat politics and public health by analyzing the framing of the issue by each respective party. Framing studies highlight how the issue is presented to the public – a public health frame of "obesity" as an urgent health concern vs. fat politics framing of large body size and discrimination against it as a civil rights issue (Nutter et al., 2016; Saguy, 2013). Saguy and Riley (2005) note that these conflicting frames may turn into contests, which then removes the possibility for sharing insights across the conflicting perspectives. These conflicts also manifest in the most basic terminology used across the two fields.

Language choices: obesity/weight vs. fatness

An important part of Fat Studies, as opposed to the study of "obesity", is the word choice around the description of larger bodies. Fat Studies scholars often put the term "obesity" inside scare quotes to denote the assumptions and "discriminatory consequences" it represents (Wann 2009: xiii). Fat Studies scholars use the term *fat* to reclaim it from its pejorative use. Fat activists like Marilyn Wann (2012) have argued for the word choice by asking "over what weight" the term overweight describes. By encouraging use of the word *fat* rather than *obese*, Wann encourages readers to shed the shame that comes with "obesity" and the control that comes from biomedicine and to instead embrace pride in describing their bodies by "taking back" the word fat. Fat activists push back against the socially constructed assumptions, especially within biomedicine, that view weight as a direct and accurate indicator of health despite research-based evidence to the contrary.

One example of this conflicting evidence is the "obesity paradox" (Amundson et al., 2010), a term describing research from public health or medicine that finds overweight or obese individuals have better health outcomes. This is a paradox, as it is assumed that they should always have worse health outcomes than thin or "normal" weight individuals. Differences in language between public health and Fat Studies have also been noted between person-first language in public health (e.g., *person with obesity*) or identity-first language used in Fat Studies (e.g., *fat person*) (Nutter et al., 2016). Some argue that person-first language is a way to reduce stigma and prejudice and builds off the legacy of disability rights movements that argue for person-first language to reduce ableism or disability stigma (Dunn & Andrews, 2015). However, others note that person-first language reproduces social norms around able-bodiedness, whereas identity-first language allows individuals to describe important aspects of themselves as a whole person (Cohen-Rottenberg, 2015; Lindemann et al., 2017).

Public health and Fat Studies also use different language to describe negative attitudes toward and mistreatment of fat people. Public health tends to use social psychology terminology such as weight bias, weight stigma or "obesity" stigma[2] continuing the trend of medical terminology language. Fat Studies generally uses the term *fat stigma* or *sizeism* when likening structural mistreatment of fat bodies to such systematic oppressions as racism or sexism. Scholars (Pausé, 2014) define fat stigma as the negative stereotypes, associations, and characteristics associated with fatness that can be experienced directly as discrimination. This can include verbal harassment, denial of healthcare services, employment, or housing. Kwan (2010) also highlights how fat stigma may be experienced indirectly through media messaging or micro-aggressions – common or everyday verbal and nonverbal slights that may not rise to the level of direct insults or harassment.

Public health body measurement critiques

Although BMI was designed as a population measure, it is often applied to individuals in medical and public health contexts. BMI has also been widely critiqued as a measure of body size and as a measure of health by both medical experts (Müller et al., 2016) and social scientists (Satinsky & Ingraham, 2014). Those groups argue that BMI does not account for differences across gender or body shape and is problematically based on White male body standards. However, the BMI is still widely used by many public health professionals to define, measure, and analyze large body size and its associated health risks (Flegal, 2012). This belief in the ability of BMI to predict health holds fast despite changes in its own classifications over the years. In 1998, the NIH changed BMI categories so that millions of people went from being "normal" to "overweight" or from "overweight" to "obese" overnight without any changes in their height or weight despite objections from many health professionals (Cohen & McDermott, 1998). Critics of BMI (Guthman, 2013) also consider it an artefact of popular epidemiological conventions that zoom into specific elements of how we conceptualize body size.

Critiques of other measures such as body line drawings used often in body image research (Gardner & Brown, 2010) or silhouette measures (Peterson et al., 2003) note that these measure drawings fail to capture true body size diversity and also erase diversity in body shape across race and ethnicity, sometimes as a part of the measure design (Satinsky & Ingraham, 2014). Fat Studies scholars argue that BMI measurement is both easily moveable and inaccurate, as was the case in the 90s shift. Furthermore, the subdivision of BMI into health categories fosters stigma by creating "us" (normal weight) vs. "them" ("overweight/obese") groups (Pausé, 2017). Both Fat Studies scholars and fat activists critique BMI and other public health strategies in several ways, including taking specific actions to protest anti-obesity health education campaigns.

Public health campaign pushback and advocacy toolkits

Health education campaigns are one of the most common forms of obesity prevention or anti-obesity campaigns in public health. These often take the form of large-scale ads on public transit or billboards highlighting a public health issue and providing brief snippets of information to educate the public and, ideally, incite behavior change around that issue (Wakefield et al., 2010). Pausé (2017) argues that, while public health recognizes the negative role of stigma on health in many other ways, it does not prevent them from using it in anti-obesity campaigns. She, like Lupton (2015), asserts that obesity campaigns rely on eliciting disgust around images of fat bodies. This further stigmatizes them based on assumptions that body size is under individual control, and that disgust is an appropriate motivator for behavior change to control body size (Vartanian & Smyth, 2013). Pausé (2017, p. 513) mentions specific examples from around the world, including the "Grabbable gut" campaign from LiveLighter in Western Australia, the Strong4Life campaign from Children's Healthcare of Atlanta focused on childhood obesity, the "Pouring on the pounds" campaign from the New York City Department of Health and Mental Hygiene focused on sugar-sweetened beverages, and the anti-obesity cheese campaign (Your Thighs on Cheese) from the Physicians Committee for Responsible Medicine.

Several scholars (Couch et al., 2017; Simpson et al., 2017) critique these campaigns that rely on fear appeals and stigma and which have been shown to be both ineffective for behavior change and a source of increased fat stigma. Some public health scholars like Callahan (2013), argue that "stigmatization lite", or relying on fear-based measures or negative views of fat bodies, can be necessary based on the health risks of obesity, much like public health has done with anti-smoking campaigns. However, this connection ignores the complicated relationship between fatness and health, to say nothing of the fact that fatness is not a singular health behavior like smoking. Other scholars (e.g., Hartlev, 2014) critique public health campaigns and argue that health policy should consider human rights alongside public health goals to avoid further stigmatization of marginalized groups.

Several scholars have also considered the ways that these public health campaigns targeting fatness also specifically target people at the intersections of multiple marginalizations – fat people of color and immigrants, specifically. For example, Dame-Griff (2016) builds on previous work (e.g., Herndon, 2005) to argue that former First Lady Michelle Obama's Let's Move! campaign that targeted Latinx and Black audiences, places blame on communities of color and Black and Brown parents specifically for the "supposedly impending deaths of legions of young Black and Brown bodies" (p. 156). This targeting of Brown bodies for public health campaign "intervention" is not unique to the United States, as scholars like McCormack and Burrows (2015) demonstrate. They argue that public health researchers in Aotearoa/New Zealand render the Brown bodies of Pasifika peoples problematic and in need of reform via weight loss. While they critique published public health research rather than a public health media campaigns specifically, they further a larger body of research that shows how public health experts position Black and Brown bodies as "ignorant" of health concerns around "obesity" and are, thus, in need of the state to provide this expertise (Boero, 2009; Saguy, 2013; Wathne et al., 2015).

One of the most prominent fat activist organizations, the National Association to Advance Fat Acceptance (NAAFA), has pushed back against public health framing of fatness by creating a series of toolkits to address fat stigma in various areas of society including education, employment and health care (NAAFA, 2016). The healthcare toolkit speaks specifically to concerns from medicine and public health that have resulted in mistreatment of fat patients in medical settings and gives providers direct advice on how to treat fat patients safely and with respect. This type of advocacy supports NAAFA's work as a social justice or civil rights focused fat activist organization that pushes for social change around acceptance of fat bodies and reduction of fat stigma (Cooper, 2016; Kwan, 2009; Saguy & Ward, 2011). While fat activists have directly targeted discrimination and fat stigma in their work since the beginning of the movement, public health has only made a more recent shift to address mistreatment of fat people.

The rise of weight stigma/bias as a public health research concern

Public health has begun to recognize the physical and mental impacts of weight stigma and weight bias in the last 20 years. Public health researchers have explored fat and non-fat peoples' experiences with weight stigma originally emanating from psychological practice concerns about its impacts on self-esteem or body image (Nutter et al., 2016; Puhl & Brownell, 2001; Puhl & Heuer, 2009). Weight stigma/bias has been found to mediate often cited correlations between weight and chronic health care concerns or weight and health-related quality of life, a common public health measure of health status (Lillis et al., 2011).

It is important to note, however, that much of the work around weight bias and weight stigma in health still utilizes an obesity frame. To its credit, it is one that advocates for less stigmatizing health education or intervention campaigns, and often describes how weight stigma is bad because it might prevent people from losing weight due to avoidance of gyms or healthcare providers (Brewis, 2014; Puhl & Brownell, 2006; Schvey et al., 2011). Pausé (2017) nods to this complexity, but continues that public health should recognize fat stigma as a driver of population health disparities (Hatzenbuehler et al., 2013) and consider it a social determinant of health.

Alternative and subversive body size movements within public health

HAES

One arm of fat politics that overlaps with public health is the concept of Health At Every Size (HAES™), a movement that includes many scholars who occupy space in both areas (Ingraham, 2018). The HAES perspective approaches health by holding a weight-neutral perspective on health. HAES advocates self and size acceptance, enhancing emotional, physical and spiritual health without focus on an "ideal weight". Other focuses of HAES include eating based on internal cues of hunger as well as individual nutritional needs, the joy of movement and an end to weight bias (Burgard 2009, pp. 42–43; see also Bacon, 2010). HAES is built on shared "principles of challenging scientific and cultural assumptions, valuing people's body knowledge and their lived experiences, and acknowledging social injustice and the role of disadvantage and oppression as health hazards" (Bacon & Aphramor, 2014; O'Hara & Taylor, 2014, p. 276). O'Hara and Taylor (2018) developed a three-point model for addressing the traditional medical model (what they and others call the "weight-centered health paradigm") by providing extensive literature review to show context, critiques, and consequences of the existing paradigm. They also put HAES forward as an alternative paradigm for consideration that centers on health and well-being rather than weight.

HAES focuses much of its attention on healthcare providers such as doctors and psychologists as well as health researchers in order to push back against the "medical pathologizing" that results in stigma and associated negative health outcomes for individuals with larger body sizes (Burgard, 2009, 45). Burgard says that "as its core, HAES is a model that reclaims the worth of our stigmatized bodies and encourages subversive acts of self-care" in its work (p. 52).

Scholars in community health (Bombak, 2014b), nutrition and dietetics (Aphramor & Gingras, 2009; Bacon & Aphramor, 2011; Humphrey et al., 2015) have all taken up HAES work within public health. This includes intervention testing with the HAES model and advocating for HAES or weight-neutral health policy. This has not been without resistance (Bombak, 2014a; Lekkas & Stankov, 2014) as "obesity" scholars agree with perspectives that reduce stigma, but are often unwilling to completely move to a weight neutral stance due to entrenched beliefs in the connection between weight and health. This certainty about the relationship between weight and health is one that Bombak describes as a discourse that "derives its stigmatizing potential, in part, from depicting its underlining science as certain" (2014a, p. e2). Nutter et al. (2016) frame HAES as a sub-discipline or model that approaches weight bias by critically examining "healthism" – the notion that health is entirely under individual control and that individuals have a social responsibility to maintain good health and strive for the perfect body (Mansfield & Rich, 2013; Petersen & Lupton, 1996; Welsh, 2011). Nutter follows other research to argue that healthism and its focus on individual responsibility also obscures social determinants of health, such as socioeconomic status, employment status, and education level, that impact access to healthy spaces and health care. Meleo-Erwin (2011) describes HAES similarly – as a project where fat activists can "simultaneously take up standard biomedical and public health calls for individuals to exercise and eat healthfully, but also reject equations between size and ill health" because HAES takes more of a harm reduction approach to health than traditional public health models (pp. 194–195).

Critical obesity studies and critical weight studies

Similar to HAES, scholars who critically approach fatness outside the biomedical lens also sometimes describe themselves as critical obesity studies or critical weight studies scholars. These terms tend to be more common outside of the United States (Sharma, 2017). Scholars note that Fat Studies as a field is often expansive enough to include these two subdiscplines, as they are all connected by a critical lens on obesity and a problemitization of obesity research (Evans, 2014). Much like Fat Studies, critical obesity/weight studies scholars draw from a variety of disciplines to advance their arguments critiquing traditional views of obesity, including social science fields and theories such as sociological, feminist, poststructuralist, queer and disability theories. Generally, these scholars (Colls & Evans, 2010) focus on challenging traditional notions of body size health as presented in research, policy, media and, most commonly, public health campaigns.

The future of public health and fatness

While it is unlikely that public health will ever shift to being fully weight neutral, the field has shifted its views of obesity and fatness over the last 20 years. The work of the Rudd Center (2012) and individual scholars in HAES, critical obesity/weight studies, and Fat Studies continue to push for health interventions and health policy that reduces fat stigma and improves the lives of fat people across the globe. Public health will likely always need some way to quantify human bodies and increased specificity in how they measure bodies has led social justice-oriented scholars in Fat Studies and other fields to contribute or, in fact, steer these conversations toward body measurement with a more value neutral stance (Satinsky & Ingraham, 2014). In many ways, it seems unlikely that fat politics will ever experience acquiescence from public health scholars that includes full abandonment of "obesity" prevention and intervention. Scholars who study the framing of these issues note that conflicts may always exist when the frames of an issue are in such strong opposition. However, I argue that HAES and other alternative paradigms are making headway in shifting conversations within public health to recognize that the current approach to large body size, as a medical problem to be solved, is doing harm. While this may not mean that conversations between fat activists and "obesity"-focused public health practitioners will be easy, it does mean they are moving toward a shared focus on the lived experiences and quality of life concerns for fat people.

Finally, another key aspect to any future public health work related to body size is the immediate and immense need to make the work intersectional. Fat Studies scholars have long called for work on fatness to be intersectional (Crenshaw, 1991; Hill Collins, 2004), acknowledging that thinness is often in close relationship to other privileges such as whiteness or higher class or socioeconomic status (LeBesco, 2004; Patterson-Faye, 2018). Patterson-Faye, LeBesco and others fighting for fat acceptance recognize fat stigma as one of many control mechanisms of "deviant" bodies that support existing power structures. Scholars arguing for an intersectional perspective on fat stigma recognize that parallels can be drawn to other differences or deviant bodies that have also been framed as biological in nature, such as race, disability, and gender (van Amsterdam, 2013). Pausé (2017) also argues in favour of intersectional thinking and perspectives in studying fat stigma as a social determinant of health. Others such as Ailshire and House (2011) consider intersectionality key in examining trends in body size and how they have been stratified among other lines of inequality over time. While fat politics and public health may never completely agree on the relationship between weight and health, adopting an intersectional approach to the study of these issues would allow each field conduct more robust and ethical research that can positively impact the lives of people around the world across body size.

Notes

1 In most cases, I use quotation marks or "scare quotes" around the medicalized terms for large body size including "overweight", "obese", or "obesity". This derives from a fat politics lens that questions these terms as medical facts. However, I chose not to use quotation marks when describing public health research on fatness (as they do not use these words critically) or when describing critical obesity studies.
2 Although bias and stigma are often used interchangeably in public health, they do have distinct meanings. Bias refers to either inclination or discrimination for one thing or group over another and is a more general term, while stigma draws from sociology (Goffman, 1963) to indicate a trait with negative associations in society. In most cases, the bias terminology in public health does refer to negative associations or attitudes towards fat people.

References

Acharya, S. D., Elci, O. U., Sereika, S. M., Styn, M. A., & Burke, L. E. (2011). Using a personal digital assistant for self-monitoring influences diet quality in comparison to a standard paper record among overweight/obese adults. *Journal of the American Dietetic Association, 111*(4), 583–588.

Ailshire, J. A., & House, J. S. (2011). The unequal burden of weight gain: An intersectional approach to understanding social disparities in BMI trajectories from 1986 to 2001/2002. *Social Forces, 90*(2), 397–423.

Allen, G., & Safranek, S. (2011). FPIN's clinical inquiries. Secondary causes of obesity. *American Family Physician, 83*(8), 972–973.

Amundson, D. E., Djurkovic, S., & Matwiyoff, G. N. (2010). The obesity paradox. *Critical Care Clinics, 26*(4), 583–596.

Aphramor, L. (2005). Is a weight-centred health framework salutogenic? Some thoughts on unhinging certain dietary ideologies. *Social Theory and Health, 3*(4), 315–340.

Aphramor, L., & Gingras, J. (2009). That remains to be seen: Disappeared feminist discourses on fat in dietetic theory and practice. In E. Rothblum, & S. Solovay (Eds.), *The fat studies reader* (pp. 97–105). New York: New York University Press.

Bacon, L. (2010). *Health at every size: The surprising truth about your weight.* Dallas: BenBella Books, Inc.

Bacon, L., & Aphramor, L. (2011). Weight science: Evaluating the evidence for a paradigm shift. *Nutrition Journal, 10*(1), 1–13.

Bacon, L., & Aphramor, L. (2014). *Body respect: What conventional health books get wrong, leave out, and just plain fail to understand about weight.* Dallas, TX: BenBella Books.

Boero, N. (2007). All the news that's fat to print: The American "obesity epidemic" and the media. *Qualitative Sociology, 30*(1), 41–60.

Boero, N. (2009). Fat kids, working moms, and the "epidemic of obesity". In Esther Rothblum, & S. Solovay (Eds.), *The fat studies reader* (pp. 113–119). New York: New York University Press.

Bombak, A. (2014a). Bombak responds. *American Journal of Public Health, 104*(7), e1–e2.

Bombak, A. (2014b). Obesity, health at every size, and public health policy. *American Journal of Public Health, 104*(2), e60–e67.

Brewis, A. A. (2014). Stigma and the perpetuation of obesity. *Social Science & Medicine, 118*, 152–158.

Burgard, D. (2009). What is "health at every size?" In E. D. Rothblum & S. Solovay (Eds.). *The fat studies reader* (pp. 42–53). NYU Press.

Callahan, D. (2013). Obesity: Chasing an elusive epidemic. *Hastings Center Report, 43*(1), 34–40.

Chrisler, J. C., & Barney, A. (2017). Sizeism is a health hazard. *Fat Studies, 6*(1), 38–53.

Cohen, E., & McDermott, A. (1998, June 17). Who's fat? New guidelines adopted. *CNN.* http://edition.cnn.com/HEALTH/9806/17/weight.guidelines/

Cohen-Rottenberg, R. (2015, Jan 13). The problem with person-first language. *The Body is Not an Apology.* https://thebodyisnotanapology.com/magazine/the-problem-with-person-first-language/

Colls, R., & Evans, B. (2010). Challenging assumptions: Re-thinking "the obesity problem". *Geography, 95*(2), 99–105.

Colosia, A., Khan, S., & Palencia, R. (2013). Prevalence of hypertension and obesity in patients with type 2 diabetes mellitus in observational studies: A systematic literature review. *Diabetes, Metabolic Syndrome and Obesity: Targets and Therapy, 6*, 327–338.

Cooper, C. (2016). *Fat activism: A radical social movement.* Bristol: HammerOn Press.

Couch, D., Fried, A., & Komesaroff, P. (2017). Public health and obesity prevention campaigns – a case study and critical discussion. *Communication Research and Practice, 4*(2), 149–166.

Crenshaw, K. (1991). Mapping the margins: Intersectionality, identity politics, and violence against women of color. *Stanford Law Review, 43*(6), 1241–1299.

Dame-Griff, E. C. (2016). "He's not heavy, he's an anchor baby": Fat children, failed futures, and the threat of Latina/o excess. *Fat Studies, 5*(2), 156–171.

Davis, N. (2008). Resident physician attitudes and competence about obesity treatment: Need for improved education. *Medical Education Online, 13*(5).

Dunn, D. S., & Andrews, E. E. (2015). Person-first and identity-first language: Developing psychologists' cultural competence using disability language. *American Psychologist, 70*(3), 255–264.

Eisenberg, M. (2015). Obesity as public policy: Creating and changing the obesogenic environment. In C. T. Morris, & A. G. Lancey (Eds.), *The applied anthropology of obesity: Prevention, intervention, and identity* (pp. 163–184). Lanham, MD: Lexington Books.

Evans, B. (2014). Fat studies. In W. C. Cockerham, R. Dingwall, & S. Quah (Eds.), *The Wiley Blackwell encyclopedia of health, illness, behavior, and society* (pp. 555–557). Chichester: John Wiley & Sons.

Flegal, K. M. (2012). Prevalence of obesity and trends in the distribution of body mass index among US adults, 1999–2010. *The Journal of the American Medical Association, 307*(5), 491.

Gard, M., & Wright, J. (2005). *The obesity epidemic: Science, morality, and ideology.* London: Routledge.

Gardner, R. M., & Brown, D. L. (2010). Body image assessment: A review of figural drawing scales. *Personality and Individual Differences, 48*(2), 107–111.

Goffman, E. (1963). *Stigma: Notes on the management of a spoiled identity.* Englewood Cliffs, NJ: Prentice-Hall.

Guthman, J. (2013). Fatuous measures: The artifactual construction of the obesity epidemic. *Critical Public Health, 23*(3), 263–273.

Hamin, J. (1999). Constitutional types, institutional forms: Reconfiguring diagnostic and therapeutic approaches to obesity in early twentieth-century biomedical investigation. In D. Maurer, & J. Sobal (Eds.), *Weighty issues: Fatness and thinness as social problems* (pp. 31–49). Hawthorne, NY: Aldine de Gruyter.

Hartlev, M. (2014). Stigmatisation as a public health tool against obesity — A health and human rights perspective. *European Journal of Health Law, 21*(4), 365–386.

Hatzenbuehler, M. L., Phelan, J. C., & Link, B. G. (2013). Stigma as a fundamental cause of population health inequalities. *American Journal of Public Health, 103*(5), 813–821.

Herndon, A. M. (2005). Collateral damage from friendly fire? Race, nation, class and the "war against obesity." *Social Semiotics, 15*(2), 127–141.

Hill Collins, P. (2004). *Black sexual politics: African Americans, gender, and the new racism.* New York: Routledge.

Humphrey, L., Clifford, D., & Neyman Morris, M. (2015). Health at Every Size college course reduces dieting behaviors and improves intuitive eating, body esteem, and anti-fat attitudes. *Journal of Nutrition Education and Behavior, 47*(4), 354–360.e1.

Ingraham, N. (2018). Health at Every Size (HAES™) as a reform (social) movement within public health: A situational analysis. In N. Boero & K. Mason (Eds.), *The Body & Embodiment Handbook.* Oxford: Oxford University Press.

Kwan, S. (2009). Framing the fat body: Contested meanings between government, activists, and industry. *Sociological Inquiry, 79*(1), 25–50.

Kwan, S. (2010). Navigating public spaces: Gender, race, and body privilege in everyday life. *Feminist Formations, 22*(2), 144–166.

LeBesco, K. (2004). *Revolting bodies? The struggle to redefine fat identity.* Amherst, MA: University of Massachusetts Press.

Lekkas, P., & Stankov, I. (2014). Framing obesity—Drawing on the margins. *American Journal of Public Health, 104*(7), e1.

Lieffers, J. R. L., & Hanning, R. M. (2012). Dietary assessment and self-monitoring with nutrition applications for mobile devices. *Canadian Journal of Dietetic Practice and Research, 73*(3), e253–e260.

Lillis, J., Levin, M. E., & Hayes, S. C. (2011). Exploring the relationship between body mass index and health-related quality of life: A pilot study of the impact of weight self-stigma and experiential avoidance. *Journal of Health Psychology, 16*(5), 722–727.

Lindemann, K., Cherney, J. L., & Ahumada, J. I. (2017). Disability. In C. R. Scott, & L. Lewis (Eds.), *The international encyclopedia of organizational communication* (pp. 1–8). Chichester: John Wiley & Sons.

Lupton, D. (2014). "How do you measure up?" Assumptions about "obesity" and health-related behaviors and beliefs in two Australian "obesity" prevention campaigns. *Fat Studies, 3*(1), 32–44.

Lupton, D. (2015). The pedagogy of disgust: The ethical, moral and political implications of using disgust in public health campaigns. *Critical Public Health, 25*(1), 4–14.

Mansfield, L., & Rich, E. (2013). Public health pedagogy, border crossings and physical activity at every size. *Critical Public Health, 23*(3), 356–370.

McCormack, J. V., & Burrows, L. (2015). The burden of brown bodies: Teachings about Pasifika within public health obesity research in Aotearoa/New Zealand. *Cultural Studies ↔ Critical Methodologies, 15*(5), 371–378.

Meleo-Erwin, Z. C. (2011). "A beautiful show of strength": Weight loss and the fat activist self. *Health: An Interdisciplinary Journal for the Social Study of Health, Illness and Medicine, 15*(2), 188–205.

Müller, M. J., Braun, W., Enderle, J., & Bosy-Westphal, A. (2016). Beyond BMI: Conceptual issues related to overweight and obese patients. *Obesity Facts, 9*(3), 193–205.

National Association to Advance Fat Acceptance (NAAFA). (2016). Education Resources. https://www.naafaonline.com/dev2/education/index.html

Nutter, S., Russell-Mayhew, S., Alberga, A. S., Arthur, N., Kassan, A., Lund, D. E., Sesma-Vazquez, M., & Williams, E. (2016). Positioning of weight bias: Moving towards social justice. *Journal of Obesity*, *2016*(2), 1–10.

O'Hara, L., & Taylor, J. (2014). Health at every size: A weight-neutral approach for empowerment, resilience and peace. *International Journal of Social Work and Human Services Practice*, *2*, 272–282.

O'Hara, L., & Taylor, J. (2018). What's wrong with the "war on obesity?" A narrative review of the weight-centered health paradigm and development of the 3C framework to build critical competency for a paradigm shift. *SAGE Open*, *8*(2), 215824401877288.

Patterson-Faye, C. (2018). When and where I always enter: An auto-ethnographic approach to black women's body size politics in Academia. In M. A. Hunter (Ed.), *The New Black Sociologists* (pp. 89–100). New York: Routledge.

Pausé, C. (2014). Die another day: The obstacles facing fat people in accessing quality healthcare. *Narrative Inquiry in Bioethics*, *4*(2), 135–141.

Pausé, C. (2017). Borderline: The ethics of fat stigma in public health. *The Journal of Law, Medicine & Ethics*, *45*(4), 510–517.

Petersen, A., & Lupton, D. (1996). *The new public health: Health and the self in the age of risk*. Thousand Oaks, CA: Sage.

Peterson, M., Ellenberg, D., & Crossan, S. (2003). Body-image perceptions: Reliability of a BMI-based silhouette matching test. *American Journal of Health Behavior*, *27*(4), 355–363.

Puhl, R. M., & Brownell, K. (2001). Bias, discrimination and obesity. *Obesity Research*, *9*(12), 788–805.

Puhl, R. M., & Brownell, K. D. (2006). Confronting and coping with weight stigma: An investigation of overweight and obese adults. *Obesity*, *14*(10) 1802–1815.

Puhl, R. M., & Heuer, C. A. (2009). The stigma of obesity: A review and update. *Obesity*, *17*(5), 941–964.

Rudd Center. (2012). Rudd Center for Food Policy & Obesity — What We Do. http://www.yaleruddcenter.org/what_we_do.aspx?id=364

Saguy, A. C. (2013). *What's wrong with fat?* New York: Oxford University Press.

Saguy, A. C., & Riley, K. (2005). Weighing both sides: Morality, mortality and framing contests over obesity. *Journal of Health Politics, Practice & Law*, *30*(5), 869–921.

Saguy, A. C., & Ward, A. (2011). Coming out as fat: Rethinking stigma. *Social Psychology Quarterly*, *74*(1), 53–75.

Samuel-Hodge, C. D., Johnston, L. F., Gizlice, Z., Garcia, B. A., Lindsley, S. C., Bramble, K. P., Hardy, T. E., Ammerman, A. S., Poindexter, P. A., Will, J. C., & Keyserling, T. C. (2009). Randomized trial of a behavioral weight loss intervention for low-income women: The Weight Wise program. *Obesity*, *17*(10), 1891–1899.

Satinsky, S., & Ingraham, N. (2014). At the intersection of public health and fat studies: Critical perspectives on the measurement of body size. *Fat Studies*, *3*(2), 143–154.

Schvey, N. A., Puhl, R. M., & Brownell, K. D. (2011). The impact of weight stigma on caloric consumption. *Obesity*, *19*(10), 1957–1962.

Sharma, A. M. (2017). Critical fat studies and obesity in Canada. *The Lancet: Diabetes & Endocrinology*, *5*(7), 499–500.

Simpson, C. C., Griffin, B. J., & Mazzeo, S. E. (2017). Psychological and behavioral effects of obesity prevention campaigns. *Journal of Health Psychology*, *24*(9), 1268–1281.

Stoner, L., & Cornwall, J. (2014). Did the American Medical Association make the correct decision classifying obesity as a disease? *Australasian Medical Journal*, *7*(11), 462–464.

Teixeira, P. J., Carraça, E. V., Marques, M. M., Rutter, H., Oppert, J.-M., De Bourdeaudhuij, I., Lakerveld, J., & Brug, J. (2015). Successful behavior change in obesity interventions in adults: a systematic review of self-regulation mediators. *BMC Medicine*, *13*(1), 84.

Vallgårda, S., Nielsen, M. E. J., Hansen, A. K. K., Cathoir, K. ó, Hartlev, M., Holm, L., Christensen, B. J., Jensen, J. D., Sørensen, T. I. A., & Sandøe, P. (2017). Should Europe follow the US and declare obesity a disease? A discussion of the so-called utilitarian argument. *European Journal of Clinical Nutrition*, *71*(11), 1263–1267.

van Amsterdam, N. (2013). Big fat inequalities, thin privilege: An intersectional perspective on "body size." *European Journal of Women's Studies*, *20*(2), 155–169.

Vartanian, L. R., & Smyth, J. M. (2013). Primum non nocere: Obesity stigma and public health. *Journal of Bioethical Inquiry*, *10*(1), 49–57.

Wakefield, M. A., Loken, B., & Hornik, R. C. (2010). Use of mass media campaigns to change health behaviour. *The Lancet*, *376*(9748), 1261–1271.

Wann, M. (2009). Foreword. Fat Studies: An invitation to revolution. In E. D. Rothblum, & S. Solovay (Eds.) *The fat studies reader* (pp. ix–xxv). NYU Press.

Ward, P., Beausoleil, N., & Heath, O. (2017). Confusing constructions: Exploring the meaning of health with children in "obesity" treatment. *Fat Studies, 6*(3), 255–267.

Wathne, K., Mburu, C. B., & Middelthon, A.-L. (2015). Obesity and minority—changing meanings of big bodies among young Pakistani obesity patients in Norway. *Sport, Education and Society, 20*(2), 171–189.

Welsh, T. (2011). Healthism and the bodies of women: Pleasure and discipline in the war against obesity. *Journal of Feminist Scholarship, 1*(1), 33–48.

PART 4

Living fat

Part 4 explores the embodied experience of fatness. The personalized narrative of the fat body situates theory as political, social, cultural and personal reality. By exploring what it means to live fat, we must explore how geography, culture, power, position, and privilege inform the lived experience of fat people's existence. There is a necessary bravery inherent in the sharing of these narratives. They demand a recounting of our family's harms, our classmates' taunts, our society's disdain for the bodies we inhabit. To tell the stories of living fat is to give the world an unearned gift. Part 4, "Living fat", asks us, "what stories live in our fat bodies and what stories are placed on us by a thin exalting world?

The opening chapter "Reclaiming voices from stigma: Fat autoethnography as a consciously political act", explores autoethnography as a salient methodology for examining the fat experience by positing that, "A rigorous fat autoethnography … must begin from the basic position that fat is a culturally constructed phenomenon intimately acquainted with broader social norms of embodiment. As such, it is always already intersectional, always in conversation with other forms of identity" (p. 183). Authors Jenny Lee and Emily McAvan remind us that fat identity is shaped and assigned by the same cultural factors that racialize, gender, and sexualize our identities. The construction of fatness cannot be fully examined without understanding the additional intersections at which fat people live and identify. In this chapter, autoethnography is presented as an inherently political and disobedient device but one that might allow us to better see each other as fellow humans. The authors offer the power of this methodology as, "autoethnography might prepare us for new ways of understanding the human" (p. 181).

Activist Kath Read's chapter opens with her reminder that, "I am the world's leading expert on life in this fat body. Yet despite growing media attention on fat bodies, actual fat people are in the minority of the people who get to speak on the topic of fatness" (p. 196). Read asks us to consider how power dynamics in academia often erase fat people from the research done about fatness or use fat people as sites of extraction, taking their stories and knowledge and offering little in return. She shares,

> Our lived experience does not belong to greater academia to investigate, disassemble or pathologise, it belongs to us. We are not whales, to be rolled back out to sea. We do not need conservation. Pity is no more welcome to us than disgust.
>
> *(p. 197)*

Read asks researchers to acknowledge that the lives of fat people are not case studies or papers to hand in, but physical and material realities of pain and triumph, realities that deserve to be treated with care and respect.

Tara Vilhjálmsdóttir examines how Western influence contributed to a national shift toward weight stigma and fatphobia on the small nation of Iceland. She writes, "Icelanders have long had national pride and it is that pride that fuels our incessant need to be better than any other nation in terms of strength, beauty, health, intelligence and conquering new grounds in economics, geothermal power and innovation" (p. 199). It is from this national pride merged with Westernized beauty ideals and products introduced after WWII that led to an increased focus on weight and health and fostered a national push toward a fatphobic media and national discourse. As a pioneering voice in body positivity and fat acceptance in her country, Vilhjálmsdóttir offers hope for those living while fat in Iceland, "While the isolation and smallness of the Icelandic nation made it a breeding ground for fat hatred and healthism, I believe those same characteristics can be useful in turning the discourse on its head" (p. 203).

In Nomonde Mxhalisa's chapter, she examines the painful intersection of fatness and Blackness in her country of South Africa. In a searing recollection of decades of experiences of verbal abuse, assault, and harm at the intersection of her size and racial identity she illuminates the dangers of being coded as ugly by a society that deems the fat body and the Black body as such and thusly, inherently disposable. "Rhodes University was where I first began to understand the poisonous ways my fatness intersected with my blackness and how that intersection meant that I moved through the world as undesirable, as ugly" (p. 206). Mxhalisa unveils how the politic of desirability is at its core about human's access to resource and support by stating,

> When I speak about desirability I'm not only speaking about sexual conquest, ego, or pleasure. Desirability is a core part of how we move in the world; how we are granted access to particular communities; how we guarantee our continued security; how we find tenderness, pleasure and care.
>
> *(p. 207)*

Mxhlisa offers that in a world that denies pleasure and care, we who are deemed ugly must cultivate our own, as a matter of survival.

Bertha Chan details the extreme cultural and familial challenges of being fat in China. In her chapter she recounts how fatness is marked as a social and family shame. Chan's "failure" to be thin is seen as a burden on her community. When she began working in Westernized contexts what was deemed extreme obesity by Chinese standards was the 'average' size of most women.

> When I work with Westerners, I rarely notice the size of my body. I feel released from the constant awareness of being "extremely obese", and people do not assume that every ailment I experience is because of my weight. I am able to live and experience different things; I'm normal in this side of society. In the West, I am of average size, a US size 14.
>
> *(p. 211)*

Chan reminds us of the social construction of fatness which can be conferred upon us and to varying degrees dependent on ever-shifting social, cultural and political factors.

The chapter by sex therapist Sonalee Rashatwar also explores how cultural pressures intensify the experience of fatphobia. Sonalee explores how growing up in an "inter-caste, upper middle class, Indian Hindu family" amplified their experience of body-policing and weight stigma.

"Diet culture created a family-wide surveillance that criminalized my fat child body. Even my younger siblings were deputized into the food police and asked to report to my parents what I would eat after school" (p. 214). Rashatwar's piece illuminates how the familial experience of fatphobia is shaped and often magnified as a result of larger social systems of oppression. "My family was enmeshed in, upholding, and representing a Hindu Indian American dream that was complicit in anti-Blackness, fatphobia, white supremacy, casteism, and Hindu fascism. This shaped how they abused me and chose to control my body" (p. 214). Rashatwar reminds us that living fat is an experience amplified by other systems of oppression and survival necessitates an end to all oppression.

In the final chapter of this section Jason Whitesel reviews the scholarship surrounding gay fat men through the lens of digital media and online communities. Whitesel explores how sub communities like the longstanding Bears, the now defunct Girth and Mirth, and others simultaneously disrupt thin gay male cultural ideals while at times reaffirming stereotypical elements therein. "Thus, the fat-gay male body is both a site of shame, and of stigma resistance and 'embodied contestation' through queer-'fat performative protest' and attempts to reclaim sexual citizenship" (p. 218). The literature elevates how fat-gay men make meaning of their lives through art, pornography, kink, and communities, while acknowledging the limitations of scholarship that is primarily white and western. Whitesel offers the reader a glimpse into definition of fat-gay life by fat-gay men, while inviting the literature of Fat Studies to welcome even more fat-gay bodies to the table.

18

RECLAIMING VOICES FROM STIGMA

Fat autoethnography as a consciously political act

Jenny Lee and Emily McAvan

Introduction

For fat readers, academic prose is often alienating and objectifying. Yet not all academic work need be so. Autoethnographic stories, as Adams et al. state, are "artistic and analytic demonstrations of how we come to know, name, and interpret personal and cultural experience" (2015, p. 1). It denotes a turn to the personal, yet one that does not discard the hard-fought insights of cultural theory and activism. As such, autoethnography has emerged as a powerful tool through which to make sense of the broader social structures that have oppressed fat people. Though we live in a world where fat people are primarily spoken about rather than speaking subjects, autoethnography can give fat writers a voice in an often hostile world. The power and privilege of thin academics often drowns out fat people, but autoethnography can give fat writers a powerful way of not only addressing everyday oppression, but making sense of broader social structures (including discourses) that stigmatise and pathologise. Holman Jones and Harris in *Queering autoethnography* suggest autoethnography might prepare us for new ways of understanding the human, asking:

> could our exercise of empathy for the known become a rehearsal for empathy for the unknown, or even the unknowable? What if that empathy gave way to a recognition of the precariousness and vulnerability of the other that allows all of us—animal, vegetable and mineral—to live out the ethical responsibility to not harm one another?
>
> *(2019, p. 11)*

Writing autoethnography in Fat Studies is an inherently political act, it can be an angry act, a vulnerable act, a scary act, and a courageous act. It is not objective or staid or quiet or obedient. It is often unruly, and exposes our culture for its damaging meta-narratives about obesity. The micro-narratives in autoethnography fight the dominant machinations of the fat hatred in anti-obesity discourse – as a kind of David and Goliath situation. Autoethnographies have power, and stories have the potential to bring forward audiences – the shamed and silenced, or angry, but without the words to express it, to create interactions between the writer and the readers, in social media, in email, sometimes in person at fat markets and community events.

This chapter discusses autoethnography as more than a methodology, but also as a way to create relationships with readers, and as a way of being present and connected in the world. In addition, the chapter considers the emergence of autoethnography in Fat Studies and links to fat activism, ethical considerations related to reclaiming lost, hidden or suppressed voices, and the importance of intersectionality as a central concern in the conversation. The therapeutic value (for readers), and dangers of, revealing vulnerable stories to the world will also be considered. What we argue here is that autoethnography allows for a more capacious understanding of body norms, in particular allowing fat writers the opportunity to address and redress the many ways fat people are denied full subjectivity. The injunction not to harm one another, fully understood, might be an invitation in fat autoethnography to understand the numerous ways that various forms of knowledge, formal and informal, are deployed against fat people as a means of disciplining and constraining the capabilities of bodies and psyches moving through culture – and to change it.

To situate ourselves: Jenny is an Anglo-Australian cisgendered queer fat academic in my early 40s. I grew up in the lower socioeconomic multicultural western suburbs of Melbourne, Victoria, Australia. My education includes undergraduate study with honours, a teaching qualification, and a PhD. Emily is a Jewish Australian transgender queer in-betweenie in my late 30s. I grew up in a lower middle-class suburb in Perth, Western Australia and my education includes undergraduate study with honours and a PhD.

Autoethnography as method

Autoethnography as a methodological practice can be a way to create relationships with readers and being present and connected in the World. We consider autoethnography as a way of positioning readership, the relationship between writer and reader, and reader expectation. Autoethnography positions the writer and reveals the distance from the events or experiences or identity being discussed in the piece.

Adams et al define the goals of autoethnography nicely. It must:

1   Foreground personal experience in research and writing
2   Illustrate sense-making processes
3   Use and show reflexivity
4   Illustrate insider knowledge of a cultural phenomenon/experience
5   Describe and critique cultural norms, experiences and practices
6   Seeks responses from audiences

(Adams et al., 2015, p. 26)

Autoethnography therefore must be understood as an intervention, one that mixes the personal with the pseudo-objective pose of most academic research.

Ethnography has traditionally relied upon the method of "thick description" (Geertz, 1973, pp. 5–6, 9–10), an accumulation of details that help to make sense of the social world. Autoethnography must therefore, in foregrounding personal experience and illustrating sense-making processes, do this through the description of the socially constructed world through which some bodies become constituted as "fat". For instance, an autoethnographic description of a plane flight might note the construction of the size of the seats, which gives rise to a phenomenological experience for some people of being "too" large for the seat as currently made – an experience which might produce feelings of rage, shame and helplessness.

Fat theorist Samantha Murray (2008) has analysed the discourses through which fat becomes legible, using a powerful mixture of Foucaultian and phenomenological inquiry. Putting scare quotes around the word "fat", Murray seeks to challenge "the notion that 'fat' is an empirical fact" (p. 3). For Murray, "'fatness' is not understood as a singular category, but rather is continually constituted and (re)constituted along a continuum of relativity that is governed by a series of gendered, classed, and raced imperatives for normative bodily being" (p. 3). In other words, fat only becomes legible *as* fat as a failure to meet a particular set of norms of embodiment whose criteria are in dialogue with the kinds of ascriptive identity markers that constitute subjectivity in late capitalist modernity. A rigorous fat autoethnography, therefore, must begin from the basic position that fat is a culturally constructed phenomenon intimately acquainted with broader social norms of embodiment. As such, it is always already intersectional, always in conversation with other forms of identity.

Autoethnography as theoretically informed

Yet as we have been making clear, description of the world in fat autoethnography must also rely upon a solid foundation of theoretical knowledge – this is what separates autoethnography from autobiography. There is not simply a choice between doing theory and not doing theory, because everything we make meaning from in the world relies in some sense on theoretical pre-suppositions. These are often strictly normative "common sense", so naturalised so as to go un-noticed *as* a theoretical position. As an intervention into broader social processes of stigmatisation and pathologisation, fat autoethnography must make use of the theoretical tools of Fat Studies, necessarily made intersectional with its roots in feminist, queer, and anti-racist theories. Some fat autoethnographers have used the theoretical framework of Lacanian (Dickson, 2015) and Deleuzo-Guattarian (Leith, 2016) tools to analyse the social experience of fat, but these far from exhaust the theoretical methods of Fat Studies.

How does autoethnography respond to and transform discourse? Fat autoethnography is arguably a response to political context – medical pathologisation, the so-called "obesity epidemic", quotidian fatphobia. This involves a complex rhetorical move on the part of the fat autoethnographer, for as queer theorist Judith Butler has put it, "the norms by which I seek to make myself recognizable are not fully mine" (2006, p. 35). For fat authoethnographers, this means grappling with a set of social norms about the morphology of bodies in which fat emerges as excessive, disgusting, pathologised. The writing of personal experience meets a broader set of social norms, and yet in the case of autoethnography, through the assertion of a fat "I", speaking in the first person, these norms can be challenged, and fat writers can seek to make themselves recognisable (as Butler argues) through a negotiation of new norms between writer and reader. In many research areas this is a political act; it is in Fat Studies.

Autoethnography as social justice

Autoethnography can therefore be considered a methodological practice that seeks to make an intervention into broader discourses of body morphology, which are necessarily experienced as moral. To put it bluntly: a thin body is a moral one, experienced as an achievement, held out as desirable and a model for imitation. In a world of diets, personal trainers and "headless fatties" on television news stories, fat bodies are talked *about*, rather than connected to selves that can speak for themselves. As Foucault argued so importantly, discourse disciplines our bodies in powerful ways, as well as the ways space is organised to discipline and correct wayward subjects. Broader social norms not only delineate an ideal body shape, but stigmatise and pathologise those bodies which least resemble those norms. As Judith Butler has put it, "sometimes the very terms that confer 'humanness' on some individuals are those that deprive certain other individuals of the possibility of achieving that status, producing a differential between the human and the less-than-human" (2004, p. 2). While for Butler, gender and sexual minorities are those groups that are most frequently classed as "less-than-human", arguably it is also the case that fat people are deprived of humanity in similar ways.

It is, sadly, often not the case that academic writing is any different from broader discourses of fat stigmatisation. Medical and psychological pathologisation still reign as the norms of the day, reducing fat people to, at best test subjects, and at worst "bad" or resistant subjects. In any case, a kind of academic ventriloquism takes place, with little space given for fat voices to speak. As a result, fat autoethnography must make an intervention into academic discourse, taking the tools of the academy and reworking them to give new voice to fat life as it is actually lived. As Toyosaki and Pensoneau-Conway state:

> For us, doing autoethnography is a life of self-emplotment. Autoethnographers engage the possible rather than settling in the actual. We do not simply accept the present as it is; rather, we continuously and critically gesture towards how the present might be differently understood in its temporality, in its coming from the past, and in its look toward the future. Autoethnography is the very labor that textures our (inter)subjective selves, the relationships in which we engage, and the communities of which we become a part through autoethnographic storytelling.
>
> *(2013, p. 563)*

Fat autoethnographic storytelling can therefore be seen as not only about telling stories about the world as it is, but of imagining new ways in which the world might be organised to more fully accord dignity and recognition to fat people. Adams et al. go so far as to argue that striving "for social justice and to make life better" (2015, p. 2) is one of the foundational ideals of autoethnographic writing. As social practices, the body norms that Butler discusses that we are thrown into as subjects – that are never entirely fully of our making – might be critically reworked and re-understood through theoretically informed narratives of the self that not only critique the world we live in, but engage collectively with other fat voices into creating a more just, body positive world.

In other words, fat authored autoethnography might raise important ethical considerations related to reclaiming lost, hidden or suppressed voices, and the importance of intersectionality as a central concern in the conversation. This will challenge the hierarchical nature of some research, even some ethnographic research, if methodologically designed and performed by a researcher of a less "othered" or stigmatised identity. It's important to consider ethical considerations around methodology, assumption, design, which questions are asked, and the discussion of data (for example, the "obesity paradox" can only exist if it is assumed that obesity is always bad for you). As Toyosaki and Pensoneau-Conway put it, "when we think of autoethnography as a research methodology, we might risk understanding it solely in epistemological terms – in terms that mark autoethnography as a way of knowing" (2013, p. 559). We can therefore see the importance and significance of autoethnography in Fat Studies, in terms of re-claiming a voice in a field where fat voices are most often left out of research – out of obesity research, out of the development of methodology on reporting "successful weight loss narratives", out of intersectional considerations of fatness, such as cultural background, sexuality, gender identity or disability. Our voices need to be present in the research, not just as quoted persons interviewed, but as the researchers who frame our stories, our experience, and how it relates to the existing research. Autoethnography can shift the hierarchy and put the research and the story/voice back into the hands of the affected group.

Most especially, autoethnography allows the writing of stories for stigmatised groups who have experienced violence and hate. In the case of fat people, this takes many forms, from being firmly entrenched in much of the medical profession to institutional biases that oppress fat subjects in adoption processes, immigration and so on. Tony Adams,[1] in the *Handbook of autoethnography* (2013, p. 21), discusses ostracism, pain and suicide around stigmatised queer identities. He found the intimate, personal and relational work important for queer people who were being harmed by ignorance and hate. In other words, autoethnographic writing is always an intervention, speaking out of the silencing of identities and parts of the self, and this is as true for fat writers as for queer. Stigmatisation, prejudice, rejection and self-hatred separate and divorce a person from engaging in the world in meaningful ways, cause social isolation, and are related to depression. Autoethnography, sharing stories and vulnerability, is essentially connecting to the world, and is a hopeful act. This is particularly important for a stigmatised group like fat people.

Paradoxically, the autoethnographic turn to the self may provide us with a more nuanced understanding of the social. For, as Toyosaki and Pensoneau-Conway say:

> This move to the constitutive nature of autoethnography is key in thinking of autoethnography as the praxis of social justice. At first, the idea of the self as fundamental to social justice may seem contradictory. However, while social justice may be fundamentally *social*, our argument for autoethnography as the praxis of social justice entails an examination of the self who engages in social justice/responds to social justice.
>
> *(2013, p. 560)*

In other words, understanding everyday experience through autoethnography allows us to see broader social structures *as* arbitrary cultural practices, and as a result to change them. The normative power structures that condition academic knowledge – the "objective" voice that very often hides a thin privilege – are able to be reworked, revised, rewritten.

Literature review

Throughout this literature review, the autoethnographies about fat and fatness that are focused on are those that are primarily concerned with the central premise of Fat Studies. The focus is on those autoethnographies that give fat people a voice, and, as stated above, those that address and redress the many ways fat people are denied full subjectivity. The literature review discusses a range of autoethnographies, and how they function to give fat readers a voice or explore fat positive spaces or reveal prejudice. Of course, these autoethnographies can also educate and pose questions for other readers. When structuring this literature review, we considered a separate section to highlight intersectional autoethnographies, and we did create a section for autoethnographies that focus primarily on intersectionality, however upon analysis, many of the autoethnographies engage with intersectionality and are written by authors with multiple intersectionalities, which include disability, queerness, people of colour and class. While some of these articles are discussed separately, others are not. At times the articles are considered by the ways in which they discuss aspects of fat identity, including when interacting in sports contexts, with the medical field or other large institutions of power like immigration authorities, or fat positive spaces and performance. To finish there is some consideration of autoethnographies that discuss fatness but don't fall within "Fat Studies", or perhaps fit better within "Critical Obesity Studies" or "Weight Stigma Studies".

Autoethnography as intervention on institutions of power

Autoethnographies with a Fat Studies focus span a broad range of topics. Some are important and direct interventions on prejudice within public institutions, such as by medical professionals. Others effectively address the history of fat activism, where institutions of power are challenged (Cooper, 2016). Some explore art practice and fat themes that express the artist's approach to a different kind of activism (Harris, 2015). These texts seek to intervene, interrupt and re-educate by giving voice to the experiences of fat people in institutions of power. This includes autoethnography and co-autoethnography written by one of the authors of this chapter. The hefty paper, "Stigma in practice: Barriers to health for fat women" (Lee & Pausé, 2016), takes the reader through the research into prejudice and stigma surrounding fat bodies, disability, the medical profession and healthcare. It was written first in a hotel room, brainstorming our own experiences with our friends, family, and the medical profession. Those life stories were then used to form a piece of writing that takes the reader through the barriers to health for fat women, and what role alternative health paradigms such as Health at Every Size, can fulfil. Among other goals, this paper aims to reveal what is set up to "help" fat people, but in fact creates barriers to their health due to the stigma and prejudice enacted (Lee & Pausé, 2016). It also discusses how fatness and disability intersect to make interacting with the medical profession particularly challenging.

An autoethnography that uses written stories, voice recorded stories and photographs, "'You will face discrimination': Fatness, motherhood, and the medical profession" (Lee, 2019), focuses on the intersection of fatness, pregnancy, motherhood, health and diabetes, and interaction with the medical profession in order to ask: "How can a fat woman have a voice during pregnancy and into motherhood?" (Lee, 2019). This also has a social justice goal – to reveal a voice that felt suppressed and lost during pregnancy and afterwards, and to publish it for other women who might be able to seek a different experience of pregnancy, childbirth and breastfeeding, and also as a therapeutic tool for women who had experienced similar prejudice (or worse), and hope-fully for medical professionals to learn from. This piece takes the reader through the negative experiences of discrimination, to a declaration of a kind of fat activism:

> I feel 'fat defiant' when I think about raising a daughter who can see her mother jiggle her fat in a naked dance, wear a swimsuit to the beach, eat chocolate without saying 'I shouldn't be eating this,' and talk about all the great things our bodies are capable of. 'Fat defiance' is raising my daughter differently.
>
> *(2019, p. 13)*

These autoethnographies, and others like them, do seek social change through the personal stories of the authors, and the theoretical underpinnings. They hope to receive reader reaction and interaction with communities and relevant professionals, as part of the goal of Fat Studies – which is to seek change, and Fat Studies scholars who also identify as fat activists – to act as agents of change in the world. There are autoethnographic examples of this that seem relevant to present here. As a result of publishing the co-autoethnography discussed above (Lee & Pausé, 2016), Jenny was asked to speak on a panel about the medical treatment of stigmatised identities at the University of Melbourne, Australia, medical student conference in 2017. The medical students responded well and there was email follow-up, with one student saying that it was the only time in her entire degree that she had been given such information and stories and there-fore had been able to reflect on her future practice as a doctor treating larger patients. Another example is from 2019, when a young woman in the US contacted Jenny and asked for a copy of a paper she wrote that was behind a paywall, and spoke about her partner being fat and recently diagnosed with diabetes. After several emails, her partner wrote to say that she had given the requested article and the co-autoethnography (Lee & Pausé, 2016) to her specialist doctor, who had been receptive to reading it to further understand the shame and fear of judgement that fat patients face when seeking medical attention, especially when it involves a disease or illness that is stigmatised and linked to fatness, such as diabetes.

A recent powerful autoethnography that also has this potential to create change is Pausé's (2019) work on being denied a resident visa in New Zealand based on her BMI. This paper tackles another large institution of power – the immigration policies in New Zealand. The notion that one's size now indicates future health, not one's current blood work or health history, that the correlation between "obesity" and health has now become a causation of ill health in the eyes of immigration authorities and medical professionals, is explored in this paper. It also reveals the educational and class judgements inherent in Pausé being eventually allowed a resident visa due to her contribution to society:

> I didn't meet the acceptable standard of health. Therefore, to gain a visa, I would need to apply for a medical waiver. A medical waiver would be granted after the immigration officers considered the circumstances of my application and whether there was compelling enough evidence to justify me being allowed to stay and work in New Zealand, even without meeting the acceptable standard of health. To facilitate this process, I hired the best immigration lawyer in the country. Luckily, I had the personal connections to get me in the door of the firm and the financial resources to pay for their services.
>
> *(p. 54)*

In other words, in addition to revealing the difficult path she was forced to take to gain a resident visa, Pausé also highlights that a struggling working class fat person without a public profile would probably not have been allowed to reside in New Zealand. This demonstrates the intersectionality between fat and class, and the increased disadvantage for fat people who are on lower incomes, or do not have university educations or careers that are deemed to contribute to society at a higher level.

Spaces: exclusionary versus fat friendly

The design of spaces for physical activity, and the exclusion of fat bodies from some of those spaces, are part of an institutional prejudice against fat bodies. Beyond this, the attitudes, beliefs and statements about fat bodies also impact other arenas of physical and outdoor activity, and the teaching of physical education at institutions of education. The irony of this is well perceived by fat people – the stereotype that fatness is caused simply by over-eating and not enough exercise, and therefore fat people should exercise, should, based on that principle, lead to fat people being welcomed and encouraged in spaces where physical activity is undertaken, however, often the opposite is true. For example, the dissertation "AbNormAll Bodies. Gender, dis/ability and health in sport, physical education and beyond" (van Amsterdam, 2014) addresses a Dutch woman's experience of sport, exercise, gender and physical education in a school system that doesn't accommodate fat bodies. It addresses the hypocrisy of a society that demands fat people exercise, yet places virtually impenetrable boundaries around accessibility of the spaces that would allow for it. Spaces are also referred to as attitudes that exclude fat people from feeling welcome, in addition to the limitations of the physical space. This discussion of hypocrisy highlights the actual situation for fat people – that there is not a universal benevolent concern for our wellbeing, health and supposed increase in physical fitness, but that, in fact, there is widespread fear of fat, fat hatred, prejudice, and discrimination, and that stereotyping fat people as being fat simply due to lack of exercise and over-eating, is an excuse to label, make assumptions, and justify the superiority and "health" of thin bodies.

As discussed above, spaces can also be referred to as attitudes that exclude fat people from feeling welcome. An excellent example of an autoethnographic article that discusses fat women and physical activity, and fear of judgement in spaces dominated by thin bodies, "Walking to heal or walking to heel? Contesting cultural narratives about fat women who hike and camp alone", by Australian scholar Phiona Stanley (2018), tells the reader stories about what it is like to be fat and to camp alone, how other hikers respond to her and her body, and how she is shamed even in "body positive" spaces. Stanley states:

> Nothing is said this time about my weight, my fitness, my femaleness, my aloneness, or my preparedness. This time: nothing. But I realise how attuned to on-trail, gendered fat-shaming I have become. I anticipate it, always prepared to defend my legitimacy even as my body says that I must be sedentary, unfit, unadventurous, and my gender says that I don't belong out here alone. Fat women's bodies have social meanings, and 'badass solo hiker' is not usually one of them. I feel I have to prove something, and I consciously and constantly perform the role of 'experienced bushwalker' and 'competent outdoorswoman'. Years ago, I was body-normative (slender, fit and athletic), and I know from that time that this on-edge anticipation of never-far-away body shaming was the last thing on my mind. Now, it is the burden that I carry along with my backpack.
>
> *(2018, p. 4)*

Stanley acknowledges that body positivity is not always about the celebration or love of a fat body, "Drawing on these latter discourses, the body positivity strand of the 'diversify outdoors' movement regards fatness neither as something to be battled ('trails not scales!' says *Fat Girls Hiking*) nor as something to be uncritically celebrated" (2018, p. 9). This is an important distinction that complicates the notion of fat acceptance or loving one's body. The fat voices that express doubt, fear, and a sense of failure at not always loving their bodies, are also important in Fat Studies autoethnography. While Fat Studies is related to fat activism, and activists tend to prefer slogans, solidarity, and more unified messages, our role as scholars is not identical to our other role as a fat activists. When we speak or act or write or talk to the mainstream media as an activist, perhaps simpler messages are preferable, to break down dominant ideas about fat, to send messages of self-acceptance and love. However, as scholars, our role as researchers and writers is to question, to complicate, to challenge, even within our own discipline area. Fat autoethnography is an especially strong form because it can marry the two – it can allow for strong voices and strong messages, and it can contextualise, question, theorise, educate, and complicate the stories we tell. Samantha Murray argues that it is not simple, and it is in fact difficult, to find acceptance or pockets of love for a fat body in a culture that hates fat. Murray counters the simplicity of the "love your body" fat activist voices. One early example of Murray's exploration of this concept is "(Un/Be) coming out? Rethinking fat politics" (2005), which takes the reader through her ambivalence towards her body, the pull of fat activist declarations about loving your body, contrasted with the desire to be slimmer, and to engage in fat denial techniques such as wearing control-top underpants.

A further complication, and demonstration of the prevalence of fat prejudice, is fat activists and scholars who work in fields that are traditionally considered to be the realm of thin people, and hence enact body policing of fat bodies. Heather Sykes and Deborah McPhail (2008) in "Unbearable lessons: Contesting fat phobia in physical education" examine fat-phobic discourses in physical education. They argue that the social constructions of fat have worsened compared to the experiences of adults who describe negative experiences of physical education as fat young people. This study is a smaller part of a much larger study which includes intersectional experiences of "heterosexism, transphobia, ableism, and body-based discrimination in Canadian physical education" (p. 68).

Lauren Morimoto (2008) examines the social construction of fat and fatness in kinesiology, researches the intersections between sport, class, fatness and ethnicity in Hawai'i and more broadly, the impact of race on sport. In "Teaching as transgression: The autoethnography of a fat physical education instructor" she discusses being a fat Asian American:

> While the students who did comment on my fatness often expressed surprise at having a fat PE teacher, they did come to see me as a competent, engaging instructor. Surprisingly, depending on what I was teaching, my race/ethnicity appeared to mitigate my fatness, positioning me as a qualified teacher from the onset, i.e. because I am Asian American, I did not have to prove/demonstrate my competence or ability in tai chi chuan.
>
> *(2008, p. 31)*

She quotes from student journals which demonstrates their prejudices, and often how those prejudices are broken down. She finishes with questions and states:

> While I do interdisciplinary work, the fact is, I choose to remain in this field, to carve out space for myself in this community of scholars. However, I am asking some of you to help me pry open the gate and allow me to enter ... not because you should accept the fat girl, but because I have earned my place.
>
> *(2008, p. 34)*

It's an interestingly non-fat-activist call out, however this was written more than a decade ago, which might have impacted the message and how it was presented. It could also be seen as a plea to value her work in the same way that any non-fat Physical Education Instructor would be valued.

In contrast to these autoethnographies that focus on ways that fat bodies and fat people are excluded by limited spaces or attitudes, are autoethnographic articles that focus on inclusive spaces, or go beyond "fat friendly" to be celebratory of fat bodies. Vicki Chalkin (2015), in her chapter, "All hail the fierce fat femmes", in *Fat sex: New directions in theory and activism* is concerned with "two embodied identities frequently marginalised in both heteronormative and queer culture, namely femme and fat", and how a fat beauty pageant event, Hamburger Queen, celebrated these identities. Hamburger Queen included camp performances that parodied both the obesity epidemic and "chubby chasers". It reveals fat activist subculture and community spaces where fat is celebrated:

> The campy parody of the beauty pageant format provided a platform for the contestants to plume and preen, exhibiting their bodies in any way they wished. In a glittering whirlwind of latex, fishnet, sequins and lace, the audience were invited to cheer, marvel, and appreciate undulating bare flesh and rolls of flab that in a world of fat shaming and hegemonic media glorification of thinness are rarely seen. For the contestants,

Hamburger Queen was an opportunity to wear outfits that may be too outrageous, too skimpy, too sexy or too brash to wear out in public in any other circumstance.

(2015, p. 87)

The chapter rightly argues that the event allowed fat femmes to assert themselves as sexual, rather than being shamed and denigrated for not being sexually attractive due to their fat. Chalkin describes her chapter as "performance autoethnography ... drawing together the value of performance as ethnographic object and method" (p. 86). This space and community that is described could perhaps be seen as a performative equivalent of having a "voice" as a fat person.

In "Big girls having fun: Reflections on a 'fat accepting space'", Rachel Colls (2012) discusses her observations as she attends Largelife, a regular nightclub event for fat people and their admirers. Colls contextualises her narrative with theory and a wider discussion of what a fat acceptance space means, however, her narrative could be considered immersive research rather than lived experience. She refers to her research as "participant observation" (p. 23) and an "empirically derived account" (p. 33) and is more concerned with describing the space and the fat women and fat admirers that move within that space than describing her own experience. She rightly points out the limitations of the space and that the event predominantly consists of cisgendered fat women and their male fat admirers. Colls states:

I also always maintained an overt researcher status during the research and told Carol and those people I talked to at Largelife that I was carrying out research on fat acceptance. Conducting research in a fat accepting space and with fat people also meant that my own body size and fat acceptance was often scrutinised and questioned. In comparative terms my body was amongst the smallest in the club space and one FA man actually asked why I was there because I didn't seem fat enough.

(2012, p. 24)

Colls is concerned with exploring spaces that give fat people a comfortable place of acceptance and admiration, to socialise and flirt, which could be considered part of giving fat people agency and a voice in the world. Perhaps articles like this are better considered as ethnography, with the author declaring her own position at times, however, it still acts as an intervention, and a discussion of a fat positive space.

Autoethnography with an intersectional focus

In addition to the autoethnographic articles that have already been discussed as intersectional, there is also autoethnography that creates links between queer and fat experiences (Wotasik, 2015). A number of scholars have contributed to queer and trans autoethnography in recent years (Nordmarken, 2014; Mesner, 2016; O'Shea, 2018), and some fat autoethnography draws on parallels between queer and fat accepting, such as the notion of "coming out". One such excellent example is "Live to tell: coming out as fat" (Pausé, 2012):

Coming out as fat allows the fat individual to embrace the identification of their physical fatness, while throwing off the stigma attached by dominant culture. I find myself drawn to Sedgwick's (1993) expression of coming out as a fat women: being out as fat means declaring and embracing a fat identity, which opens the opportunity to have your body read in new ways, on your own terms.

(Pausé, 2012, pp. 44–45)

As stated, the notion of coming out is borrowed from the queer community, and while fatness can't be "hidden" physically in the way that some cisgendered queerness can be invisible, Pausé discusses the notion of "covering" as a way to contextualise how a fat person could be "in the closet", or assimilate to avoid judgement in a thin-positive, fat-condemning, culture:

> Covering by dieting is only one type of covering performance fat individuals may engage in. Fat women engage in covering when they accept that they do not deserve the same rights as others. Fat people engage in covering when they are willing to endure discrimination, because it is what they believe they deserve as fat people. They are working to make it easier for the fat hating society that surrounds them to tolerate their fatness.
>
> *(p. 48)*

This paper gives voice to an experience that many readers, including fat readers, would not have realised or articulated – that to move through a fat phobic, sometimes fat hating and fat condemning culture, you can do it with shame, or you can throw off the shackles of self-recrimination, throw off acceptance of dieting as a way of life and self-flagellation of a fat identity, and stop using self-judgment as a bargaining chip to gain acceptance as a moral human being who rejects the fat self as an inadequate contributor to society, a drain on healthcare, an insult to mainstream aesthetics. This is an article that is deeply concerned with social justice, and the deconstruction of self-loathing and self-hatred, towards the individual happiness of fat people within a larger fat accepting community, as a social justice issue.

Jenny has at times focused on autoethnography around fat and queer identities, and sexuality (Lee, 2014, 2015). However, in hindsight she considers these articles to fit in a category more like "culturally informed memoir and commentary". Sharrell D. Luckett (2017) in *Young, gifted and fat: An autoethnography of size, sexuality, and privilege* writes the autoethnographic experience of a fat Black American woman with a history of weight loss and gain. It documents the author's attempts to "perform" thin in real life and on the stage and considers intersections of size politics, race and sexuality. It uses a series of confessions, memories and diary entries as well as theoretical writing. The author is a performer and academic, and specialises in African American studies, Fat Studies and acting/directing, and shows the experience of an insecure young Black girl.

There is a real need for further autoethnographies that focus on how fatness and intersectional identities co-exist, that go beyond white, middle-class, able-bodied, predominantly cisgendered female narratives. Unfortunately, the fat scholars with the privilege to have an academic or tenured position, and who are funded to research and write in Fat Studies, are more often white and middle-class, owing to major barriers and discrimination against other identities and cultural backgrounds within the academy.

Other ways of talking about fat

There are autoethnographic narratives about fatness and weight loss that don't utilise the Fat Studies paradigm, such as Santoro's (2012) "Relationally bare/bear: Bodies of loss and love". This autoethnography explores the position of the fat, hairy male body in gay culture and gay bear culture, body image and body love, the desire of other large hairy bodies, and weight loss as part of that narrative. While many of the themes intersect with those of a Fat Studies autoethnography, narratives that include weight loss in order to fit into a culture or feel better about the self don't fit within the Fat Studies discipline area. These autoethnographies are still a valuable contribution to the discussion of the body, however they lack the central premise that we are concerned with here, that of Fat Studies autoethnography as a way for fat scholars and fat allied scholars to have (and publish) a voice that is not "pseudo-objective", is not attempting to eradicate "obesity", is not discriminatory or seeking change in order to better fit within society's expectations or to avoid judgment from the surrounding culture. There are other places where those aims and voices are published and given plenty of airspace.

Then there are autoethnographic papers that fit within Critical Obesity Studies or consider weight stigma as their central premise, for example, Andrew Dickson's (2015), "Re:living the body mass index: How a Lacanian autoethnography can inform public health practice". He discusses how autoethnography can be utilised as a methodology to conduct public health research. The argument is structured around an application of Lacan's psychoanalytic theory which supports and extends a critical understanding of the so-called obesity epidemic and related issues. He refutes the effectiveness of the BMI system and challenges commonly held beliefs about weight and fat in the public health system. These autoethnographic accounts are valuable, however they often don't position the voice of the fat person as central. Another example is Zanker and Gard's (2008) "Fatness, fitness, and the moral universe of sport and physical activity", which describes itself as autoethnography, yet is theoretically framed by Gard and Zanker with sections of life story written by "Lindsey":

> This article represents the culmination of a collaboration between three people: two academics and a woman who, for the purposes of this article, we will call Lindsey. For personal reasons, Lindsey does not wish to appear as an author of this article.
>
> *(2008, p. 50)*

In addition, despite "fatness" being the first word in the title, the stories of Lindsey are about a woman afraid to become fat and living as severely underweight for most of her adolescence and adult life. While there are intersections with Fat Studies, and we considered many such autoethnographies (also see Leith, 2016), we have focused here on autoethnography that gives fat scholars a direct voice to tell their stories and also to frame and contextualise their own stories and voices with Fat Studies theory, and with a social justice focus.

Conclusion: Contextualising the challenge

Autoethnography produces a profound therapeutic value for readers. In its combination of the theoretical and the personal, autoethnography is able to show the place of the subject amidst broader social structures in ways that challenge both dispassionate "objective" academic prose and the dismissal of memoir as "just" stories. For activists, who often (necessarily) seek progress in society, autoethnography can contextualise the ongoing struggle for self-determination and recognition. Moreover, the exposure of vulnerability has a distinct role in creating empathy in and for activism. Vulnerability leads to more meaningful experiences and helps to form deep connections with others. As Judith Butler has put it, "Let's face it. We're undone by each other. And if we're not, we're missing something" (2004, p. 19). Adams et al. (2013) refer to autoethnographic works presenting an intentionally vulnerable subject:

> secrets are disclosed and histories are made known. Given that we ground our stories in personal experience, we write, dance, paint, and perform the ways we have lived. As such, autoethnographic texts open the door to criticisms that other ways of knowing do not.
>
> *(p. 24)*

By opening up and telling stories, being vulnerable, connections are created.

Or to put it another way:

> World-making and having faith in humanity are critical ingredients of doing autoethnography … We get excited about the idea that autoethnography becomes our way of life, an ethical code of being *in* the world, being *with* others, and being there *for* others. In other words, we get excited about the idea of autoethnography as social justice. We wonder how different the world would be, how differently we would move through such a world, if autoethnography were a way of being in the world.
>
> *(Toyosaki & Pensoneau-Conway, 2013, p. 559)*

Autoethnography thus understood produces a profound ethical responsibility to the other – to all others. The vulnerability of storytelling opens its readers to an empathy and what Butler calls *"ways of being dispossessed*, ways of being for another or, indeed, by virtue of another" (2004, p. 19, italics in original).

And yet not all forms of dispossession are equal, and there are some ways in which the loss of self that Butler valourises can be seen as problematic or even harmful. Though academic work requires the privilege of education and the time to write, academic privilege doesn't cancel out vulnerability or the triggering trauma in one's past. Fat Studies academics who are also fat activists will often face judgment, from threats from the public to hostile media coverage. Jenny's concerns over the personal costs of doing media as a fat woman were dismissed as unimportant, as it was "too good for your career, the fat cause, and the university". The mask of "calm" performance, the avoidance of being perceived as an "angry fat feminist", which is reinforced in neoliberal academic settings, might have served Jenny well on national television, for instance, but this had a psychological cost in the aftermath.

As a result, the practice of autoethnography poses certain risks for writers in exposing vulnerabilities – first and foremost in losing the power of "objective" academic authority. "Autoethnographic writing reveals multiple layers of consciousness, connecting the personal to the cultural" (Ellis & Bochner, 2000). Exposing a "vulnerable self" is considered an indulgence on the researcher's part whose unempirical dwelling on his/her own subjectivity/emotions/ignorance/self-doubt/exclusion is conventionally considered unscientific. Positivism, in its "rigorous application" of "instruments" to "generate" objective "data" by "eliminating bias" and arriving at "dispassionate" findings has its obvious uses (Tomaselli et al., 2013, p. 580)

And yet, we can say in the end that, even with the risks that autoethnography might pose for writers, as an academic practice it creates important and significant opportunities for fat researchers. Autoethnography is a powerful tool for writers, and "a way to orient ourselves towards the world as both an enactment of social justice and a response to social injustice" (Toyosaki & Pensoneau-Conway, 2013, p. 559). For activists and writers, the structures arrayed against fat people can be overwhelming at times. But in telling our stories, in exercising our voices, and in seeking ways to uncover other marginalised voices, we can talk back to marginalising and stigmatising discourses in order to create, and build upon, a new discourse.

Authors note

The authors thank Sean Ryan, PhD candidate at Victoria University, researching "fat boys in young adult literature", for his research assistance on this chapter.

Note

1   Though this is a multiple authored introduction, the particular section being discussed is solely authored by Adams, in a move designed to signal the specificity of autoethnographic writing.

References

Adams, T., Holman Jones, S., & Ellis, C. (2013). Introduction: Coming to know autoethnography as more than a method. In S. Holman Jones, T. E. Adams, & C. Ellis (Eds.), *Handbook of autoethnography* (pp. 17–47). Walnut Creek: Left Coast Press.

Adams, T., Holman Jones, S., & Ellis, C. (2015). *Autoethnography*. Oxford: Oxford University Press.

Butler, J. (2004). *Undoing gender*. New York: Routledge.

Butler, J. (2006). *Giving an account of oneself*. New York: Fordham University Press.

Chalkin, V. (2015). All hail the fierce fat femmes. In H. Hester, & C. Walter (Eds.), *Fat sex: New directions in theory and activism* (pp. 85–98). Farnham: Ashgate Publishing.

Colls, R. (2012). Big girls having fun: Reflections on a "fat accepting space". *Somatechnics, 2*(1), 18–37.

Cooper, C. (2016). *Fat activism: A radical social movement*. Bristol: HammerOn Press.

Dickson, A. (2015). Re:living the body mass index: How a Lacanian autoethnography can inform public health practice. *Critical Public Health, 25*(4), 474–487.

Ellis, C., & Bochner, A. P. (2000). Autoethnography, personal narrative, reflexivity. In N. K. Denzin, & Y. S. Lincoln (Eds.) *Handbook of qualitative research*, 2nd ed. (pp.733–768). Thousand Oaks, CA: Sage.

Geertz, C. (1973). *The interpretation of cultures: Selected essays*. New York: Basic Books.

Harris, R. D. (2015). My fat body: An axis for research. In R. Chastain (Ed.), *The politics of size: Perspectives from the fat acceptance movement Vol 1* (pp. 55–70). Westport, CT: Praeger.

Holman Jones, S., & Harris, A. M. (2019). *Queering autoethnography*. New York: Routledge.

Lee, J. (2014). Flaunting fat: Sex with the lights on. In C. Pausé, J. Wykes, & S. Murray (Eds.), *Queering fat embodiment* (pp. 89–96). Farnham: Ashgate Publishing.

Lee, J. (2015). Hidden and forbidden: Alter egos, invisibility cloaks and psychic fat suits. In H. Hester, & C. Walters (Eds.), *Fat sex: New directions in theory and activism* (pp. 101–112). Farnham: Ashgate Publishing.

Lee, J. (2019). "You will face discrimination": Fatness, motherhood, and the medical profession. *Fat Studies, 9*(1), 1–16.

Lee, J., & Pausé, C. (2016). Stigma in practice: Barriers to health for fat women. *Frontiers of Psychology, 7*, 2063.

Leith, V. M. S. (2016). An autoethnography of fat and weight loss: Becoming the Bw0 with Deleuze and Guattari. *The Robert Gordon University Sociological Research Online, 21*(3), 7.

Luckett, S. D. (2017). *Young, gifted and fat: An autoethnography of size, sexuality, and privilege*. New York: Routledge.

Mesner, K. (2016). Outing autoethnography: An exploration of relational ethics in queer autoethnographic research. *Qualitative Research Journal, 16*(3), 225–237.

Morimoto, L. (2008). Teaching as transgression: The autoethnography of a fat physical education instructor. *Proteus. A Journal of Ideas: Sports, exercise and recreation, 25*(2), 29–36.

Murray, S. (2005). (Un/Be) coming out? Rethinking fat politics. *Social Semiotics, 15*(2), 153–163.

Murray, S. (2008). *The "fat" female body*. Basingstoke: Palgrave MacMillan.

Normarken, S. (2014). Becoming ever more monstrous: Feeling transgender in-betweenness. *Qualitative Inquiry, 21*(1), 37–50.

O'Shea, S. (2018). This girl's life: An autoethnography. *Organization, 25*(1), 3–20.

Pausé, C. (2012). Live to tell: Coming out as fat. *Somatechnics, 2*(1), 42–56.

Pausé, C. (2019). Frozen: A fat tale of immigration. *Fat Studies, 8*(1), 44–59.

Santoro, P. (2012). Relationally bare/bear: Bodies of loss and love. *Cultural Studies ↔ Critical Methodologies, 12*(2), 118–131.

Sedgwick, E. (1993). *Tendencies*. Durham: Duke University Press.

Stanley, P. (2018). Walking to heal or walking to heel? Contesting cultural narratives about fat women who hike and camp alone. In P. Stanley, & G. Vass (Eds.), *Questions of culture in autoethnography* (pp. 129–141). London: Routledge.

Sykes, H., & McPhail, D. (2008). Unbearable lessons: Contesting fat phobia in physical education. *Sociology of Sport Journal, 25*(1), 66–96.

Tomaselli, K. G., Dyll-Myklebust, L., & van Grootheest, S. (2013). Personal/political interventions via autoethnography. In S. Holman Jones, T. E. Adams, & C. Ellis (Eds.), *Handbook of autoethnography* (pp. 576–594). Walnut Creek, CA: Left Coast Press.

Toyosak, S., & Pensoneau-Conway, S. L. (2013). Autoethnography as a praxis of social justice: Three ontological contexts. In S. Holman Jones, T. E. Adams, & C. Ellis (Eds.), *Handbook of autoethnography* (pp. 557–575). Walnut Creek, CA: Left Coast Press.

van Amsterdam, N. (2014). *AbNormAll Bodies. Gender, dis/ability and health in sport, physical education and beyond* [Doctoral dissertation] Utrecht: Utrecht University.

Wotasik, J. (2015). Come out come out wherever you are: Queering as a fat identity. In R. Chastain (Ed.), *The politics of size: Perspectives from the fat acceptance movement Vol 1* (pp. 131–138). Westport, CT: Praeger.

Zanker, C., & Gard, M. (2008). Fatness, fitness, and the moral universe of sport and physical activity. *Sociology of Sport Journal, 25*(1), 48–65.

19

SAVE THE WHALES

An examination of the relationship between academics/professionals and fat activists

Kath Read

In the world I grew up in, girls were considered an inconvenience on a family. Ugly girls were considered an embarrassment as well as an inconvenience. And ugly, fat girls were considered a punishment. It was believed intellect was wasted on girl children, and considered stolen or unlawful in an ugly, fat girl child, as though she had somehow robbed one of the other children of what was rightfully theirs.

I fought for every scrap of my education. It was rarely encouraged, regularly discouraged. My voracious hunger for reading was ridiculed and often blamed for my fatness. Consequently, I barely scraped through my senior year of high school, believing the barrage of messages at home and in school that told me that I was worthless because of my fat, female self.

I don't have a string of letters after my name. I have never attended a fine university. The years that many young people spend working hard to fill their heads with an education, I spent scraping a life up on my own from whatever tools I had at hand – elbow grease, that voracious hunger for reading and a base of kind friends who believed in me all along, even when I didn't believe in myself.

But what I have done, is spent a lifetime in this fat body. I have spent almost 40 years learning exactly what the world thinks of fatness. I have lived in this fat body, loved in it, laughed in it, cried in it and tried to erase it through almost every method available. I have spent most of my 40 years being one of the fattest bodies in any given room.

I am the world's leading expert on life in this fat body.

Yet despite growing media attention on fat bodies, actual fat people are in the minority of the people who get to speak on the topic of fatness. People who have no connection to fatness, either personally or professionally are given forum to express their opinions on fatness. While we have Phil (not his real name) the marketing executive denouncing fat people for being angry and aggressive while not taking responsibility for their bodies, and Ryan (not his real name either) the lecturer in politics declaring that fat people are unwilling to "conform to the societal standards of eating" and therefore earn discrimination, we have very few actual fat people who are given space to tell their stories and speak their truths, and when they are, vitriol is poured on them with no support or even acknowledgement of this vitriol from the media that published them.

With this growing media attention on weight and health, more and more opportunities arise for grassroots fat activists like myself to collaborate with academics and professionals in these fields. These can be powerful projects that shed positive light on life in a fat body, and can also open up a world of opportunities for fat activists. But there is still a chasm between how academics and professionals in these fields are treated in comparison to how fat people are treated. To start with, it is as if, for any information about life in a fat body to have merit, it must be validated by an academic or professional, preferably a thin one.

There is a direct relationship between the amount of power and privilege an academic or professional has and how valid their voice is in the media, regardless of any motive or bias that the academic or professional may have.

In the words of Dr Lindo Bacon, author of *Health at Every Size: The surprising truth about your weight*, "People seem to give more credence to my words than if they were spoken by a fatter person – after all, I'm not just saying them to rationalize my existence" (2012, para 1).

For fat activists and fat people in general, these topics are deeply personal and often emotionally charged. Our passion for the topics of life in fat bodies are borne of how deeply we carry the societal assumptions about our fatness. When fat people are vilified or dehumanised, it is personal and we are justified in our emotional reaction to the highly toxic messages that are sent to us about our bodies.

When our voices are dismissed in favour of academics or professionals with thin privilege, it further stigmatises us as human beings, yet even further damage is done when those academics or professionals dismiss us themselves, ignore their privilege and treat our lives and realities as case studies or mere data. Even when making the same arguments that we fat activists make ourselves, the failure to acknowledge their privilege does harm. It gives agencies like the media unspoken permission to dismiss the voices of fat people as well.

It is important for academics and professionals to acknowledge that they are also often in a position of power when working with fat activists. They usually have the decision as to what is published, the ability to choose which media outlets they engage with and resources that grassroots fat activists do not have access to. It is important for academics and professionals to regularly "check in" with fat activists they are working with, to ensure that they are comfortable with the way they are portrayed in the media, that they consent for personal information to be shared at any time and that they have the right to choose what level of engagement they make.

After all, this is not just research to us, this is our lives. Our lived experience does not belong to greater academia to investigate, disassemble or pathologise; it belongs to us. We are not whales to be rolled back out to sea. We do not need conservation. Pity is no more welcome to us than disgust.

But most importantly, no human being wants to feel discarded, and once the research or project is over, and the academics or professionals move onto their next body of work, they must acknowledge that we fat activists do not get to hand in the paper and walk away. We must continue on fighting for our right to a life of dignity and respect. We must continue on, living in a body that general society treats as diseased and defective.

Collaborations between grassroots fat activists and academics or professionals, when conducted ethically, with clear communication and understanding, can result in powerful changes to the quality of life of not just fat people in general, but the activists themselves. But academics in positions of power and privilege must be conscious of, and acknowledge that power and privilege.

After all, it is not their stories that are being told. They are ours to tell.

In the words of the character Aminata Diallo from Lawrence Hill's book *Someone knows my name* in reference to the scholars supposedly fighting for her liberation,

> They [the abolitionists] may well call me their equal, but their lips do not yet say my name, and their ears do not yet hear my story. Not the way I want to tell it. But I have long loved the written word, and come to see in it the power of the sleeping lion.

This is my name. This is who I am. This is how I got here. In the absence of an audience, I will write down my story so that it waits like a restful beast with lungs breathing and heart beating.

(2007, p. 117)

References

Bacon, L. (2012). Because of thin privilege, I am seen as an authority on the fat experience. *This is Thin Privilege* [Tumblr Post] https://thisisthinprivilege.tumblr.com/post/24581541934/because-of-thin-privilege-i-am-seen-as-an

Hill, L. (2007). *Someone knows my name.* New York: W. W. Norton & Co.

20

FAT HATRED AND BODY RESPECT

The curious case of Iceland

Tara Margrét Vilhjálmsdóttir

How do you go from fat hatred to radical fat acceptance activism when you live in a small remote island in the middle of the Atlantic inhabited by a monolith nation of around 350,000 people? A nation that believes it is one of the healthiest nations in the world, but is at the same time a nation in the throes of dieting culture, healthism and fat hatred? (Daníelsdóttir & Jónsson, 2015; Matthíasdóttir, 2009; OECD, 2017).

Iceland is one of the Nordic countries; an island situated in the North Atlantic with a population of 348,850 and an area of 40,000 square meters, making it the most sparsely populated country in Europe (United Nations, n.d.). Most people know Iceland by its rugged nature consisting of black sands, volcanoes, lava fields, geysers, glaciers and harsh climate. The word geyser is actually derived from Iceland's most famous one, Geysir. The weather is windy, wet, and famously unpredictable. In fact, a common saying of ours is "If you don´t like the weather, just wait five minutes". The winters are cold, dark, and long, giving natives optimal views of the aurora borealis, while the summers are mild, short and known for almost continuous daylight. Until the twentieth century, Iceland was among the poorest nations in Europe, relying heavily on fishing and agriculture (Hansson, 2013). While World War II had a devastating impact on most European countries, to Iceland it was the beginning of an economic boom. As a matter of fact, natives adoringly called it "the blessed war" (Hansson, 2013). When British soldiers docked in our harbors on the morning of May 10th in 1940, intent on occupying and denying Iceland to Germany, they were not met with any resistance, nor were subsequent Canadian and American troops. The occupation signaled a long-awaited breach from isolation, introducing foreign objects and customs to natives such as Coca-Cola®, gum and dating etiquette (Hansson, 2013).

Icelanders have long had national pride (Byock, 1992) and it is that pride that fuels our incessant need to be better than any other nation in terms of strength, beauty, health, intelligence and conquering new grounds in economics, geothermal power and innovation. Visitors and tourists can testify that locals are desperate to boast about Iceland being one of the safest, peaceful, and most self-sufficient countries in the entire world! They get to hear how our women are the most beautiful, our men the strongest, and how our national soccer team is the most resilient, making

Iceland the smallest nation ever to qualify for the World Cup finals. They will get a speech on our air and water being the cleanest, our nature being the most breathtaking, and our food being the best but weirdest at the same time. We truly are a nation of extremes. There is, however, one thing they will probably not hear us boasting about: our supposedly record-breaking and expanding waistlines. In 1990 the prevalence of "obesity" for Icelandic women was 9.5 percent and for men it was 7.3 percent (Valdimarsdóttir et al., 2009). According to the OECD's latest publication of *Health at a Glance* (2017) the corresponding number for both sexes in 2017 was around 19 percent, reaching its highest in 2015 at 22.2 percent (OECD, 2015). It was seen as a shame for a nation that prides itself on being the best, the strongest, the most beautiful and the healthiest in the world! As soon as we began gaining weight a national frenzy ensued, spurred on by alarmist headlines in the media. In Daníelsdóttir's 2006 article on the war against fat in Iceland, she did a content analysis of Morgunblaðið, our oldest and most prominent newspaper, examining how news articles shaped Iceland's war on "obesity". The first mention of "obesity" as a serious health threat appears in the paper in 1948 and for the next 30 years no more than seventeen articles were added to the list. Then suddenly in the 1990s, over a hundred articles on "obesity" were published, and in a 5-year span between 2000 and 2005 almost 300 were published. Daníelsdóttir (2006) also noted a change of tone in the articles over time, adding that public anxiety about an "obesity epidemic" did not start to really escalate until the late 1990s when the scare-mongering got worse and statements such as "obesity poses a serious threat to mankind", "obesity is a national disaster", and "obesity spreads at an alarming rate" became a fixture in the media.

This is where our nationalistic pride gets us in trouble and results in social control that can only be achieved in small populations like Iceland. Coupled with our tendency for going to the extremes, the weight loss industry became a booming business avenue in Iceland as the "obesity epidemic" came to life in the media, headless fatties and all (Daníelsdóttir, 2006)! Soon, everyone had to be on that new diet until a newer diet came along the Monday after that. My grandfather only ate fruit for a 6-month period in the 1980s and lost 60lbs (yes, he put them all back on), my grandmother tried all kinds of exotic diet drinks from meal substitutes to aloe vera gels. My mother has never known a time where she wasn't watching her figure. In 1996 one of the most popular domestic television programs involved a 375lb man trying out various diets and slimming methods before coming back to the studio where he stripped naked and went willingly on the scale on live television every week, as if to atone for his sins and hope for a salvation. Sure, he lost a lot of weight and became a national hero. But he also became bulimic (Bjarnar, 2016). You can't sit for a cup of coffee in the break room at work without hearing how we are all doomed to die from gluttony, sloth, and sugar addiction. These days everybody and their grandmas are cutting sugar out of their diets or going on a juice fast trying to "cleanse" their systems, causing headaches and sick days off from work (as shared in many Facebook groups). It seems our biggest threat in the fight against drugs has become sugar instead of marijuana and opioids. Our small country even has its own "The Biggest Loser"-franchise generating record-breaking ratings! (Biggest Loser með mest áhorf, 2016). And if you do not partake in the frenzy you risk being subjected to harsh social penalizations.

I was born in August of 1987, while the great epidemic of "obesity" was picking up its pace. For as long as I can remember, I have been surrounded by societal messages telling me that I could never be happy, healthy, or successful if I was not thin. Everything in my life was doomed to fail as long as I lived that life in a fat body. And everyone and everything around me further solidified that message. I was 11 years old when I was enrolled in my first fat burning boot camp hosted by the guy who lost all those pounds on live television and was eager to spread the gospel. It mostly involved spinning, learning to count calories and keeping a food diary. The kid that lost the most weight by the end of the camp was declared the winner. At the age of 12 years old I started drinking meal substitutes and chewed only one meal per day. At 13 I enrolled in an 8-week weight loss challenge at my local gym. I ended up doing the challenge three times. In my teenage years I didn't sneak out to meet my friends at night. Instead I'd spend all my free time in the gym, going to the classes that burned the most calories. Every single night before bed I went through my Victoria's Secret catalogues, scanning the models' bodies, promising myself that one day I would become just like them. In the end I developed an eating disorder at age 16. I would then become a patient of the psychiatric departments until I was 20 years old.

I was not alone in the belief that my life was worthless if I spent it in a fat body. In 2009, 72 percent of Icelanders aged between18–79 believed that they needed to lose weight, and half of them had tried to in the previous 12 months (Matthíasdóttir, 2009). That means almost three quarters of the nation is dissatisfied with their bodies and are actively trying to "fix" them, at any given time. This is mirrored in the nation's weight stigma. In the most extensive study of weight stigma in Iceland, almost half of the participants with a BMI of, or over, 30 had experienced teasing because of their weight, one third had been treated unfairly and 25 percent had been the victims of discrimination (Daníelsdóttir & Jónsson, 2015). Seventy-five percent of those asked said they knew a friend or a family member who had experienced teasing or been treated unfairly because of their weight, and that same percentage recognized teasing and bullying on the grounds of weight as a common and serious problem among children. Almost 90 percent of the sample believed that lifestyle factors such as lack of exercise, fast foods and overeating, were the most important causes of "obesity", while only around 50 percent believed hereditary factors were important. Women endorsed lower levels of weight bias than men and were also more likely to support legal actions trying to combat weight stigma. They were also much more likely to say they had experienced discrimination because of their weight. Those who showed higher levels of weight stigma were significantly less likely to support legal actions. Thinner participants and those who did not have a personal experience with weight stigma also showed higher levels of weight stigma and less support for legal actions combating weight stigma than those who were heavier and who did have that experience (Daníelsdóttir & Jónsson, 2015). In sum, we see all the typical characteristics and predictors of weight stigma which have been established throughout decades of research, i.e. dispositional attributions, gender differences and the effect of personal experiences on levels of weight stigma (Crandall & Horstman, 2005; Puhl et al., 2008; Schwartz et al., 2003).

It doesn't matter that as a nation we have never been "healthier", at least according to health markers derived from healthism. Healthism refers to the neo-liberalistic trend of situating the problem of health and disease at the level of the individual, meaning that solutions to health problems are also situated at that level. It assigns moral value to the concept of "health" and the "lifestyle choices" we are supposed to undertake to gain optimal "health" e.g. dietary choices and exercise (Cheek, 2008). The mortality rate from coronary artery disease has gone down dramatically since the 1980s and the incidence of coronary thrombosis has dropped nearly 60 percent during that same period (Hjartavernd, 2008). Icelandic nutritional surveys since the 1990s show how our nutritional intake has consistently been getting better and more in line with national guidelines, as consumption of dietary fat decreased while the consumption of fruits, vegetables and water increased (Steingrímsdóttir et al., 2003). Average caloric intake has not changed in the slightest since the 1950s (Daníelsdóttir, 2006) and our leisure-time activity has increased (Hjartavernd, 2008). Our life expectancy has risen from the average of around 74 in 1970 to 82.5 years in 2015 (OECD, 2017) and is expected to keep rising (Hagstofa Íslands, 2017). Only 5.7 percent of the Icelandic population perceive their health status as bad or very bad (OECD, 2017).

Our panic about the "obesity epidemic" is therefore purely a moral one and it is bolstered by our nationalist pride and arrogance. The rules our society has created for fat people, on the grounds of prejudice and stigma, are written in stone. Those rules dictate that all fat people should hate their bodies and that they should do everything in their power to make them smaller. Every and any means to reach that goal are acceptable, whether it involves systematic starvation, wiring our jaws shut, planting a device in our stomach that lets us mimic bulimia or take drugs that help us lose 5–10 pounds at the most, but increase our risk of "obesity-related" diseases, such as high blood pressure. Eating disorders are acceptable and even encouraged in fat people. I remember how my therapist vehemently tried to get me to reject the "delusions" I was so plagued by, during my eating disorder treatment. Those ideas and attitudes were the same ones that were supposed to serve as my thinspiration when I was fat; that I could never be happy in a fat body. The further fat people take their dieting attempts and the more open they are about how they need to "get a grip", the more approval they can expect to get from society at large. That is why so many of us are active participators in our own repression. "Good" fat people are simply trying to gain approval within a society that calls them freaks, an "epidemic" that needs to be eradicated and declared war upon. Indeed, in our healthist society, where health/diet behaviors are assigned a higher moral value than others, "good fatties" can expect more acceptance in society than "bad fatties" (those who do not adhere to societal rules for fat people) (McMichael, 2013; Tidgwell et al., 2017).

When my body eventually started fighting my self-imposed famine, I began gaining weight. Exhausted from fighting my body for most of my life, a body that had become a prison, I started looking for other role models than the Victoria's Secret models. Shortly after, in 2011, I became acquainted with new ideas and new approaches to health and weight. I learned about fat phobia and weight stigma, and how those forces sustain a status quo and serve a highly profitable industry. I stopped interpreting systemic discrimination as a sign that something was wrong with my body and started seeing it as a sign there was something wrong with the system. I educated myself in Fat Studies, wrote articles for newspapers and the internet, met courageous women with whom I founded the Icelandic Association for Body Respect in 2012 and wrote my MA dissertation in social work on fat phobia and the discrimination it entails. I became fat again, came out as a proud fat woman and began challenging the rules society had created for fat people.

In disobeying those rules, I have become a social pariah. In true Icelandic fashion there is no middle ground when it comes to me; people either love me or hate me. Most love to hate me as is evident from the comments section every time I am used as a click-bait in the media. I have been threatened and harassed and been told I belong in the psychiatric ward for daring to utter the fact that long-term weight loss is unsustainable for 95 percent of people. We have invested too much money, sweat, and tears, in the thin ideal and it will take a whole lot of effort for us to come to terms with the fact that it is okay to be fat. Over time my activism has become more intersectional and radical. I truly believe that when marginalized groups come together something amazingly powerful happens. The strength and the courage that survivors of systematic discrimination bring to the table can never be underestimated. It is indescribable. For the past year I have also been reading up on the history of the fat acceptance movements. It has been illuminating, depressing, infuriating, and inspiring, all at the same time. It has been an emotional roller coaster learning that fat acceptance movements go as far back as the 1960s, and how much effort so many people before me have put into the fight. Sometimes I feel like it is hopeless, especially when I see that so many of our new "solutions" to the "obesity epidemic" are actually being recycled over and over again. They are never successful, and they are always harmful, but still it seems like people never learn. That is how deep our society's fat hatred goes.

They would rather see us suffer; they would rather amputate a perfectly healthy organ from our bodies; they would rather see us dead than fat. This battle is not fought in the name of "health", it never has been. In fact, the entire healthcare system has utterly failed us in their endeavor to slim us down. Turns out the Hippocratic oath is only valid when the patients are not fat.

The fat acceptance movement had made pretty good headway in the U.S. and the U.K. when the concept of the "obesity epidemic" appeared just before the millennium leading us to be inundated with prophecies of doom and death, slowing it down considerably. There was just no way to keep up with the train of Obesity.inc at the time. However, at this time in history I feel like we are finally making some strides again. The advent of the internet and social media has helped enormously and recently we have made amazing gains in the fight here in Iceland. As an example, the words "body respect" and "weight stigma" were literally unheard of just 5 years ago, while today they have become a part of our daily vocabulary. In fact, the Icelandic translation of "body respect"; "líkamsvirðing", was one of ten words nominated by the Icelandic National Broadcasting Service and the University of Iceland to be voted as the "word of the year 2017" (Þráinsdóttir, 2017). Sadly, it did not win but the nomination shows the impact it has had on Icelandic culture. In 2015 Sigrún Daníelsdóttir, weight stigma activist and the founder of the Body Respect movement in Iceland, hosted the Weight Stigma Conference marking even bigger shifts in the conversation on weight stigma in Iceland. It was sponsored by the City of Reykjavik as part of the celebration marking 100 years of women's suffrage in Iceland (Weight Stigma Conference, 2016). The following year Reykjavík included weight as a protected category in its human rights policy, following in the footsteps of only a handful of other cities worldwide (Weight Stigma Conference, 2018). This inclusion has opened a door for further activism and the possibility to take it to the next level. In October 2019 I was invited to attend a meeting of Reykjavík City's Council for the Prevention of Violence (Ofbeldisvarnarnefnd Reykjavíkurborgar). There I got the chance to speak on the systemic discrimination fat people face and how that can result in violence, especially pertaining to bullying, domestic abuse and sexual violence. My speech was very well received and met with enthusiasm on behalf of the city to fight weight stigma and the violence it begets (Ofbeldisvarnarnefnd, 2019). I have already been invited to educate professionals as well as non-professionals working with vulnerable groups on this particular type of violence. While the isolation and smallness of the Icelandic nation made it a breeding ground for fat hatred and healthism, I believe those same characteristics can be useful in turning the discourse on its head. And so, we will keep fighting and hopefully one day Icelanders will break yet another record – managing to reduce the rate of weight stigma dramatically, making us the model nation for human dignity and respect. Now, that is going be something to boast about!

References

Biggest Loser með mest áhorf. (2016, 15 March). Mbl.is. https://www.mbl.is/folk/biggest-loser/2016/03/15/biggest_loser_med_mest_ahorf/

Bjarnar, J. (2016, Sept 10). Uppgjör Gauja litla við offituna og sviðsljósið. http://www.visir.is/g/2016160909751

Byock, J. (1992). History and the sagas: The effect of nationalism. In G. Pálsson (Ed.), *From sagas to society: Comparative approaches to early Iceland* (pp. 44–59). London: Hisarlik Press.

Cheek, J. (2008). Healthism: A new conservatism? *Qualitative Health Research, 18*(7), 974–982.

Crandall, C. S., & Horstman, A. R. (2005). Attributions and weight-based prejudice. In K. D. Brownell, R. M. Puhkl, M. B. Schwartz, & L. Rudds (Eds.), *Weight bias: Nature, consequence, and remedies* (pp. 83–96). New York: The Guilford Press.

Daníelsdóttir, S. (2006). The obesity war in Iceland. *Health at Every Size, 19*(4), 207–216.

Daníelsdóttir, S., & Jónsson, S. H. (2015). *Fordómar á grundvelli holdafars í íslensku samfélagi*. http://www.landlaeknir.is/servlet/file/store93/item28261/Holdafarsfordómar_ skyrsla_des.2015.pdf

Hagstofa Íslands. (2017, Oct 30). Íbúar verða 452 þúsund árið 2066 [Press release]. https://hagstofa.is/utgafur/frettasafn/mannfjoldi/mannfjoldaspa-20172066/

Hansson, R. D. (2013). Áhrif hernáms Breta á Reykjavík, Akureyri og Seyðisfjörð. *Skemman*. https://skemman.is/handle/1946/16442

Hjartavernd. (2008). *Handbók Hjartaverndar*. http://www.hjarta.is/Uploads/document/Timarit/Handbok%20Hjartaverndar.pdf

Matthíasdóttir, E. (2009). *Sátt Íslendinga á aldrinum 18–79 ára við eigin líkamsþyngd*. https://www.landlaeknir.is/servlet/file/store93/item11598/m_lokaeintak_15_6_09.pdf

McMichael, L. (2013). *Acceptable prejudice? Fat, rhetoric and social justice*. Nashville, TN: Pearlsong Press.

Ofbeldisvarnarnefnd. (2019). Item 1: Kynning á fitufordómum og ofbeldi. In *Minutes of Reykjavík's city council for prevention of violence 14 October 2019*. Reykjavík City: City Hall.

Organisation for Economic Cooperation and Development (OECD). (2015). *Health at a Glance 2015* (OECD Indicators). https://doi.org/10.1787/health_glance-2015-en

Organisation for Economic Cooperation and Development (OECD). (2017). *Health at a Glance 2017* (OECD Indicators). https://doi.org/10.1787/health_glance-2017-en

Puhl, R. M., Andreyeva, T., & Brownell, K. D. (2008). Perceptions of weight discrimination: prevalence and comparison to race and gender discrimination in America. *International Journal of Obesity, 32*(6), 992–1000.

Reel, J. J., & Bucciere, R. A. (2010). Ableism and body image: Conceptualizing how individuals are marginalized. *Women in Sport and Physical Activity Journal, 19*(1), 91–97.

Schwartz, M. B., Chambliss, H. O., Brownell, K. D., Blair, S. N., & Billington, C. (2003). Weight bias among health professionals specializing in obesity. *Obesity Research, 11*(9), 1033–1039.

Steingrímsdóttir, L., Þorgeirsdóttir, H., & Ólafsdóttir, A. S. (2003). *The Diet of Icelanders* (Dietary Survey of The Icelandic Nutrition Council 2002 Main findings). https://www.landlaeknir.is/servlet/file/store93/item11603/skyrsla.pdf

Tidgwell, T., Friedman, M., Rinaldi, J., Kotow, C., & Lind, E. R. (2017). Introduction to the special issue: Fatness and temporality. *Fat Studies, 7*(2), 115–123.

United Nations. (n.d.). World Population Prospects – Population Division – United Nations. https://population.un.org/wpp/DataQuery/

Valdimarsdóttir, M., Jónsson, S. H., Þorgeirsdóttir, H., Gísladóttir, E., Guðlaugsson, J. Ó., & Þórlindarson, Þ. (2009). *Líkamsþyngd og holdafar fullorðinna Íslendinga frá 1990 til 2007*. https://www.landlaeknir.is/servlet/file/store93/item11583/Holdafar.skyrsla.25.sept.pdf

Weight Stigma Conference. (2016, Oct 18). News: Reykjavik protects against weight discrimination in new legislation. https://stigmaconference.com/2016/10/18/news-reykjavik-protects-against-weight-discrimination-in-new-legislation/

Weight Stigma Conference. (2018, Mar 22). Reykjavik adds "weight" as a protected category to equality regulations. https://stigmaconference.com/2018/03/21/reykjavik-adds-weight-as-a-protected-category-to-equality-regulations/

Þráinsdóttir, A. S. (2017, Dec 18). Hvert er orð ársins 2017? http://www.ruv.is/frett/hvert-er-ord-arsins-2017

21

DESIRABILITY AS ACCESS

Navigating life at the intersection of fat, Black, dark and female

Nomonde Mxhalisa

My first year at Rhodes University I loved partying at a dingy but fantastic spot on campus called the Union. Coyote Ugly was brand new and a massive hit and just about every white girl on the planet was dancing on tables as a consequence. The Union is where I, ecstatic and gleeful, joined them in the table dancing. I was still incredibly naïve about my place in the world. I had been a child in the 80s, been tear gassed several times by the Apartheid police before the age of 8, but my parents had made it a priority to create a cocoon around us at home where race and racism rarely touched us. When it did it was jarring, ugly, and violent but I was always able to retreat from those moments. And so, my greatest hurt, the thing that wounded me worst in those early years, was my fatness. The attacks on my fatness were made by family and community members, friends and loved ones. My fatness was the tragedy of my young life – the hideous failure nobody would let me forget. My race, even though I was raised in such an incredibly politically charged and dangerous situation, was a distant worry because the ones attacking my blackness were large, white men perched atop giant, grey caspers, rolling through our streets carrying guns. They were not my family or community. Most times they barely felt real. From my childish perspective they were almost mythically dangerous – like boogeymen that every now and then would inconveniently materialise and wreak havoc.

And so I knew absolutely that I was despised for my fat body and that this revulsion was felt by everybody, no matter the race, gender, or age. During Physical Education at school I did a forward tumble and landed badly on my neck. I still remember the piercing nature of the pain in my neck and back. It winded me and I lay on the little green rubber mat gasping, trying to hold the tears back. The other children laughed hysterically and when I asked why, the teacher who was giggling along with them, said "Well you looked so funny folded over like that cos you're so fat. Don't worry when you lose weight they won't laugh at you anymore." I remember being 10 and drinking from the water fountain at school. You had to bend forward fairly far to sip at the water and queues always formed around the fountains as there were not many on school grounds. The girls behind me were giggling – I heard them as I drank – and then suddenly a cold, sharp nailed finger stabbed at the fat roll on my neck. "Eeww that is disgusting! Why is your neck like that? It is so black and fat! You need to scrub your neck you're so dirty!" I clutched a protective hand over my nape, drowning in the hot rushing ache of shame, and walked away. That night I rubbed at my skin with methylated spirits till the little folds of my fat neck bled and crusted over. When I was 17 a boy I really liked held the door open at the movies for my friend to walk through and when I went to follow her he slammed it in my face. He and his friends looked at me through the glass and laughed till they were bent over with glee. By age 8 my general state of being fat and revolting was an accepted fact in my mind and soul. It was only when I went to Rhodes University that I truly began to understand how utterly despised I was for my race too.

Rhodes was where I first learned that racism did not just manifest as the white boys spitting on us on the bus to the library or the other white boys trying to run us over with their motor-bikes in the park. Racism was subtle and insidious and incredibly hard to name at times but I still knew it and I still felt it. Rhodes University was where I first began to understand the poisonous ways my fatness intersected with my blackness and how that intersection meant that I moved through the world as undesirable, as ugly.

One night my friends had gone home earlier than I wanted to and I remained at the Union on my own. The Union was a laid-back oasis of bare foot dancing and revelry. It wasn't safe. Rhodes University Campus was not safe for women as a whole – but nights at the Union were so easy and spontaneously joyful that I didn't think about safety when I was there. Also, because our campus was tiny, I knew several of the girls still dancing it up, as they were in my residence, and so I didn't feel alone even after my own group departed. Creed was blaring out the speakers. I was singing at the top of my lungs, every bit of me consumed in ecstasy, just lifted in that way when music and movement come together to give you a glimpse of heaven. And then this huge, blonde, white boy grabbed me and stuck his tongue in my mouth.

It was a moment and then it was over. It left me reeling. I felt sick. The slime of his saliva on my lips, the taste of beer and ash left in my mouth. I gagged, staggering away from him and climbing down off the table. I had never been kissed before and I had never expected it to feel like an assault. One of the girls I was in residence with grabbed my arm. "Why'd you stop dancing? Are you ok?"

I shook my head no, feeling stupidly tearful. "That boy kissed me and he did not ask," I responded, blinking the wetness away.

She looked at who I was pointing at. He was with a group of other boys. They were laugh-ing, hysterically, their eyes wide with malicious delight, and I felt this sinking awfulness from knowing absolutely that they were laughing at me.

She turned back to me; eyebrow raised sceptically. "Are you sure it was that guy? His girl-friend is really pretty."

I turned and hurried away then, something cold and heavy sitting on my lungs.

It was the first time somebody dismissed a moment of sexual violence against me as untrue because I am ugly. It was not the last.

When I call myself ugly, I would like to assure you that I am not waiting, heart aquiver, for reassurance from somebody, anybody, that I am not ugly. I really love the way I look. When I call myself ugly, I mean that I move through this world in a fat, black, dark skinned, female body and those elements combined mean that I am constructed as ugly because none of the things that I am fit our society's white supremacist ideals and standards of beauty. I understand that to many, my physical body is hideous and as a consequence, many of my interactions begin from this place of physical ugliness. As a child and a teenager I struggled with what moving in this body meant for my self-esteem and joy but as I became more and more aware of privilege – the privilege I have and do not have – I realised how my perceived ugliness and lack of desirability could impact not just my self-confidence and fuckability – but my safety, my financial opportunities, and my access to competent and concerned medical care, health, and longevity.

What happens when people still believe that rape and sexual violence is motivated by desire and desirability is that people who are ugly become liars when we speak on our experiences of unwanted sexual advances.

One evening as I was heading home from work the driver of the taxi I was in tried to kidnap me. He refused to drop me at home and drove past my stop. This avalanche of rage and terror blindsided me when I realised what was happening. I yelled – the sound felt like it was coming out of my soul – and hit him over an over with my hand bag and my fists while he was driving. He raised a hand to try to stop me while keeping us on the road and I bit hard into his arm, spitting out the blood that welled from his wound. He finally came to a screeching halt on the side of the road and I rushed out of the vehicle, sobbing hysterically. I told my employer about it the next day, tears and rage still lodged in my throat, and she said I should enjoy the attention because I would get less and less of it as I got older.

Desirability does not only mean access to sex and pleasure, which is why I roll my eyes for days when I speak on desirability as access and people respond with: "You cannot say I'm oppressing you just because I don't want to fuck you." When I speak about desirability I'm not only speaking about sexual conquest, ego, or pleasure. Desirability is a core part of how we move in the world; how we are granted access to particular communities; how we guarantee our continued security; how we find tenderness, pleasure and care. And speaking on it is not a condemnation of people who won't have sex with those of us who are ugly. It is a condemnation of the way we are denied security and validation. It is a judgment of a system that makes us vulnerable outsiders and then mocks, trivialises, and violates our attempts at building communities of love and safety for ourselves. Our ability to survive and thrive is based on how our various privileges and oppressions come together or intersect and this is why the concept of intersectionality is so crucial in conversations about desirability.

Intersectionality is a framework created by Kimberlé Williams Crenshaw, an American civil rights lawyer and a leading scholar of critical race theory. Intersectionality speaks to the fact that we are not an identical group with identical histories, contexts, privileges or realities. Intersectionality allows for a clearer view of our differing and varied identities and the ways in which those identities meet and overlap to create our unique perspectives of, and engagement with, society (Crenshaw, 1994). Coming to an understanding of intersectionality was how I finally began to make sense of the ways I moved in the world and the way people reacted to and treated me. It was critical to my unpacking years of voiceless, nameless pain and the beginning of being able to give words and sound to my resistance to my oppression.

The first time somebody made fun of my dark skin was when I was 5. He was an old acquaintance of my father's and I remember him roaring with laughter when he saw my face. "Meneer!" he chortled, poking my nose, "And then this dark, ugly little one! You ruined her! She inherited everything about you! How is she going to cope in this world with her sister so pretty and her looking just like you! She's dark dark! Man! And that nose!"

I sat there wondering why my tummy and throat suddenly hurt so much. I kept wondering why my dad was laughing with him. I looked at my sister then and for the first time compared our skins. Hers was yellow and mine dark – gone a kind of green-black from days spent in the summer sun. That is the first memory I have of hating my skin. I dreamt for months after that of taking a pair of scissors and cutting off my nose.

Whenever I go to get my hair done, the owner of the salon my hair lady works at is always trying to get me to buy her skin bleaching creams. It has turned her a raw kind of pinky-yellow and she assures me that since she transformed her skin, she transformed her life. She is dating a wealthy man now who helped her to finance her hair shop and she says, often, that she never would have gotten him if she had remained as dark as I am. She regularly proclaims: "My sister, the men love a big woman but you cannot be big and dark my sister – you need to be big and fair! Then you won't be able to keep them away!" I constantly assure her that I am content with my love life and my complexion and she laughs and promises me that until I have a ring on my finger and a baby on the way there is no such thing. I confess I love seeing her joy. She bought it with bleached skin and the risk of cancer, yes, but she is a joyful, fat, black woman realising her dreams and I cannot feel grief when I am with her. I celebrate her victory even as I mourn what she had to do to win it.

Nothing makes me angrier than the way desirability has impacted my pocket. If you have lived even one day as an ugly human being you know that creeping sense of being denied and dismissed because you are too fat or too dark or both. The worst thing about this feeling is that most times it is impossible to prove that you have been discriminated against based on your looks. Several years ago, a friend at an executive level encouraged me to apply for a position in the company she worked for. She did not inform her colleagues on the interview panel of our relationship. I arrived the next day, perfectly polished and loving my new dress and heels, glowing with confidence. The moment I walked into the room I felt the ice settle over the gathered panel. I shook off the odd sense of gloom, decided it was my imagination, and proceeded to blow them away. The interview went extremely well and the writing test I submitted afterwards clearly impressed them. However, I did not get the job. I was bewildered because I had been fantastic – modesty is not a problem I suffer from – but I bit my tongue, bided my time and waited for her to call me. We met, two weeks later, over lunch and she told me, with rage glinting in her eye, that the panel had decided not to employ me based on the fact that they doubted my ability to perform the job because my size caused them to question my energy levels. They had said: "We don't want her getting sick or sleepy on the job. We really need somebody who can bring vigour to the role."

It hurt to hear what she said. It felt like reopening an old wound just barely healed. But it was also oddly satisfying because finally, I knew that all those times I had a sneaking suspicion that I did not get the job or promotion because of my fatness or blackness or both was real, it was true. I was not imagining the prejudice or the judgment. I was not fabricating the ways my perceived lack of desirability had doors slamming in my face.

At least during job applications, they have to pretend. Doctors and nurses don't even pretend to not disdain fat patients. As a fat person in need of medical care you are not afforded even the façade of good manners. When I was 15, I had a cough that turned into bronchitis. My dad took me to the doctor to get me checked out and medicated. I remember it was right after school and I was wearing our summer uniform. We wore these little blue dresses with white ankle socks and black shoes. I was already wearing the largest size uniform they had, an 18, and it was tight on my breasts and arms. It had a zip on the side and the zip stuck sometimes so I was a little anxious about getting it zipped up again when the doctor was done with the exam. I walked into the examination room and I remember the chill and the smell of rubbing alcohol. The doctor was this tiny blonde lady with her hair cut in a curly bob. I smiled and greeted her cheerfully. She did not return the greeting.

"Take off your clothes," she said, her back to me as she scribbled on her chart. I wriggled out of the top of the dress and let it pool at my waist. She turned back and said, coldly, "No take it all off."

That was weird but I shrugged mentally and stepped out of the dress.

She looked me over silently and so I began to speak. "I've had a cough now for – "

"My God do you see how big you are? How old are you? You're enormous! I just saw a 60-year-old gogo smaller than you!"

I was in shock. I giggled nervously. I had no idea how to process what she was saying or how to react. My stomach clenched, pain lancing through it as humiliation rose to my throat.

"Your chart says you weigh 80kgs! By the time you're 30 you'll be too fat to be weighed on a normal human scale. We'll have to take you to the train station and weigh you on those scales they weigh cargo on – or the zoo where they weigh elephants! Do you want that? Do you want to weigh the same as an elephant?"

"No," I whispered, my mouth like the desert.

"Do you have a boyfriend? Don't bother I know you don't. Nobody wants to touch a body like that. Don't you want children and a family? Don't you want a husband? How are you going to find one looking the way you do? You're going to die alone."

She stared at me, mouth curled into this vicious little smile. The silence went on. I finally looked away and put my dress back on.

"Lose the weight. You still have a chance. Next time I see you I want you to be at 50kgs."

She gave me a prescription sheet. I said, "Thank you doctor," and I left. She never examined me. She never touched me. I carried her revulsion around inside me for years. I still hate visiting doctors. Every time is a battle. Every time I know I have to advocate for myself and insist that they focus on my actual health and not the fat they despise so much. It is truly terrifying how many medical professionals are willing to ignore even fatal health issues in favour of talking weight loss when the problem has nothing to do with the patient's weight. If you are fat or black or both do not let doctors kill you. Do not let them ignore your pain. Do not allow them to trivialise your hurts. Demand fair treatment. Only you can fight for your health and longevity.

Ugly is not easy. But ugly is also not all that I am. It is not all that you are. The world constructs and categorizes us but we are also responsible for the creation of our realties. You have to believe in your own magic; in your own wildness; in your own wanton wonderfulness. I survive this world because I try very hard not to lie to myself about people and situations and my own motivations. I *thrive* in this world because I give myself permission to be miraculous; to be sexy and spectacular. I claim all the ways I am unique and marvellous. I savour all the ways I am unspeakably, deliciously beautiful. I have grown into and crafted the woman I am and I love every contrary, juicy, tender, raw part of myself, no matter what anybody who is not me might feel about that. I understand and recognise the way the world sees me but, ultimately, I know that my construction of myself is the only one that matters.

References

Crenshaw, K. W. (1994). Mapping the margins: Intersectionality, identity politics, and violence against women of color. In M. A. Fineman, & R. Mykituik (Eds.), *The public nature of private violence* (pp. 93–118). New York: Routledge.

22

THE IMPACT OF BEING A FAT CHINESE WOMAN IN HONG KONG

Bertha Chan Hiu Yau

I am one of the very few fat acceptance and body positivity advocates in Hong Kong. Struggling to reach a "healthy" weight and BMI my whole life, I face discrimination in many aspects of my daily living. Be it finding a job, looking for a spouse, or finding clothes to wear. Everything is telling me that I am abnormal, being a fat Chinese woman in Hong Kong. I am not thin enough to be normal, not fat enough to be plus size, or not fit enough to be called curvy; but from the doctor's point of view, I am obese in Hong Kong. At the same time, I am considered average size in the West.

Why do I emphasise on being a fat "Chinese" woman in Hong Kong, and not just a woman in Hong Kong? It is because being fat in Hong Kong is different from being fat somewhere else. According to the Hong Kong government website – Centre for Health Protection, it states that "For Chinese adults living in Hong Kong, BMI from 23.0 to 25.0 kg/m2 is classified as overweight, and BMI 25.0 kg/m2 or above is classified as obese" (Centre for Health Protection, 2019, para 1).

As a Chinese person, we are already classified as obese at a BMI of 25 or above, and not 30 as designated by the World Health Organisation (2018). It means that a person who is 5'5 (165cm) and weighs over 150.5lbs (approximately 68kg), will not just be overweight, but obese. And for me, being 5'5 and around 200lbs, I am extremely obese and it's apparently life-threatening and I may die any minute, according to the BMI measurement in Hong Kong.

According to the Centre for Health Protection, "Obesity increases the risk for a number of chronic diseases, such as hypertension, heart diseases, hypercholesterolemia, diabetes mellitus, cerebrovascular disease, gallbladder disease, osteoarthritis, sleep apnoea and some types of cancer (breast, prostate, colorectal and endometrial)" (2019, para 2). Most people accept this warning and believe that being fat or "obese" is the same as being unhealthy. That it leads to an early death. That fat people, essentially, are worthless.

I have been told my whole life that I am an irresponsible person, I am unhealthy because I am fat. This is not because I have an illness or a disease or am unwell, but because potentially I am going to have all of the above diseases mentioned, as I am "extremely obese". Which means I am going to suffer when I get older, and I should not expect to live a normal lifespan. My knees are going to give up on me and I will be a burden for the people who love me. I won't be able to take care of my elderly family members as expected, because I will be the one needing care instead. I need to get health insurance because nobody else will take care of me and I do not wish to become a burden to my family. No, I am not being negative, these are not my own words. These are not my original thoughts, these are words and thoughts that I hear constantly, spoken by my family, by strangers, by healthcare workers, and people in the society and now they are in my head as if I planted them in there. Health and weight are some of the most popular topics for gossip. Commenting on someone's weight is common in Asia, even when that someone is a stranger.

They all keep reminding me that I am going to die sooner than everyone else and suffer a horrible death. And they believe this because the government and society have told them so, too. Comments like this, born of misconceptions and government propaganda, cause me great distress and pressure. They have stopped me from living a life I enjoy; interfered with my development since I was a child. I did not have a normal childhood, adolescence, or emerging adulthood.

I became fat late in my childhood, and before that, no one ever focused on my size or how I looked; I was just a kid. At one point, though, my body became bigger. My family demonstrated their love by providing me and my siblings with a helper (a nanny), and that helper believed in feeding. My parents, in the entertainment business, were rarely home, especially in the evenings and on the weekend. We had a running tab at the store downstairs, that our Dad paid off every month. I could walk in and take whatever I wanted; candy, chocolate, ice cream. Anything I wanted. This formed my habits and relationship with food. I underwent puberty early, so that contributed to my body being different, and more developed, than my classmates and friends. As my body became bigger, I became a target for sexual harassment from strange men in public, especially while riding public transport. Leering, sexually hostile language, groping; these were common occurrences for me as a teenager. I changed my style to that of a tomboy, to try and protect myself from unwanted sexual attention. I only began dating in my thirties, stunted by these earlier experiences with how men interacted with my fat body.

During my teen years, I was often told that I needed to be thin in order to find a rich husband. My Mom purchased me replacement shakes and diet pills; my first diet started when I was 12. The goal was to convince my stomach that it was full and did not need real food. I did lose weight and received lots of praise from my family for how thin I managed to become. But the weight came back, and through this process, I developed an eating disorder. I learned strategies and developed a community through engagement with pro-ana websites. That eating disorder was a normal part of who I was until I discovered body positivity.

But even being happier with myself and less invested in thin culture, I still experience fat discrimination. I find it harder to get jobs with local companies, and if or when I do, I get bullied constantly because of my weight. Even though I am an active person who works hard, I am constantly the one being called out for being slow. I've found that if I work for Westerners, things are better, so I try to avoid working for companies with Chinese bosses. When I work with Westerners, I rarely notice the size of my body. I feel released from the constant awareness of being "extremely obese", and people do not assume that every ailment I experience is because of my weight. I am able to live and experience different things; I'm normal in this side of society. In the West, I am of average size, a US size 14. I am considered petite, cute, and beautiful to many people. I have more success in romance, I can date a large portion of the singles in the pool. I started to realise that I am a sexual being. In the West, many more doors are open to me.

I'm not fat by white Western standards. But when I step outside of those Western parts of Hong Kong, I am back to being a fat Chinese girl again. And I live in a city that is really small; the most expensive thing in Hong Kong is space. It is a premium and shapes everyone's life here.

Wherever I go, the space between the people around is limited. On the tram and other forms of public transportation, especially, my larger body takes us more space than everyone else. The designated seats on the tram have been designed with small bodies in mind; my body spills over. My ass encroaches on the seating area next to me. I am double the size of most people, especially other women, so I cannot move around as easily; I need more room to get through or move through the door. Being a 200lbs woman in Hong Kong I really stand out; I may as well be Godzilla. The stereotype that Asian women are all petite, with tiny bones, is internalised. I'm not supposed to be this big. I know this. Others in Asia know this. I am the elephant in the room.

This struggle contributes to my confusion about who I am, who I want to be. It makes me question how healthy I really am. It makes me fight against falling back into old destructive patterns with food and exercise. At almost 40, I am getting older, and my body is showing normal signs of ageing. My periods are unpredictable. I have a sneaking suspicion that I may struggle to get pregnant when my partner and I decide to take that step. It is hard not to blame these issues on my weight. Or *maybe* my decades of dieting. But anytime my knees hurt, or I get winded when walking up the hill, it's hard not to blame my size and wish it was different. Sometimes I think that I'm likely to die younger than those around me. Every sign of ageing or ill health only reminds me of my impending death. These thoughts stay with me every single day and often result in panic attacks. Being fat in my society has caused my mental illness. It will surely shorten my lifespan if I have anxiety like this across my adulthood.

Tomorrow, I am going to have my first therapy session, where I will finally talk about this fear. It is my hope that I can shift these thought patterns; that I can stop overthinking things and start healing.

References

Centre for Health Protection. (2019, May 9). Obesity. Department of Health. https://www.chp.gov.hk/en/healthtopics/content/25/8802.html

World Health Organisation. (2018, Feb 16). Obesity and overweight. World Health Organisation. https://www.who.int/news-room/fact-sheets/detail/obesity-and-overweight

23

SURVIVING AND THRIVING WHILE FAT

Sonalee Rashatwar

It was 1995. I was 7 and excited for my first jazz recital where my class was performing to Pat Benatar's 'Hit Me with Your Best Shot.' I was a pudgy little Indian girl living in a small blue-collar town in southern New Jersey. My younger sister was standing next to me dressed as a lion for her performance. We were ready. This is one of the few moments I can remember before diet culture took hold of what my body was allowed to look like. In photos I am standing with my chubby arms outstretched way over my head, double chin cheerfully haloing my wide open-mouthed grin. My rosy cheeks were full of excitement. Peeking through my half-unzipped fire engine red costume, was a sequined black bandeau, belly outstretched and thighs abundant. I remember being so proud of all the hard work and sweat it took to learn that dance. I lived my life as a fat kid, and things were fine.

I started being put on non-consensual diets at the age of 9. At first it started by encouraging me to eat less.

I became the kind of fat kid who enjoyed elaborate imagination games like house, but I was mostly interested in feeding my playmates saccharine delights like cakes and pies. Even my school-based imagination projects involved ornate hundred-layer ice cream sundaes, which could only be eaten using a golden spoon. I had a healthy relationship with pleasure. Food was my pleasure. Before I learned about Indigenous history, I enjoyed Thanksgiving, when dozens of my family members would gather to play games, eat turkey, candied yams, buttery stuffing – just celebrate life. This was one of the few times a year when my eating was not policed. I was not discouraged from wearing elastic clothing to the dinner table or getting up to arrange a second helping of gravy and mashed potatoes. The purpose of the gathering was to prepare rich, delicious foods and no calorie was spared.

Looking at photos from ages 10–13, I was gaining an appropriate amount of weight during puberty. It feels strange to scrutinize my prepubescent body, as if there exists any kind of abnormal weight gain. But the attention I received for this weight gain, was specific to my gender and desirability. My younger sister was thin, had a petite frame, and ate daintily. She was offered access to traditional femininity and her eating was not regulated. In fact, she was often praised for eating "bird-like." My younger brother was fat like me, but he was not monitored, because boys are allowed to be fat while they are developing.

My fascination with food probably started when I was experiencing food restriction at home. Despite living in a mixed caste Indian suburban home with abundant food access, I experienced a specific kind of food scarcity because I was the fat eldest daughter. At first, I was discouraged from eating as much as my younger siblings or friends. The restrictive food abuse occurred mostly at mealtime, in kitchen spaces, house parties and public spaces like restaurants. My father had a hand signal to pump the breaks and a derisive look he'd give me, as he'd follow me to the buffet table to surveil what I was putting onto my plate. This was how he told me he did not trust the decisions I'd make about my body. Food policing existed to disconnect me from my own body, to ignore my hunger cues and the satisfaction of fulfilling food cravings.

Diet culture created a family-wide surveillance that criminalized my fat child body. Even my younger siblings were deputized into the food police and asked to report to my parents what I would eat after school. Every November, our parents would hide our collective Halloween candy. My Dad would tell my younger sister that I was so sick in the head, that my fat body was unable to control itself. Shame was the primary tool used to teach me that both my body and the food it required were too much. And South Asians, we know a thing or two about shame. Shame was the foundational method to terrorize, harm, and control women who defied patri- archy. "Log kya kehenge?" (What will people say?) was my parents' motto.

Some of my most shame-filled memories come from my father rifling through the trash can in my bedroom during my early 20s, searching for evidence. I eventually learned to crumple snack wrappers in newspaper, hide food in my underwear drawers, and throw all takeout con- tainers in public trash cans so I wouldn't get caught eating anything other than home cooked, nutritious, fat-free Indian food. No offense to my Mom, but Indian food deserves some of the oil, cream, butter, and luxurious ingredients that makes it delicious.

When I was first pressured to have weight loss surgery (WLS) in 2009, the only thing I worried about was my immense shame at the thought of my friends or family finding out I had failed so horribly at being able to control by body size, that doctors had to cut my healthy guts open. Shame dictated my life. It was woven into the fabric of my everyday life.

In my mixed caste Indian Hindu family, money was used to manipulate my body auton- omy. Being an Indian American, means that my body was policed in the canon of upper caste Brahmanical Hindu Indian values. Caste has existed in South Asia for over 6,000 years, as one of the oldest systems of domination that is now institutionalized throughout my Indian Hindu community. Coming from an upper-class family that prided itself on being Indian, Hindu, and successful, meant that white supremacy, casteism, and heteropatriarchy were embedded into their ways of being in the world.

My family was enmeshed in, upholding, and representing a Hindu Indian American dream that was complicit in anti-Blackness, fatphobia, white supremacy, casteism, and Hindu fascism. This shaped how they abused me and chose to control my body. Brahmanical patriarchy was the dominant culture that determined my worth, and I learned through the ways my fatness was policed, how upper caste bodies represent the epitome of glory for my people. I was the un-glorious fat daughter, who brought shame to my family.

Fat on my body queered both my gender and sexual orientation. In college, I learned being fat meant I was not feminine enough to be conventionally attractive to heterosexual men. My parents were more interested in fitting into the existing hegemony, like good Indian immigrants, rather than standing up for my fat body. I had to be as small possible, to be able to make Indian cis-heterosexuals love and value me in order to fit into their model of conformity.

Over two decades, my parents spent close to $100,000 on weight loss products for me, which made them great customers to the $66 billion diet industry. When Jenny Craig failed at age 13, there was an ayurvedic shaman with non-FDA approved herbal supplements for me. When Isagenix juice fasting failed, there was Structure House residential weight loss facility. When one predictably flawed weight loss product failed, diet culture was ready to offer them another opportunity to throw their money at the problem of my fat body. Long term weight loss has a higher failure rate than not getting pregnant from pulling out during sex and the prediction of the season change by a groundhog.

I was never able to have a stress-free relationship with my parents, whom, if I haven't mentioned already, were also fat. For my mother, my fat body was a project of surveillance and obedience. Marriage pressure is an important part of class and caste maintenance in Hindu families. I was not the skinny Indian girl who they would have the honor of giving away during an extravagant wedding, and I wouldn't bring honor and dignity to my parents. My sexual desirability, and therefore marriageability as a thin cisgender heterosexual Hindu Indian woman was more important to my family than giving me the time and space to figure out who I was and what I wanted.

Fatphobia affected the way I experienced my body, which is why it impacted my sexuality. I became grateful for the emotionally abusive, callous, and unkind attention I would receive from men, because my parents told me from a young age it would be unlikely I would experience authentic romantic attraction. This led to my experience of many non-consensual and inappropriate sexual experiences, sometimes with men much older than me. My internalized fatphobia made it difficult for me to understand what my rights to sexual pleasure and sexual freedom were.

I was in an abusive relationship in my early 20s that reflected this residual commitment to assimilation. I pretended to be straight. My abusive boyfriend demanded a dress code where I performed my femininity and desirability by wearing dresses and skirts only, shapewear, makeup, and long straight hair. I was praised for keeping my hair long and straight and wearing high femme makeup to compensate for my fatness. Before this relationship, I did not know where to purchase dresses that came in my size, because before this abusive relationship I was most comfortable in a pair of bootcut jeans.

The second and final time I was pressured by my parents to have WLS again was in 2014. I was 26. The process I went through to become eligible for WLS was shockingly easy, while also being time consuming. My parents wanted me to have the surgery before we were slated to visit India that December, in hopes that I would experience less fatphobia and therefore less shame. It was a rush to visit a parade of doctors that summer, including a pulmonologist, cardiologist, gastroenterologist, psychologist, and even a dietitian.

In retrospect, this process was an investigative journey; I was deeply curious about these doctors, who would do ultrasounds, electrocardiograms, barium swallows, endoscopies, colonoscopies, blood panels, and mental status exams on me. Each would give a resounding approving head-nod that my insides were super healthy. I thought to myself: "Wow, my insides were healthy enough to have this surgery." This evidence flew in the face of what my parents had been trying to convince me for the better part of my life: that I was an obesity time bomb ready to die from fatness at any time. These contradictions in the medical field informed my journey.

It was only when I met the dietitian who showed me what my quality of eating would be like post-op that I was able to firmly hear the record scratch. Nope. I could not see a future where I could only eat one quarter to a third cup of food in a meal. When I had to consciously decide if I was willing to trade thinness for the pleasures of basic humanity, I said no. I was not going to devote my entire life post-op to thinking *even more* about food and my body than I already did. I would have had to mix protein powder and vitamins and supplements into all of my food for the rest of my life because my stomach couldn't digest the amount of food I'd need to meet basic nutrition standards. The surgery would have essentially meant voluntary malnutrition. And the saddest part was that my parents were offering me long sought-after praise and validation after every additional doctor signed off in approval of my having this surgery.

This might not come as a shock to you, but saying no to voluntarily removing healthy gut tissue was the healthiest decision I was able to make for myself. It meant choosing my fat body over my family's obsession with thin supremacy. And I would not have been able to make that decision without having the queer fat community and my sister's deep concern for my life when she learned one in 200 die on the table during surgery. I am grateful for my fat life. I have gained lots of weight in the past 5 years.

That trip to India was the last time I may ever go to India. While I never got WLS, my parents forced me to have hair extensions installed so that my short boyish haircut could be hidden. But what happened while traveling within the subcontinent was something I could have never predicted. Fatphobia in places where there is a highly normalized standard of social conformity felt amplified to me. People would covertly take photos of me in the airports. Children would run behind me and laugh at tourist sites. Strangers would point and stare in the villages. It was such a horrifying silent trauma to endure because no one in my family would acknowledge the harm I was experiencing, nor would they step in to protect me from it.

TheFatSexTherapist took all of her traumas and shaped it into a political canon. Young Sonalee informs all of my endeavors as a therapist, coach, and activist. Body image trauma should be considered any pressure from a romantic or intimate partner, family member, or significant other to manipulate body size using tactics of power and control. Both my parents and abusive ex-partners were clear that I was too fat and that I had to take steps to monitor my body because I did not deserve good things until that was achieved. I was offered conditional acceptance, love, and praise. This communicated to me that my body had less value and deserved the abusive treatment it received.

This is the primary function of diet culture and healthism. It offers consumers the veil of belief that they have the ability to control their body size, when actually bodies are more complicated. As a fat sex therapist, I work to unlearn internalized fatphobia with my clients to reframe the reason our bodies are fat by looking at things like genetics, family diet history, ancestral lineage, intergenerational trauma, and Set Point theory. Set Point theory explains why my body regained weight every time I attempted intentional weight loss. For unexplainable reasons, the weight range my body was programmed to function within optimally is one that my body has fought to maintain. And when I look at people in my family, while I am the fattest, I belong among these other fat brown people.

Now in my 30s, I have been in therapy to really sit and inspect what it is I've survived. Only after a year of guided introspection did I realize the parental rejection of my fat body was just a projection of the rejection they experienced of their own fat bodies. Sometimes that rejection happens in childhood, and sometimes it happens in adulthood. As fat adults who grew up as thin adolescents, my parents had a textured understanding of structural fatphobia. My immigrant parents were so anxious about me growing up fat because they did not want me to experience hardship. Their concern comes from a place of deep love, and also deep anxiety caused by social nonconformity. I remember having conversations late into the night with my parents. I was a confused small-fat teenager sitting across the kitchen table wondering why I was awake past my bedtime to have the same painstaking conversation about my inability to lose weight. I had to sit and listen silently as I held the tears in my throat while they would explain how being fat would affect the way my body would experience sexual desirability, fertility, racism, and career advancement.

Daring to love my fat self was my teen rebellion. I demanded to live in a world where I could be happy with my fat body, where I could have sex in my fat body, where I could have a fat fulfilling life. My parents told me it was not worth trying to change the world, that it would be impossible to be happy and successful by staying fat. And every day I walk towards my life's purpose, I prove them wrong.

24

REVIEW OF SCHOLARSHIP ON FAT-GAY MEN

Jason Whitesel

Introduction

This chapter provides a survey of the scholarship on gay men who belong to fat-affirming subcultures. It also considers big-gay-men's media, sidelined by mainstream gay tastes. It offers an overview of how the literature on big gay men and different media outlets for them address fat-gay shame and big-gay-men's responses to stigmatization at the intersection of size and sexual orientation. It is one of the first pieces of writing to comprehensively chronicle research and media that focus on fat-gay men's issues. A caveat to the relatively small body of literature on fat-gay men available and reviewed in this chapter is that many citations are not firmly situated in the Fat-Studies paradigm. To review what is out there on fat-gay men by only considering work by avowed Fat Studies scholars would quickly lead to a dead-end. Herein, I err on the side of going farther afield than Fat Studies scholarship alone, and also incorporate allied perspectives that remain *somewhat* in the spirit of Fat Studies, though not calling itself such.

A quick Google Scholar search for "gay male body image" yields studies in clinical psychology, social work, health communications, public health, men's health, sexuality studies, and sociology – all disciplines which consistently demonstrate heightened body-image concerns among gay men. Anti-fat bias becomes particularly poignant among gay males, with empirical analysis of psychological item pools completed by respondents that indicate gay men are unhappy with their own bodies and they are likely to fat shame one another (Foster-Gimbel & Engeln, 2016). Likewise, qualitative content analysis reveals that anti-fat attitudes crop up even toward big gay men who are contestants on *RuPaul's Drag Race* (Pomerantz, 2017), a reality television show that openly embraces drag queens, yet appears less "tolerant" of the wider brethren among them. Moreover, cyber-ethnographers have documented how gay men brazenly dole out sizeism toward those with fat physiques on social networking, dating, and hookup sites (Conte, 2018). Thus, fat-shaming is even harder on big gay men who encounter anti-fat bias, as they feel the pressure of the ideal gay body on, for example, gay dating apps where men can be intimidated as bodies are compared and quantified (Robinson, 2018). In all, a strong correlation exists between promoting body ideals within the mainstream gay male community and inculcating a sense of body shame for those who strive to belong.

In reaction to gay fatphobia and to being ostracized, collectivities such as Girth & Mirth developed as an organized network of social groups with international reach for big gay men and their admirers to assuage their social injuries (Pyle & Loewy, 2009; Whitesel, 2014). Girth & Mirth promotes size acceptance and is suspicious of weight-loss surgery or other body modifications to cope with the gay-thinness imperative or the incessant compulsion for muscularity (Whitesel & Shuman, 2016). Likewise, sociological ethnography has described a vibrant subculture of hirsute big gay men, the Bears, which is debatably kinder to those who are full-figured and getting on in years (Hennen, 2008; McGrady, 2016; Pyle & Klein, 2011).

Within these subcultures, media-and-cultural-studies scholars have documented "chubs" (big gay men), "gainers" (gay men who seek to "bulk up" intentionally), "chasers" (admirers of chubs and gainers), and "encouragers" (those who support gainers' intentions to loosen up the restrictions on their waistlines) (Adams & Berry, 2013; Textor, 1999). Sociologist Lee Monaghan (2005) referred to such gay men in the UK as "big handsome men" who reconfigure the politics of fat male embodiment. They provide alternative, mostly positive representations of fatness in both actual and virtual environments (Monaghan, 2005). Such online worlds include Bigger-City, the largest online community for gay chubby men and their chasers to form a "collective identity" (Pyle & Klein, 2011, p. 82) or smartphone apps like Scruff "targeted primarily at bears and their admirers … a generally older, larger-bodied … demographic" (Roth, 2014, pp. 2113, 2124). They also include Grommr, a contraction for "growth community," a social network/dating site for gay and bi men self-described as being "into fat and fatter bellies, chubby men, beer guts, big muscle and chunky muscle, bears and non-bears, and so much more" (Grommr, n.d).

Thus, the fat-gay male body is both a site of shame, and of stigma resistance (Whitesel, 2019; McGrady, 2016) and "embodied contestation" (Pyle & Klein, 2011) through queer-"fat performative protest" and attempts to reclaim sexual citizenship (Whitesel, 2019). For example, as Whitesel (2014) observes, Girth & Mirth's activities, from the everyday to the carnivalesque, provide an opportunity to examine how a stigmatized group negotiates visible and less visible forms of discrimination via a playful reconfiguration of their sullied identities through sex; gender and sexuality; social-class positioning; and fashion and performance (see also Whitesel & Shuman, 2013).

Fat-gay men, in their efforts to democratize and diversify desire, trend toward the "art of sexual transgression, and in particular the sexualized art of the body" in their visual culture (McNair, 2002, p. 13), which includes the now-defunct *Bulk Male* magazine, Bears addressing body image concerns through digital art communities, and the Chubby Guy Swag blogging community founded in response to the lack of body-positive "fatshion" for plus-size males. *Bulk Male* at one time thrived as a 1990s specialty magazine, which catered to big-and-hairy gay men with erotic photos and personal ads (Whitesel, 2017a). "Bear Art" aims to re-present fat-and-hairy gay men as having desirable bodies worthy of sexual attraction (Beattie, 2014). Even mainstream television shows, such as HBO's short-lived series, *Looking* (Lannan, 2014), cast a fat-gay actor, Daniel Franzese, to play a big-and-hairy HIV-positive Bear, who appeared completely naked on screen, shown in a romantic relationship with a man who had an "ideal" body, making him "more than a comic sidekick," not unlike fat men in specialty and user-created gay-porn (Highberg, 2011). Chubby Guy Swag was co-founded in 2010 by Zach Eser and Abigail Spooner as a "safe space for plus-size men . . . to include them in the conversation on body positivity and fat acceptance" and "to promote body diversity and body positivity amongst men" (Eser & Spooner, n.d.). This community has international reach, providing a safe space for big men who do not fit the mass media's image of the "ideal" body type. It provides room for those who still aspire toward becoming fashionable, and who therefore appreciate the information and wisdom users share on this site. In fact, several users submit selfies in their favorite outfit, i.e., posts and photos by men of size who are queer, disabled, people of color, and/or "just plain broke," most of whom are young adults who are underrepresented in both mainstream and queer media (Whitesel, 2015).

Buddhist activist Ganapati Durgadas (1998) argues that fat-gay and bi men are poignant "reminders of the feminine stigma with which heterosexism" still haunts queer men (p. 370). Sociologically speaking, Hennen (2008) argued that Bears seek to recuperate "regular-guy" masculinity. Interdisciplinary sociologist of gender and sexuality studies and body politics, Whitesel (2019), suggests that Girth & Mirth activities make room for gender maneuvering, and give members creative license for deconstructing masculinity through campy performances of fat queerness. Society feminizes fat men and gay men, yet some of the playful, campy-queer performances of fat-gay sexuality among Girth & Mirthers do not fully seek to disavow effeminacy, as Bears are wont to do. Rather, a few chubs seem open to embracing a performative resignification of femininity as an integral component of an active fat (and gay) sexuality. Among the Girth & Mirthers whom Whitesel (2014) interviewed for *Fat gay men: Girth, mirth, and the politics of stigma*, one big man commented that the group fosters a space where members do not have to put on the "butch" act (p. 135). That is to say that clubs like Girth & Mirth allow for a wider range of gender performances that go into producing legible forms of fat-gay subjectivity.

Yet another response to fat-gay stigma is drag, which embraces the shared wisdom of the overlapping subjectivities of gay men and fat women. For example, take the dialogue between queer theorists Michael Moon and Eve Sedgwick in 1990–91 about "Divine," John Waters's "cross-dressing diva," to use their lingo. In this dialogue, Moon promises on behalf of Sedgwick and himself that they both will speak to their combined wisdom which involves Michael's "experiences of divinity as a fat woman, and Eve's as a gay man," destabilizing both categories through the lens of fat-positive drag (p. 15). The authors remind us of the sometimes "divine" coming together of the fat diva and the gay man.

A couple of studies provide an overview of organized groups and clubs for fat-gay men and their admirers. Among them is Alex Textor's (1999) taxonomic history of the community-organizing features of various subgroups that fall under the big-gay-men's umbrella and the media they produced. In addition, Lee Monaghan's (2005) Goffman-esque *Body-and-Society* article is based on his 10-month ethnographic observation of 15 websites, chatrooms, and seven e-mail exchanges with key informants involved in the eroticization of expansive male bodies online. These sources were primarily, though not exclusively, gay-identified, and Monaghan systematically analyzed them through the *ATLAS.ti* qualitative data-analysis software. Others studied specific groups for big gay men, including Bears, Girth & Mirth, and Gainers. These groups and the scholarship about them are presented below.

Bears: a well-established subculture in the gay community

By far the largest literature on groups for fat-gay men is devoted to big-and-hairy gay men, the Bear community, who celebrate and eroticize larger, masculinized (though not necessarily muscularized) male bodies. In 2007, an estimated 1.4 million gay Bears existed in the US (Mann, 2010), while David Moskowitz and his colleagues (2013), who conducted two large-scale surveys, estimated the Bears comprise 14–22 percent of the gay/bi men's community. For further reading, interested readers can refer to *The bear book* (Wright, 1997), *The bear handbook* (Kampf, 2000), *The bear book II* (Wright, 2001), *Bears on bears* (Suresha, 2002a), "Understanding the bear movement in gay culture" (Manley et al., 2007), *Guide for the modern bear* (Smith & Bale, 2012), and "A concept analysis of bear identity" (Quidley-Rodriquez & De Santis, 2019).

Operating from the vantage point of critical and qualitative approaches to health and social psychology, Gough and Flanders (2009) ask: How do Bears discursively manage their subjectivities in a healthist/sizeist culture? The authors conducted 10 semi-structured, in-depth interviews with self-identified Bears from a white British cohort in the North of England. Nine participants met the medicalized BMI criteria for "obese" and four as "severely obese." One of the authors, a Bear himself, accessed the participants as an insider to their networks. Themes from Gough and Flanders's interview transcripts were generated using grounded theory and analyzed through a synthesis of approaches to discourse analysis. The authors found Bears draw on various interrelated interpretative repertoires in their interviews to make sense of their bodily experiences. First, the interviewees chronicled anti-fat abuse and negative stereotyping in childhood, medical settings, and the wider gay community. Second, they reported finding supportive and sexualized acceptance of a diverse range of plus-sized bodies and shared bodily attributes. Large bellies and body hair within the Bear community was often used to construct the Bear body as *more* desirable than the culturally "ideal" gay body. Third, the research participants caricatured and emasculated "twinks" who perpetuate the thin-ideal of gay beauty as "prissy"– the oppositional anchor to the Bears' "regular-guy" masculinity (Hennen, 2005). Gough and Flanders find evidence of Bears' twink-shaming and *othering* thin gays as shallow; countering dominant assumptions that pathologize ample size; equating "fatter" with "healthier and happier"; expressing discomfort with their thinner selves as looking unhealthy with reference to HIV/AIDS-related stigma; projecting self-confidence through the Bear ideal; drawing on "My body, my choice" in defiance and rebelling against social- and media pressures to look a certain way; suggesting that widespread use of BMI is not without criticism, and arguing for more balanced perspectives on personal wellbeing and sex appeal.

Similar themes appear in sociologist Patrick McGrady's (2016) content analysis of 20 issues of *A Bear's Life* magazine coupled with 21 life-history interviews with Bears where he traces a stage model of men "feeling weight stigma," "finding bears," "embracing the bear body," and "emulating the bear body," including recent anxieties around the "muscle bear phenomenon," which revives some Bear men's feelings of being self-conscious about their weight around other Bears converting body mass into building muscle and bulking up.

Drawing on related disciplines of public health, health education, community psychology, nursing, and clinical psychology, Quidley-Rodriquez and De Santis (2017) synthesize the health-research literature on Bears, which they contend is exploratory and still in its infancy. In 2016, these same authors published a similar paper in the *Journal of Clinical Nursing*, "Physical, psychosocial, and social health of men who identify as bears: A systematic review." Using Health Risk Appraisal/Assessment as their lens, they conducted a literature review in 2015 of eight texts on health issues for Bears. Their research question asks: What are the clinical implications for healthcare providers working with Bears whose weight plays a significant role in their self-identification, and, having experienced weight-related stigma, their self-esteem? The authors find that existing research on Bear health suffers from convenient samples in order to recruit a hard-to-reach population. Most participants are white men, hardly diverse, and most research on Bear health does not use biomarkers other than physical appearance and BMI, making it difficult to draw firm conclusions. Existing research tends to approach Bear health from a psychosocial perspective *versus* the physical health of the community's members. Quidley-Rodriquez and De Santis (2017) also cite some prior work which finds that Bears engage in high-risk sexual behavior (e.g., anal sex with multiple, casual partners without a condom) and in a more diverse range of sexual behaviors, many of which signal masculinity, as does their larger frame.

Edmonds and Zieff (2015) utilize "a transdisciplinary [and holistic] approach that brings together … queer studies, critical obesity studies, fat studies, physiology, public health, gender studies, psychology, and sociology" (p. 417). Trained in kinesiology, the authors who do not identify as Bears, conducted in-depth interviews (with seven Bear-identified men with BMIs in the "obese" category) and participant observation (among the Bear community) in San Francisco. In the spirit of Fat Studies, they understand "obesity" and "the problematic and reductive measure of Body Mass Index" as oppressive terms and prefer "politically resistive deployment of alternative terminology that reintegrates the fleshy corporeality of lived experience" (p. 417), simply using the descriptive term "larger bodies" (ibid.). They draw on Goffman's (1963) Stigma Theory, extend it to include Meyer's (2003) Minority-Stress Perspective to look at Bears doubly stigmatized as fat and gay, all the while connecting this back to the exercise physiology literature on the detrimental effect discrimination and shaming have on one's well-being. The authors recognize that the gay community could offer a site for building resilience to sexual-minority stress, but Bears feel side-lined in this community that valorizes thinness. Moreover, the Bear community struggles with a wider discourse that depicts fat as "feminizing filth" and responds by parlaying their bigger build into masculine capital as burly lumberjack- or football-player types (p. 419). The Bear community serves as a buffer, providing resilience in the face of fat- and sexual-minority stigma, and promotes a healthy skepticism of fatphobic health messages, though sometimes uneven.

Overall, Edmonds and Zieff (2015) find evidence of the Bears' biopolitical resistance to body ideals, fat stigma, and mainstream gay values. Moreover, Bears find themselves in a "double bind" – their community becomes a safe space to build resilience, but they have not necessarily dealt with the effect of fat stigma on their beliefs and actions, sometimes still reproducing sizeist and healthist norms. Several themes emerge in Edmonds and Zieff's research. First, Bears suffer from *compounded stigma*. In adolescence, one respondent conflated his developing sexual orienta-tion with body-image issues: he hated his body, coveted other men's slim-and-muscular bodies and wanted to look like them, which this desire then explained away his own developing sexual orientation as simply envious of the culturally ideal male body versus any burgeoning same-sex romantic interest. College-level experiences of respondents revolved around lacking erotic capital as "a Bear trapped in a Twink's experience" or not knowing where one fits in the "social hier-archy of the gay community," its spaces, and popular representations (p. 423). Other respondents spoke of their bodies becoming ampler while finding themselves unable to transition into the gay scene, yet still feeling reticent to identify with the Bear community. Another theme involves *avoiding stigma*. Bears bypass mainstream gay spaces where their access to size-friendly furniture and accommodations as well as support for their intellectual and social contributions becomes diminished because of their size. One respondent reported a love of expressing himself physically through dancing with his shirt off, but only at Bear dance events where he feels safe from being judged. Other Bears said they avoid the gym, despite finding physical activity pleasurable, for fear of the same. Yet another said he enjoys surfing at the beach, but he goes less often than he desires because he feels self-conscious around fellow surfers because of his belly. According to the authors, physical activity for Bears appears to be "a space of both desire and defeat" (p. 430). Other themes chronicled by Edmonds and Zieff (2015) include *internalized sizeism, accepting net-works, border wars,* and *changing times*. Some Bears internalize the belief that their weight impinges on their quality of life; others buy into the narrative that their fate comes from their lack of phys-ical discipline, and still others bemoan falling short of the ideal muscle-Bear masculinity (re: the latter, see also McGrady, 2016). Nevertheless, Bear spaces increase erotic capital in favor of bigger bodies; and mentors ease new members through the social undoing of fat- and sexual orientation stigma. Finally, greater awareness of the need to diversify gay male (body) images is changing the way younger cohorts envision more democratic participation in the queer community.

Gay men in the Girth & Mirth subculture

Little scholarly work has been published on big men and their admirers who belong to Girth & Mirth, notwithstanding my (2014) book, *Fat gay men: Girth, mirth, and the politics of stigma*, and its spinoff chapters, blogs, and (co)authored articles that bring together Folklore, Queer, and Soci-ological Theory with Fat Studies and ethnographic research. These works discuss how Girth &

Mirthers trouble and interrogate the thin-and-muscular body ideal in the gay male community through their performative play and redefine themselves as embodied, sexual beings, motivated by the desire for, and of, other men.

Girth & Mirth started as a national social movement organization in the mid-1970s in reaction to weight discrimination and big men's need for acceptance in the gay community (Whitesel, 2014; Pyle & Loewy, 2009; Textor, 1999). Local clubs provide a safe haven for men who are doubly stigmatized, both by body size *and* by sexual orientation, allowing members to stake a claim to be ordinary in a society that sometimes regards them as misfits. Worldwide, the organization offers a friendship circle to bring big gay men out of social isolation as members help one another deal with their "wounded attachment" to the gay community (Brown, 1993). The activities sponsored by the group involve mainly the ordinary – ordinary people attending ordinary events, like a potluck with friends (Whitesel, 2014).

Members of local chapters of the club also attend annual pan-Girth & Mirth weekend reunions. One of these is the Super Weekend, a regional event that takes place yearly at a gay motel in Oklahoma City. This venue provides a fat-affirming sanctuary for the big men where they can express their sexuality without fear of ridicule or rejection. Another annual event is Convergence, coordinated through the hub of the Big Gay Men's Organization. In US society, size often intersects with a class-based assumption that being fat equals being "lazy" and "poor"; therefore, some of the big gay men in Girth & Mirth take a class-elevating route toward reducing fat stigma, feeling compelled to become middle-class consumers. Converging at a mainstream luxury hotel, they attend seminars, a dance, sightseeing excursions, and outings to museums. All of these activities are about gay big men seeking class validation (Whitesel, 2014; Pyle & Loewy, 2009). Those who attend Convergence differ from the "uncouth" Super Weekenders, who mostly make a mockery out of status-seeking behavior.

Today, versus post-Stonewall, Girth & Mirth does not appear all that political to insiders and to insider academics like Michael Loewy. In their co-written chapter on Girth & Mirth, "Double stigma: Fat men and their male admirers" (Pyle & Loewy, 2009), he and his coauthor explain that the group does not have an activist agenda, except as it pertains to identity politics. Though club members may not think of what they do, e.g., getting together for a potluck, as a political statement, nevertheless, group organizers understand the Girth & Mirth movement in identity-based terms (Whitesel, 2014). As the board of directors for the 1996 anniversary of the San Francisco chapter wrote, "gay and bisexual bigmen, and those who prefer bigmen, have cast off the shackles of hiding and insecurity and now revel in their proudly accepted identity" (Textor, 1999, p. 219); others find Girth & Mirth to be a "queer ghetto too small" and cramped (Giles, 1998, p. 356), identifying bigotry in some of the chubby-chasers' sexual preferences (Blotcher, 1998). Nevertheless, Ron Suresha, who identifies as a bisexual "Wolf" moreso than Bear (2014, p. 27), exhorts big men's groups to keep the faith as "gay pioneers' initial work with Girth & Mirth was not simply to socialize; it was part of a whole culture of liberationist activity. Girth & Mirth was active before any mainstream fat-acceptance groups" (2002b, pp. 63–64). Therefore, Girth & Mirth is not just a manifestation of the gay scene divided, but also about politics in a minor key, a softer, less perceptible fat activism. This politic co-exists alongside the well-established big men's erotic media, another collective communication outlet that has "provided the backbone of the big men's movement's social networks" (ibid.).

Gaining subcultures: gay-fat kink

Gay-fat kink includes fat-gay men and their admirers who engage in debatably "queer" bodily practices such as belly rubs, pro-weight-gain fantasies and behaviors, encouraging one another to expand physically, and events where big bellies are positively celebrated and flaunted. This "gaining" subculture offers "alternative ways of living and being in the world" that enables members to "disrupt culturally prevalent ideas about size and sexual attractiveness" (Boylorn & Adams, 2016, p. 93).

John Campbell (2004), working from the framework of communications and Cultural Studies to conduct a three-year ethnographic study of social scenes for gay men online, builds on Michel Foucault and Judith Butler's theories, arguing that online gaining communities discursively re-configure and re-conceptualize what constitutes "sexy" (p. 136). Gaining – intensely pleasurable for some gay men, while incomprehensible to most – often involves slim gay men who come to these online worlds seeking someone to mentally and sometimes physically nurture them to build a bigger body of fat, sometimes combined with muscle (Campbell, 2004, p. 137). This online communication can involve physical exploration or may solely exist in the realm of mythmaking and fantasy, for "as with any sexuality, it makes no difference whether the desire is actually fulfilled in reality" (Oliverio, 2016, p. 232).

Traditionally, the word "gut" registers as a failure on a man's part to keep his body healthy, resulting from being *inactive*. Paralleling this outlook on male fatness, virtual communities privilege thin/fit/youthful bodies. Even researchers, when they foreground large/hairy/big-gay men, focus solely on their being big men. Attention is not necessarily given explicitly to men who intentionally put on weight and/or encourage other men to do so, neither to men who are bound together by eating or "obsessed" with being big. Yet here, in the online world of pro-weight-gain communities, guts are showered with messages of adoration and achieved through *actively* putting on weight. Borrowing from Adams and Berry (2013), their behavior is "counterintuitive," because desiring to inhabit a fatter body unsettles the reasoning that one becomes fat because one "lets oneself go" (p. 140). Gaining weight intentionally troubles the dominant narrative that people must manage their weight for health reasons; bodies should be small versus large; and should they expand, it should *not* be the result of enthusiastic, unapologetic choices, for those bodies would be understood as illogical and bodily excess would engender social fear (Adams & Berry, 2013).

Following Butler, Campbell (2004) understands gainers as an example of the sexed body that is socially informed, with some gay men expanding it to include gaining/guts as erotic/erogenous. They reconfigure how the sexed body acquires its social significance and what constitutes sexiness (pp. 144–145). Moreover, Campbell compares gainers to cyber-feminist Donna Haraway's (1986) postmodern cyborgs (i.e., "freak" bodies) who delight in transgressing bodily boundaries in their discussion of fat embodiment that supposedly would correspond with a physical body with which one engages offline: "virtual body bending," as it were (p. 176).

Textor (1999), a doctoral candidate in American Cultural Studies at the time of his research, examined the cultural histories of various groups that fall under the umbrella of big gay men. He provides a genealogy of this subset of fat-gay men, gainers, and their "encouragers," beginning with the launch of gaining/encouraging newsletters from the 1980s and 1990s, followed by a 1–900 phone line for men to record gaining fantasy ads. In 1992, an erotically charged weight-gain convention started, called "EncourageCon," and the print and phone media moved to internet sites for men to meet, such as GainRWeb founded in 1996. The contemporary website, Grommr, continues to chronicle this unfolding history on its webpage entitled the "Abridged Gainer History Project."

Key issues that Textor explores include how these men "concern themselves with a particular kind of weight gain" (1999, p. 228). Many gainers rely on the ex-jock trope. This image appeals to not only weight gain, but also references muscle mass, bodybuilding, "the gym," a football-playing past, or having "put on a beer belly." Citing these signifiers thereby masculinizes "non-muscular weight gain" (ibid.). In some cases, this amounts to "frat-boy fetishism"

(Johnson, 1998), gay men eroticizing the boorish, belching, unceasing appetite imbued in the frat-boy trope, consuming this image despite a history of fraternities sometimes being hetero-sexist and homophobic. The "frat-boy-on-boy *tópos* haunts the homosexual male pornographic imagination" (ibid., 200), with gainers who cite frat-jock histories, reveling in the chance to build hypermasculine sexual capital, even as they subvert it. They redefine fetishized masculinity from gym-toned bulk to a beer belly loaded as a masculine signifier. Dan Oliverio (2016) equates gainer/encourager groups to kink communities, which organize around divergent sexual tastes and erogenous zones, often splitting into various subgroups. He insists that erotic *ideas* drive kink fantasies moreso than fetish objects, with participants needing permission to explore socially "deviant" bodily and sexual desires without guilt or shame.

Public transgression remains central to gainers' narratives, whether it be "pigging out" at a buffet or having people be disgusted/amazed by them, from which they would derive some pleasure (Textor, 1999, p. 229). Similar to Bakhtin's (1965) idea of the "carnivalesque," gainers symbolically invert overdetermined ideas through "grotesque realism" and hybridization, their inversion being not a recasting of "fat is beautiful," but a hybrid that is invested in the abjection of fat bodies, that fat taboo adds to pleasurable gaining. HIV/AIDS also contributed to gay and bi men celebrating generously fleshed bodies, making ample size a counterpoint to sickness and the gradual wasting of the body (Textor, 1999, p. 230; see also Kruger, 1998). The HIV-AIDS era follows a post-Stonewall backdrop, where gay men valorized sameness (e.g., gay "Castro clones"), then re-evaluated this desire for sameness with oppositional pairings (Textor, 1999, p. 235), e.g., chubby/chaser, gainer/encourager.

Communications professor Tony Adams and his colleagues work from the vantage point of the ethnography of communication to consider whether gainers truly offer a queer counter-culture, taking on the unjust body-fascist system or, in fact, reinforce body shaming, gender stereotypes, and social privilege. They confront the privilege of "being able to live in queer ways . . . in terms of body size, sexuality, and desire" (Boylorn & Adams, 2016, p. 96). Adams is an "insider" to the discursive system he seeks to study, being fond of big gay men. Taking a queer perspective in Communication Studies through qualitative critical auto-ethnography, he self-reflects on whether he, as a white gay man from the rural Midwest, can fully incorporate a queer-intersectional approach into his research/writing on pro-weight cultural performances. He analyzes his personal experience of attending "Belly Rub Weekend" (BRW) over Labor Day 2015 in Chicago and wonders whether the event is "queer." Gay men fret about gaining weight. Therefore, those who find bigger men attractive and find fat bodies more desirable than they find thin bodies register this event, on some level, as queer. In this way, the BRW disrupts the thin-and-fit, gay-male aesthetic and advocates beliefs and practices others might consider "wrong."

However, in a "quare" framework as articulated by E. Patrick Johnson (2001), which draws on Black vernacular to counteract the whiteness of queer studies, Adams focuses on the inter-sectionality of race/gender/sexuality/class at BRW. He notes BRW is a "predominantly white space" where "white, gay, male privilege" might allow participants to "maneuver the event with ease" (Boylorn & Adams, 2016, p. 93). In such spaces, one has to question the absence of Black men, whether they would "pass" as "just regular guys" were they to attend, or would they become hypersexualized objects reduced to the "*big* Black cock" and "*big* Black ass." As for social class, participants learn about this event via their access to its companion online community. Attendees need money to spend on the event; and they need such social capital indicators as interpersonal skills and able-bodied-ness to flirt among attendees. Thus, those who lack social desirability and online access/travel options for financial or geographic reasons may not feel welcome at the BRW gathering of members of the gaining/encouraging community, or may not attend at all due to feeling excluded because of class discrimination.

Thus, "BRW espouses queer sensibilities ... that ... disrupt ... norms of body size, desire, and sexuality ... celebrating bigger, expanding bodies" (Boylorn & Adams, 2016, p. 95). However, the authors wonder if a queer theory take on this event overlooks social privilege. This nagging suspicion leaves Adams speculating about how BRW for mostly white males grants him the privilege as such not to think about who can gain weight and then maneuver social interactions with relative ease. Certainly, white women would not have the same leeway as straight white men gaining. For example, some white hetero-men put on weight after becoming fathers and no longer maintain a fit physique. People find these "dad bods" cute, but there is no equivalent fuss over "mom bods."

Adams, and to a lesser extent his co-author, also conducted four years of virtual ethnographic insider research on "FatClub.com," a pseudonym they used for a website for the gay gainer community. He and a co-researcher clocked more than 1,000 hours of covert fieldwork, not introducing themselves as researchers when going on the site, but being careful to use a pseudonym for the site and other users' screen names. Adams and his colleague merge "ethnography of communication ... communicative practices that comprise a speech community" (2013, p. 310) *à la* Dell Hymes (1968), whereby speech acts including ecstatic/performative language and communal norms become the ethnographer's focus. The idea of performativity is a common paradigm used to theorize fat-gay men, as is qualitative research, especially ethnography, a common method to study groups for such.

"FatClub.com" started in 2003 and continued until 2011, when its administrators faced trouble keeping the site going. Of the approximately 1,500 members, most were white and identified as gay or bi in this safe virtual environment to explore men who are into weight gain. As Adams and Berry (2013, p. 308) observe, this "counterintuitive cultural scene" supports "pro-weight cultural performances ... that ecstatically cite, dis-identify, and play with normative health and beauty ideals" – an "online community of mostly gay men who collectively pursue bigger bodies." Among the themes Adams and Berry (2013) cover in their ethnography is the unique naming practices central to the FatClub.com community. "Gainer" signals a desire to get bigger, and any size man can identify as such. "Encourager" refers to someone who motivates gainers; again, any size man could identify as such, but it is usually thinner men. "Bloater" describes someone who expands his stomach, albeit temporarily, often with excessive fluid intake. Such men rarely desire to gain weight, but get pleasure on their own, or through the adoration of others, from abdominal distention.

In his book, *Transgressive bodies: Representations in film and popular culture*, Niall Richardson (2010), a scholar of film, media, and Cultural Studies, writes about "stuffing" or bloating oneself. He suggests that belly expansion often exists in the realm of representation, watching an online film or reading amateur erotica produced for self- or communal pleasure, sometimes profit, often about an offseason bodybuilder or ex-jock who is a conventionally attractive man who extends his belly to erotic proportions to have a rock-hard stomach that hangs down against his genitals. He achieves this effect by chugging weight-gain supplements/protein shakes, which make his gut hard, to mimic bodybuilding aesthetics. Some stories entertain male pregnancy fantasies, finding pleasure in queering gender dynamics by looking like one is about to give birth – being turned on by getting attention from others for their big belly; or they find "sensual pleasure" in "abandon[ing] restraint" on the abdominal muscles so that "a butch enough gay man" may like letting his belly "stick out" versus "sucking it in" (Stoltenberg, 1998, p. 406).

Katariina Kyrölä (2011) writes about how the slim body "before" looks boyish, while the rock-hard belly "after" resembles feminized pregnant embodiment, but then again masculinized, with the men often pushing the limits of how much their stomach can hold as it expands. Bloaters move less against gendered norms, as they become creators of their own growth, whereby size signals masculinity. Still, this behavior could represent a hybrid of both expansive queer desires with the pleasure of a body "exploding," so to speak, a metaphor for orgasm, and submitting to masochistic pleasure of testing one's intake limits (Richardson, 2010). According to Kyrölä, circulating images online of members' pre-gain bodies shown sideways, going from slim to protruding, both performs hyper-masculinity that commands space and sexualizes it, and simulates male pregnancy, also breaking with the infantilization of the fat male body. In all, gaining and its subspecialties rely on both a performance of masculinity and of polymorphous perverse pleasure. It is queer in the sense of pleasure distributed across the entire body that is changing over time. Queer theorists such as Jack Halberstam (2005) have written about queer temporality, which blurs boundaries; in this case, questions arise about "normal" adult gay male embodiment versus taking pleasure in the body changing over time, which disrupts normative understandings of growing "up" to be adult versus an unruly body that is still growing and filling "out" (Kyrölä, 2011).

Adams and Berry (2013) also explore privileging big bodies/bellies through online users posting photos of their bodily transformation/weight-gain progression. Circulating photos, videos, and stories or chatting about belly worship/objectification while images of genitalia are strictly prohibited on the site reinforces that "It's all about the belly, baby!" (Whitesel, 2014, p. 122), meaning the belly is the sex object/center of attention, in which to take pride. Likewise, users' nonconforming social practices both "reinforce and subvert normative ideals of gender, sexuality, and health" (Adams & Berry, 2013, p. 318). The authors find both subcultural reinforcement of "the desire to look and feel like a 'real' man" and an "attempt to work against the stereotype of the youthful, thin-and-fit gay male ... 'twinks'" (ibid.). Moreover, some members of Fat.Club.com disregard the public-health narrative on obesity, taking a nonconformist stance. By framing "big" as "masculine," they reflect the status quo in the online community, while going against the twink aesthetic and even resulting in twink-shaming. In fact, members post pics of themselves struggling to fit into their clothes from their "twink days."

One final theme in Adams and Berry (2013) is erotic self-pleasure one derives from eating and growing. At the same time, eating also becomes erotic *relational* pleasure, meaning that dining together, interacting with bigger men, or mutually feeding one another can be "hot," thereby sharing in one another's body projects. What drives all of this is personal, relational, and sociocultural for members of the Fat.Club.com community, where "big" does not equal diseased or disgusting, but rather implies counterintuitive pro-weight pleasure. According to Adams and Berry, the gaining community cites strict/cruel beauty norms to support what they are doing. They are committed to "play" – i.e., gainers introduce flexibility into the rigid social system, experimenting with an alternate reality. The late queer theorist, José Muñoz (1999), might frame this as an example of "dis-identification." These men would certainly take a minority position and are disempowered by the existing representational hierarchy. They have identified exclusionary messages within the gay community when it comes to body shape and size and then come up with new strategies for representing themselves – with subject positions unthinkable to the dominant culture and most gay men alike.

Adams and Berry (2013) note that gaining practices are not without criticism. This growth community requires social privilege insomuch as members would require access to abundant food and clothes as their weight fluctuates/climbs. Moreover, these men are not oblivious to "health concerns," but resemble other fetish communities (e.g., BDSM) where participants manage enacted/weighted risks, not so different from skydiving, smoking, or riding a motorcycle. Then there are questions of "out-ness" – are members out to others beyond this community about their desires and weight-gain fantasies (e.g., vorarephilia)? According to the research, gainer communities cite normative masculinity and dis-identify with the thin/fit gay male ideal. These men enact socially constructed "risks" with regard to not managing their weight under the Foucauldian panoptic gaze, and promote "big is beautiful" as the requisite mantra for inter-acting with their community, based on sublimely abject body adoration.

Visual culture: Artwork, digital media, pornography

Artwork

In 2014, Digital-Media-Studies scholar and specialist in the sub-fields of media/internet/technolo-gy-law Scott Beattie interviewed artists who create Bear Art. This genre "opens up wider fields of erotic possibility beyond that of the conventionally hard phallic body" (p. 115). Bear historian Les Wright (2001) equates Bear Art to "erotic folk art" (as cited in Campbell, 2004, p. 138). Bear folk erotica, according to Beattie, "queers" representations of the body with its disruptive power in depict-ing ordinary bodies: big hairy "regular guys" who fit within the comfortable bounds of everyday life versus the contoured gym body that gives gay men an Adonis complex. Bear Art relies on a creative counterpublic that circulates images of men who have "meat on their bones" (Beattie, 2014, p. 117). It resists beauty and health industries by representing diverse gay male bodies and forms of intimate relations, tactile expressions like bear hugs or nuzzling another man's ample furry chest. Such imagery has been censored in gay representation in the main and emerged in zine culture. A contemporary example of a zine, *The little book of big black bears* (2015) created by Ajuan Mance, English professor at Mills College, lightheartedly pays tribute to same-gender-loving big Black men.

Bear Art and Chubby Art both make room for a rounder aesthetic, with images of gay men that diverge from the Grecian ideal of the hard body in classical art. Men with squeezable curves contradict beauty socialization in the contemporary white Western imagination where a chise-led jawline, square pecs, and a v-shaped torso exemplify idealized male beauty; not "man boobs" or a "beer belly" (Whitesel, 2017a). Beattie (2014) finds art depicting Bear and chubby men's bodies as inspiration for sexual alternatives that may cause a paradigmatic shift in the viewer's own erotic politics: haptic Bear Art involves a sense of touch, inviting one to imagine fondling flabby, round, dimpled parts of the body, which are generally off limits to touch or admire. Such art turns big men's bodies into sites of production of extraordinarily polymorphous pleasures – whole-body sensuality, with the fat body becoming a field of erotic play, versus phallic pleasures as the be-all, end-all of gay sex (Whitesel, 2017a; Beattie, 2014; Hennen, 2005). Beattie reads Bear Art as a form of queer-fat activism in its diverse imaginings of the body, alternative expres-sions of masculinity based on mutual touch, and its special techniques created to represent fat bodies. Viewers may include an ample-bodied audience, but also those who may *not* be big gay men, those attracted to bigger men, whereby such art allows them to not feel socially deviant, to feel okay for having such desires. As one such artist puts it, elevating fat-gay men to the level of art "reflects how I see my own position in a world that tells me I should find skinny women attractive and I happen to find fat men attractive" (Whitesel, 2017a, p. 5).

Beattie (2014) finds that Bear Art reaches beyond big men's subcultures, having found its way into galleries. For example, UK artist James Unsworth's fourth solo show at the RawArt Gallery, "Girth and Mirth" in 2017–2018, represented scantily clad fat-gay men once featured in the erotic magazine, *Bulk Male* (Whitesel, 2017a). Likewise, James Gobel, an artist at California College of the Arts, San Francisco, uses felt/yarn/fabric – all supple and highly tactile mate-rials associated with feminine handicrafts – to celebrate the unsung sensuality of big gay men, inspired by the same pinup magazines that Unsworth reimagines, questioning which bodies are acceptable and which are not (Blake, 2000). Or NYC artist, Nayland Blake (using they/them pronouns), a bearish, bi-racial queer artist, depicts body weight/fat/food as erotic signifiers in *Starting Over* (2000), a video of the artist struggling to dance with taps on their shoes in an oversized bunny suit stuffed with 140 pounds of dried beans – a weight equal to Blake's partner of 12 years. Blake's 1998 video, "Gorge," featured the artist sitting shirtless, being handfed copious amounts of food for an hour by a shirtless Black man (Russeth, 2019). Later staged live, Blake invited the audience to feed them. Similarly, Campbell (2004) included pictures of Gainer Art he found circulating in his online ethnographic study of the embodied sensual experiences of gay men. Examples were also featured in a documentary, *Hard Fat* (2002), by media artist and film educator, Frédéric Moffet – a film about beauty not defined by social conventions and pressures, wherein clichés of before-and-after transformations become reversed.

The point is, returning to Beattie (2014), that the iconography of Bears and big handsome gay men seems to no longer be contained in the Bear and Girth & Mirth scenes alone. Such artworks come with their own techniques for how to render fat as abject or desirable, depending on their message. Art's transformative powers help shift sexual interests, placing Bear and big men on the menu of desires.

Digital media

Gay men who possess or desire a body that does not conform to the gay male beauty myth find mainstream and gay media dissatisfying. Therefore, they construct and consume imagery of male bodies that transcend, yet do not fully reject, the idealized images of "attractive and desirable" male bodies (Campbell, 2004). Using semiotic analysis, I (2010) explored "fatvertisements" that recreate commercial images by recasting fat bodies for the models or by photoshopping existing images to give the male model a paunch. Often, media hype around male celebrities – whose photographs "need" airbrushing to hide their love handles – served as inspiration for these eroticized images (Whitesel, 2010). Gay men's preoccupation with thinness was complicated by the AIDS crisis, which occasioned revisiting the ideal gay body and body types that signify "health" (Hennen, 2005). Thus, fat became sexy, transforming the standards for what qualifies as a desirable male body, thereby also compensating for the gay body wasting with HIV/AIDS. Fatvertisements appeared to be a mixed mode of resistance, as they still relied on the worship of other idealized male qualities such as facial attractiveness, or babyfaces that signal youth. Haraway's (1986) cyber-feminism applies here, with image-makers challenging bodily boundaries, deconstructing/reconstructing advertisers' obsession with men's rock-hard abs: fatvertisements turn the funhouse mirror on airbrushed ads and build cyborg imagery, with both imagination and material reality, floating between reality and computer artifice. They equate fat male bodies with bodies of homoerotic celebrity hunks or sports and/or porn stars, with a certain amount of "baby fat" signaling a "healthy" weight for gay men (Whitesel, 2010).

Likewise, websites have formed in response to lack of fashion for queer men who do not possess an "ideal" body. For example, a blog on Tumblr, "Chubby Guy Swag," supports those defeated by the fashion industry, looking to get their swag back. Followers describe this site as a confidence booster with style references for not only fat-gay men, but also fat trans men, fat gender-queer people, and people with Down Syndrome who may have a short, stocky body. It is clear that the democratization of fashion starts from do-it-yourself looks, forging creative style from a lack of extended size options, and then sharing it with others (Whitesel, 2015).

Pornography

Framed both as damaging/transgressive and as free speech, different kinds of porn appeal to different kinds of analysis. While garden-variety heterosexual porn can be viewed as offensive/abusive to women, specialty genres of porn are particularly important to those with nonnormative bodies and desires, who cannot find their sexual/romantic lives depicted elsewhere. In the latter case, chubby-gay porn could offer a venue where gay men with ample builds have their body type taken seriously, thereby rendering them sexual citizens (Highberg, 2011). Porn, like being gay or being fat, is often treated as shameful, yet chubby-gay porn is a performance that constitutes itself outside of "official" public opinion, i.e., a "queer counterpublic" (Berlant & Warner, 1998, p. 558). Access to some films requires disposable income with some offerings behind a paywall versus free content available in digital commons (Highberg, 2011). Free-flowing content has become less accessible in popular online venues, with Silicon Valley blocking and removing adult content.

Gender-and-Technology-Studies scholar Nels Highberg (2011) explores the social utility of chubby-gay porn online – both user-generated videos and longer films produced by small suppliers accessed for a fee. He melds together four perspectives – Trauma Theory: insidious, everyday forms of trauma *à la* queer theorist, Ann Cvetkovich (2003); Porn Studies: in particular, benefits of publicly accessible sexual culture *à la* Lauren Berlant and Michael Warner (1998); Fat Studies: reframing ample weight as a form of bodily diversity *à la* Marilyn Wann (2009); and Performance Studies: particularly visibility politics – by which he means being seen and heard. The author's relationship to the material is that of a somewhat-ambivalent insider; he is a big gay man weighing 250 pounds, who grapples with reclaiming labels like "fat" as simply factual, while he knows all too well the sting of the judgment the term carries.

Highberg (2011) writes about men intimately and erotically engaging with other men of various shapes and sizes; he is particularly enamored by "real-life" porn that often begins with interviews of those in the erotic film, so that their personal, private histories become social, cultural, and public histories of sexuality. In the films he analyzes, "unconventional" (i.e., fat-gay) pornographic performers are shown as couples in fulfilling relationships, making the films not simply about sex, but also about a real relationship. Highberg also finds that fat-gay men have a place within other pornographic genres like sadomasochistic and fetish porn, providing a much-needed venue for them to express sexual desire and feel pleasures that might otherwise be denied to them in a thin, straight world. In films and television shows, big and middle-aged gay men are portrayed as shoulders to cry on or as the comic relief, rarely, if ever, playing the love interest or being taken seriously as adult sexual beings.

Still, anthropologist Matti Bunzl (2005) questions whether chubby-gay porn really makes much of a progressive statement for fat and queer people. Building off the work of Laura Kipnis (1996), he engages with a mid-1990s strand of Fat Studies that uses a cultural-criticism framework to argue that fat-admiration pornography takes society's aesthetic prejudices and socially sanctioned disgust to task. Kipnis argues that porn desires to be seen, fat desires to be hidden, and fat/queer porn wants gay/chubby sexuality to be known, naked, in all its glorious sexual sharing, publicly defiant. Chubby-gay porn films like Maximum Density Productions' infamous *Bustin' Apart at the Seams* in 1998 or *Bulk Male* magazine, the fat/gay equivalent to *Playboy*, feature those weighing 200–300 pounds. They cater to the tastes of chasers, defined by their desire for bigger men, and not necessarily by being thin. Yet Bunzl finds that although such media may be sexually liberating, it is far from providing sexual equality, with superchubs, those weighing significantly more than chubs, often absent from the imagery, indicative of power differentials still at play. Little racial/ethnic diversity exists in fat-gay pornographic media in general (Bunzl, 2005).

Sociologist Natalie Ingraham (2015) conducted in-depth interviews and ethnographic fieldwork with the San Francisco Bay area's queer-pornography producers/directors/performers, among them, two queer- and fat-identified gay men who were romantic partners with large Bear bodies. Fully aware of the tendency in older Bear pornography to primarily feature white men of size, they created a series called "Real Bears of Color." Ingraham found that most who participate in queerer porn eroticize fat sexuality that's usually excluded from widely circulated porn or "ghettoized" into fetish porn. Moreover, fat/queer porn is built from improvization, as two larger men or a larger man having sex with a mid-build actor require cinematographers/producers to think anew about sexual positions and lighting issues.

Recent developments

Adams's (2016) co-authored reflection on the need to "*quare*" Fat Studies speaks to the historical development of ideas in this field, where white/male privilege has not been critically examined in prior work on fat-gay men. Those looking to the future of the field will find themselves well to follow Adams's example and better articulate the intersectionalities of size, sexual orientation, and gender identity with regard to race, class, age, ability, and nationality.

In "On being different and loving it," Nadav Antebi (2015), a public-health practitioner and psychotherapist, ponders on his 14-year-old self: "I was fat, fem, and a fag. Too much? Maybe?" (p. 214). The future of Fat-Studies scholarship on fat-gay men will more thoroughly explore the "intricate double marginalities that fat-and-femme queers must navigate," as Gender and Sexuality Studies scholar, Matthew Conte (2018) does in his autoethnography. For example, Conte writes about his negative experiences with the dating app, Grindr, wherein he felt "fatness was deemed as gross and unattractive," his "femininity was devalued and degraded," and fat/femme/racialized queer people were relegated to the "queer unwanted" (pp. 25–26). In fact, Conte could not even find the category to check "fat" or "fem" from the "body type" or "tribes" checkboxes on Grindr. These identity markers are not only subordinated within gay culture, but also fetishized as sexually submissive, seen only as "more cushion for the pushing." Future research should further explore fat/fem as they intersect with race/ethnicity among dominant cisgender gay males.

Fat bodies in drag also merit further research. Using a Fat Studies framework, Ami Pomerantz (2017) conducted qualitative content analysis of the representation of fat drag-queen contestants on the reality television show, *RuPaul's Drag Race* (RPDR). He explores how this queer show that should approach sizeism and fatphobia in transgressive ways instead sends conflicting messages to contestants of size. Sometimes it supports fat pride, but it is often reluctant to embrace "big girls" and has never awarded its top prize to a fat contestant. Pomerantz refers to this tension as a "polyphonic discourse" surrounding fat men in drag that simultaneously supports bodily diversity while also discriminating against larger queens. The show typecasts fat contestants as comedy queens who bring up fried/caloric foods and make fat jokes in their shticks, even as it exploits contestants' storylines about body image and weight struggles/loss to tug at viewers' heartstrings. Polyphonically, the show feigns size acceptance, even as it condemns fatness. Nevertheless, after 11 years of RPDR on television, big girls at least have been given more air time as the seasons have progressed (Pomerantz, 2017).

Pomerantz (2017) categorizes strategies RPDR contenders deploy in various combinations to weather the shame of fat stigma and resist sizeism. First, some queens capitulate to the sizeist stereotypes, which the judges reward. Second, fat queens walk a thin line between campy empowerment and self-deprecating jokes that cooperate with fatphobic hegemony. Third, queens of size form oppositional identities, with fat pride positioned against the slim/muscular hegemonic body ideal (i.e., "Fuck dem skinny bitches, it's a big girls' world!"). A fourth strategy claims "fat is beautiful," drawing from people-of-color and feminist traditions of women's resistance to rigid beauty standards. A fifth strategy sexualizes fatness as feminine, whereby fat queens accentuate their curves, breasts, and ample buttocks. The last strategy emphasizes traits other than body shape and size, with the tokenized big girl offering more than just an ample figure. Overall, Pomerantz (2017) underscores the struggle over compliance with, and resistance to, fat oppression.

Interdisciplinary Feminist/Queer/Trans Studies scholar Emmanuel David and demographer Christian Cruz (2018) demonstrate the need for greater cross-cultural work in Fat Studies. Their ethnographic research on fat *bakla* contestants in a plus-size beauty pageant, *Miss Gay: Queen-size Edition*, takes place in an urban-poor neighborhood in Manila, Philippines. *Bakla*, a reclamation of a derogatory term in Tagalog, refers to people birth-assigned "male," but "whose gender identities/expressions and/or sexual orientations do not conform to conventional gender norms or heteronormative society" (David & Cruz, 2018, p. 42). This contest is open to gay, bi, and trans people who are chubby, with the 2012 contest under study having 24 contestants vying for the win. Embodying multiple, subordinated statuses, big/brown/queer bodies onstage renegotiate global beauty ideals. The authors frame the pageant scene – performers and audience – as a queer "counterpublic" *à la* Warner (2005), building on the history of racial integration into pageants. Fatness, to Manila's urban poor, registers as wealth and access to resources; it symbolizes overconsumption without regard to those suffering economically. Yet the pageant contestants' fat, taken as a wealthy affront, occurs in bodies of sexual and gender minorities, making for a complex intersection between big bodies "taking up too many resources" and marginalized *bakla* identities. David and Cruz (2018) find that like many fat and LGBTQ people, the contestants contend with moral evaluations of their bodies and identities, and they must negotiate fat's class-inflected association with wealth on the Manila stage. They approach the pageant light-heartedly as they sexualize food, consumption, and fatness. They engage in fat-is-beautiful advocacy, incorporating race/ethnicity to claim "big, brown, bakla, and beautiful" (p. 38). Despite outsiders' opinion of the scene, contestants display pride in their fat shame, salvaging their right to dignity and respect – appeals that would "register with fat activists' size-acceptance discourse" (p. 40). Their performances redefine fat with sexual and aesthetic currency; showing skin, being sexy and glamourous. Most of the queen-sized drag performers powder their faces to appear fairer-skinned, sometimes impersonating white, skinny Westerners, while a smaller minority of queens celebrate "brown is beautiful," combining fat embodiment with makeup matching their complexion (David & Cruz, 2018).

Seldom expanding beyond US borders for its material, Fat Studies of gay men should also consider how body shape and size affect people across nations, races, ethnicities, and religions in its research and reporting. In 2014, Pranta Patnaik, sociologist specializing in Cultural and Media Studies, conducted open-ended, semi-structured interviews on- and offline with 12 gay/bi men in Delhi. They were comprised of five Hindus (three Brahmins, no untouchables), five Muslims, and two Sikhs. All but two were married men, ages 30–52, identifying as fat, chubby, or Bear, most being "in the closet." The dating site that these men frequent depicts itself as a welcoming space, yet user demand remains highest for disciplined, hard bodies, thus posing an equal-representation problem. Patnaik (2014, p. 93) therefore asks, where does the fat-gay body fit on these websites?

Patnaik's (2014) interviewees affirm having internalized dominant discourses by citing their disproportionate weight-to-height ratio, body type, genetic predisposition to fat, indulgence in deep-fried street food, and frequent ridicule they endure. They speak of grappling with terminology, some partial to embracing the cute, cuddly Bear identity, others finding the term too Western, and still others resisting the unclean-animal image of a bear (*bhallu* in Hindi), which also means "dumb," making this symbolic identity even less appealing. Using an intersectional lens, Patnaik found fat to be crosscut by family/gender/class/religion. One respondent commented on fat's visibility versus gay's invisibility: his family knew about his body weight, but not his struggles with sexuality. Another respondent lamented his wife admiring the looks of other men, mentioning to him that fatness diminishes the size of his penis, which made him feel emasculated beyond sometimes feeling devalued on gay websites. In terms of caste/class, an older, fat-gay man had the monetary resources to wine-and-dine younger gay men, who were viewed as admirers rather than predatory types. As for religion, one fat-gay Sikh felt that potential partners were turned off by his wearing a turban and having long hair – associated with effeminacy. Some of the men in the study reported being emasculated because of their male breasts or rendered as figuratively impotent on this dating site. Others felt they amounted to teddy bears sought out to cuddle or play with, but not taken seriously as sexual beings. Thus, the internet provided a safe space for Indian gay/bi men to interact with one another, yet gay enclaves tended to still form online around traditionally ideal male bodies, designed to keep "less-desirable" users off the site, or pushing them to form affinity subgroups. Patnaik (2014) concludes that online dating sites are rife with profiles of users who state "no fatty uncle"-types, yet the men in his study are glad that a subgroup of fat admirers does exist.

Recent studies on fat-gay men focus on gay Bears in East and Southeast Asia (Lin, 2014; Tan, 2016, 2019). Chichun Lin (2014), US trained in couples and family counseling, collected quantitative (N = 217 questionnaires) and qualitative (N = 12 Skype interviews) data on gay Bear men in mainland China, Hong-Kong, Taiwan, and Malaysia. Lin found the gay-bear-identified men he surveyed and interviewed were pursuing an "idealized gay bear appearance" (heavier, hairier, hypermasculine) to achieve higher status (p. 188), wanting to become popular within the Chinese gay Bear community. While they reported having higher self-esteem than did non-bear-identified gay men (N = 429), they also reported being teased because of their appearance and feeling isolated in mainstream gay male communities. Yet, according to Lin (2014), they did not create diverse "personal styles" like Western gay Bears do, but lived up to the collectivist, "stereotypical Chinese gay Bear look" (pp. 189–190).

Chris Tan (2016, 2019), Associate Professor of Anthropology specializing in central academic domains: gender, sexuality, and bodies, extended Lin's above study with his ethnographic articles about how Taipei gay Bear men use their bodies and clothes to increase their erotic capital. Tan's study illuminates how their desirability gets stratified within group (2019). Tan (2016) self-identifies "as a gay Bear of Chinese ethnicity and Singaporean nationality" (p. 848). He attributes the homogenized Taiwanese Bear look to interpersonal competition.

According to Tan (2016), Taiwanese gay bears reject the Orientalizing label of "Panda" used in the US to describe Asian gay Bear men. Instead, they use the label *xiong*, meaning "bear" in Mandarin. US gay Bears' popularity was diffused in the 1980s first to Japan, represented in fantasy drawings of *gatchiri* men or "G-men" eroticizing blue-collar strongly built bodies, and next to the rest of Northeast Asia, blossoming in Taiwan. At first, fat-gay men and Bears were one and the same; by the late 1990s/early 2000s in Taiwan, the *xiong* differentiated themselves from the *zhu*, meaning "pig," a pejorative term for a fat person, as in English. The muscle-bear body became the look to emulate. This was compelled, in part, by competition to differentiate oneself from the Bear pack by being bulky and muscular versus fat. Nevertheless, fat-gay men continue to try to self-identify as Bear, capitalizing on the label's fuzzy definition as to whether one registers as "Bear" or "Pig," which Tan found mostly depends on one's popularity and vice versa.

Tan (2016) notes that most shops in Taiwan do not carry extended sizes, which drives fat-gay men to shop online on websites that cater to the Bear community. However, the choices there, too, are limited, which results in Taipei Bears becoming gay clones, criticized for their homogenized look. This somewhat flies in the face of the big men's and Bear movements in the US in reaction to Castro clones, desiring to celebrate somatic diversity. Moreover, as the muscle-Bear dominates the Taipei Bear circuit, it becomes a "meat market" where outsiders who visit for Pride events find the scene competitive and alienating.

Tan (2016) connects his ethnographic study to the literature on "gaydar," demonstrating how one might "spot" a gay Bear in Taipei by his homogenized Bear look. Tan's findings on the ability to notice someone is gay also give insight into the notion of the ways in which "gaydar," like "selective hearing," is a form of "selective seeing," where Taiwanese Bear men tune out those they consider not worth looking at. In the US, gay Bears might blend into the suburbs as "regular" guys; but in Taipei, Bears stand out based on the time they spend in the gym, or by the tank tops with Bear emblems that they don. This speaks to the Bear indexing changing global gay masculinity. While the gay Bear subculture set out to celebrate bodily diversity, it is rendered quite the opposite in Taipei.

Conclusion and future directions

Existing research on fat-gay men is mostly written by white Western men. It often involves insider research by fay-gay men or members of fat-affirming communities, or sometimes by an ally-outsider-within, gay, but thin-privileged, and white, like myself, when I wrote *Fat gay men* (2014). Future research into fat-gay men should continue to broaden its investigation into subjectivities beyond US borders, engaging in greater cross-national comparative research. For example, in the late 1990s/early 2000s, attempts were made to document Bear groups around the globe, mostly Euro-Bears (McCann, 1997) or Bear groups formed in Oceanic countries like Australia (Hay, 1997; Hyslop, 2001) and New Zealand (Webster, 1997). Ron Suresha (2002c) tried to assemble voices of different Bears from around the world by publishing a 23-page focus-group discussion that included Western Bears and three interviewees from Bear clubs in the Global South (Mexico, Argentina, South Africa) and one from Turkey (re: Turkey, also see Sahin, 2001). To my knowledge, little-to-no effort has been made to establish research into social networks for fat-gay men in Latin America/Africa/Middle East. Virtually absent are studies of self-identified big gay men in Asia.

On the horizon should be robust literature on the ways big men's racial or ethnic identities mutually construct their fat-gayness or position them differently within some of the subcultures chronicled herein. See my own writing (2017b & 2019) on race-based problems with representation in US big mens' communities that overlook same-gender-loving big men of color in their event advertising and erotic imagery. In reaction, big men of color in the US have created their own weekend runs like Heetizm Myami, Big Boy Pride Orlando, and Heavy Hitters Pride Houston. In response to other gay Prides and circuit parties across the nation that reinforce the mainstream gay media's narrow focus on young, hairless, thin or muscular, white men, these annual gatherings place men of size and color at the fore. For example, the 2017 theme for Heavy Hitters' weekend was "My Presence Matters." The group describes itself as "a place where EVERY pound has a story" and where attendees come to "celebrate the urban man of size, his admirers and allies" (Heavy Hitters Pride, 2017). If imagery like that put out by Heetizm, Big Boy Pride, and Heavy Hitters did not exist, then same-gender-loving big men of color might find it difficult to recognize themselves in existing white-dominant big-gay-men's imagery (Hennen, 2005), and thus might internalize the message "You are not welcome" (Whitesel, 2017b & 2019).

Topics on fat-gay men that remain unexplored might include: 1) groups for same-gender-loving big men of color, 2) big gay men beyond Western boundaries in East and South Asia, and 3) special risks for those multiply marginalized as fat/gay/fem. Additionally, sexologists are just beginning to untangle the particular risks confronted by men who are multiply marginalized by their size, sexuality, and gender identity.

References

Adams, T., & Berry, K. (2013). Size matters: Performing (il)logical male bodies on fatclub.com. *Text and Performance Quarterly*, *33*(4), 308–325.

Antebi, N. (2015). On being different and loving it. In R. Chastain (Ed.), *The politics of size: Perspectives from the fat acceptance movement* (pp. 207–216). Santa Barbara, CA: Praeger.

Bakhtin, M. (1965). *Rabelais and his world*. Cambridge, MA: MIT Press.

Beattie, S. (2014). Bear arts naked: Queer activism and the fat male body. In C. Pausé, J. Wykes, & S. Murray (Eds.), *Queering fat embodiment* (pp. 115–129). New York: Routledge.

Berlant, L., & Warner, M. (1998). Sex in public. *Critical Inquiry*, *24*(2), 547–566.

Blake, N. (2000). James Gobel [Exhibition essay]. Los Angeles, CA: Hammer Museum. https://hammer. ucla.edu/exhibitions/2000/hammer-projects-james-gobel/.

Blotcher, J. (1998). Justify my love handles: How the queer community trims the fat. In D. Atkins (Ed.), *Looking queer: Body image and identity in lesbian, bisexual, gay, and transgender communities* (pp. 359–366). New York: Harrington Park Press.

Boylorn, R., & Adams, T. (2016). Queer and quare autoethnography. In N. Denzin, & M. Giardina (Eds.), *Qualitative inquiry through a critical lens* (pp. 85–98). New York: Routledge.

Brown, W. (1993). Wounded attachments. *Political Theory*, *21*(3), 390–410.

Bunzl, M. (2005). Chaser. In D. Kulick, & A. Meneley (Eds.), *Fat: The anthropology of obsession* (pp. 199–210). New York: Penguin.

Campbell, J. (2004). *Getting it on online: Cyberspace, gay male sexuality, and embodied identity*. New York: Harrington Park Press.

Conte, M. (2018). More fats, more femmes: A critical examination of fatphobia and femmephobia on grindr. *Feral Feminisms: Queer Feminine Affinities*, 7, 25–32.

Cvetkovich, A. (2003). *An archive of feelings: Trauma, sexuality, and lesbian public cultures*. Durham, NC: Duke University Press.

David, E., & Cruz, J. (2018). Big, bakla, and beautiful: Transformations on a Manila pageant stage. *Women's Studies Quarterly*, *46*(1–2), 29–45.

Durgadas, G. (1998). Fatness and the feminized man. In D. Atkins (Ed.), *Looking queer: Body image and identity in lesbian, bisexual, gay, and transgender communities* (pp. 367–371). New York: Harrington Park Press.

Edmonds, S., & Zieff, S. (2015). Bearing bodies: Physical activity, obesity stigma, and sexuality in the bear community. *Sociology of Sport Journal*, *32*(4), 415–435.

Eser, Z., & Spooner, A. (n.d.). Chubby Guy Swag was founded by bodyposi activist and dj/producer, zacheser, in 2010. https://chubbyguyswag.tumblr.com

Foster-Gimbel, O., & Engeln, R. (2016). Fat chance! Experiences and expectations of antifat bias in the gay male community. *Psychology of Sexual Orientation and Gender Diversity*, *3*(1), 63–70.

Giles, P. (1998). A matter of size. In D. Atkins (Ed.), *Looking queer: Body image and identity in lesbian, bisexual, gay, and transgender communities* (pp. 355–358). New York: Harrington Park Press.

Goffman, E. (1963). *Stigma: Notes on the management of spoiled identity*. Englewood Cliffs, NJ: Prentice-Hall.

Gough, B., & Flanders, G. (2009). Celebrating "obese" bodies: Gay "bears" talk about weight, body image and health. *International Journal of Men's Health*, *8*(3), 235–253.

Grommr (n.d.). Abridged gainer history project. https://www.grommr.com/Home/Community

Halberstam, J. (2005). *In a queer time and place: Transgender bodies, subcultural lives*. New York: New York University Press.

Haraway, D. (1986). A manifesto for cyborgs. Science, technology, and socialist feminism in the 1980s. In D. Meyers (Ed.), *Feminist social thought: A reader* (1997, pp. 502–531). New York: Routledge.

Hay, B. (1997). Bears in the land down under. In L. Wright (Ed.), *The bear book: Readings in the history and evolution of a gay male subculture* (pp. 225–238). New York: Haworth Press:

Heavy Hitters Pride. (2017). My presence matters empowerment summit. https://www.facebook.com/events/1809292522725796.

Hennen, P. (2005). Bear bodies, bear masculinity: Recuperation, resistance, or retreat? *Gender and Society*, *19*(1), 25–43.

Hennen, P. (2008). *Faeries, bears, and leathermen: Men in community queering the masculine*. Chicago, IL: University of Chicago Press.

Highberg, N. (2011). More than a comic sidekick: Fat men in gay porn. *Performing Ethos: International Journal of Ethics in Theatre & Performance*, *2*(2), 109–120.

Hymes, D. (1968). The ethnography of speaking. In J. Fishman (Ed.), *Readings in the sociology of language* (pp. 99–138). The Hague, Paris: Mouton.

Hyslop, S. (2001). The rise of the Australian bear community since 1995. In L. Wright (Ed.), *The bear book II: Further readings in the history and evolution of a gay male subculture* (pp. 269–283). New York: Harrington Park Press.

Ingraham, N. (2015). Queering porn: Gender and size diversity within SF Bay area queer pornography. In H. Hester, & C. Walters (Eds.), *Fat sex: New directions in theory and activism* (pp. 115–132). Farnham: Ashgate.

Johnson, E. (2001). "Quare" studies, or (almost) everything I know about queer studies I learned from my grandmother. *Text and Performance Quarterly, 21*(1), 1–25.

Johnson, F. (1998). Frat-boy fetishism: When the goods get together. In the Bad Subjects Production Team (Eds.), *Bad subjects: Political education for everyday life* (pp. 196–200). New York: New York University Press.

Kampf, R. (2000). *The bear handbook: A comprehensive guide for those who are husky, hairy, and homosexual and those who love 'em.* New York: Harrington Park Press.

Kipnis, L. (1996). Life in the fat lane. In L. Kipnis, *Bound and gagged: Pornography and the politics of fantasy in America* (pp. 93–121). Durham, NC: Duke University Press.

Kruger, S. (1998). "Get fat, don't die!": Eating and AIDS in gay men's culture. In R. Scapp, & B. Seitz (Eds.), *Eating culture* (pp. 36–59). Albany, NY: SUNY Press.

Kyrölä, K. (2011). Adults growing sideways: Feederist pornography and fantasies of infantilism. *Lambda Nordica, 16*(2–3), 128–158.

Lannan, M. (Creator, Co-Executive Producer). (2014). *Looking* [Television series]. New York: HBO.

Lin, C. (2014). Chinese gay bear men. *Culture, Society & Masculinities, 6*(2), 183–193.

Mance, A. (2015). *The little book of big black bears.* 8-Rock Press. https://8-rock.tumblr.com/post/111129223148/the-little-book-of-big-black-bears-a-zine-by

Manley, E., Levitt, H., & Mosher, C. (2007). Understanding the bear movement in gay male culture: Redefining masculinity. *Journal of Homosexuality, 53*(4), 89–112.

Mann, J. (2010). Bear culture 101 (no prerequisite). *The Gay & Lesbian Review Worldwide, 17*(5), 22–24.

McCann, T. (1997). Atlantic crossing: The development of the eurobear. In L. Wright (Ed.), *The bear book: Readings in the history and evolution of a gay male subculture* (pp. 251–259). New York: Haworth Press.

McGrady, P. (2016). "Grow the beard, wear the costume": Resisting weight and sexual orientation stigmas in the bear subculture. *Journal of Homosexuality, 63*(12), 1698–1725.

McNair, B. (2002). *Striptease culture: Sex, media and the democratization of desire.* New York: Routledge.

Meyer, I. (2003). Prejudice, social stress, and mental health in lesbian, gay, and bisexual populations: Conceptual issues and research evidence. *Psychological Bulletin, 129*(5), 674–697.

Moffet, F. (Producer). (2002). *Hard Fat* [Documentary film]. Montréal, QC: Vidéographe.

Monaghan, L. (2005). Big handsome men, bears and others: Virtual constructions of "fat male embodiment." *Body & Society, 11*(2), 81–111.

Moon, M., & Sedgwick, E. (1990–91). Divinity: A dossier, a performance piece, a little-understood emotion. *Discourse, 13*(1), 12–39.

Moskowitz, D., Turrubiates, J., Lozano, H., & Hajek, C. (2013). Physical, behavioral, and psychological traits of gay men identifying as bears. *Archives of Sexual Behavior, 42*(5), 775–784.

Muñoz, J. (1999). *Disidentifications: Queers of color and the performance of politics.* Minneapolis, MN: University of Minnesota Press.

Oliverio, D. (2016). *The round world: Life at the intersection of love, sex, and fat.* West Hollywood, CA: The Antrobus Group.

Patnaik, P. (2014). Bearly Indian: "Fat" gay men's negotiation of embodiment, culture, and masculinity. In R. Dasgupta, & K. Gokulsing (Eds.), *Masculinity and its challenges in India: Essays on changing perceptions* (pp. 93–105). Jefferson, NC: McFarland.

Pomerantz, A. (2017). Big-girls don't cry: Portrayals of the fat body in *RuPaul's Drag Race.* In N. Brennan, & D. Gudelunas (Eds.), *RuPaul's Drag Race and the shifting visibility of drag culture: The boundaries of reality TV* (pp. 103–120). Cham, Switzerland: Palgrave Macmillan.

Pyle, N., & Klein, N. (2011). Fat. hairy. sexy: Contesting standards of beauty and sexuality in the gay community. In C. Bobel, & S. Kwan (Eds.), *Embodied resistance: Challenging the norms, breaking the rules* (pp. 78–87). Nashville, TN: Vanderbilt University Press.

Pyle, N., & Loewy, M. (2009). Double stigma: Fat men and their male admirers. In E. Rothblum, & S. Solovay (Eds.), *The fat studies reader* (pp. 143–150). New York: New York University Press.

Quidley-Rodriquez, N., & De Santis, J. (2016). Physical, psychosocial, and social health of men who identify as bears: A systematic review. *Journal of Clinical Nursing, 25*(23–24), 3484–3496.

Quidley-Rodriquez, N., & De Santis, J. (2017). A literature review of health risks in the bear community, a gay subculture. *American Journal of Men's Health, 11*(6), 1673–1679.

Quidley-Rodriquez, N., & De Santis, J. (2019). A concept analysis of bear identity. *Journal of Homosexuality, 66*(1), 60–76.

Richardson, N. (2010). *Transgressive bodies: Representation in film and popular culture.* Farnham: Ashgate.

Robinson, B. (2018). The quantifiable-body discourse: "Height-weight proportionality" and gay men's bodies in cyberspace. *Social Currents, 3*(2), 172–185.

Roth, Y. (2014). Locating the "scruff guy": Theorizing body and space in gay geosocial media. *International Journal of Communication, 8,* 2113–2133.

Russeth, A. (2019). Serious play: Nayland Blake's gifts from the department of transformation. *ARTnews, 118*(1), 80. http://www.artnews.com/2019/04/09/nayland-blake/

Sahin, M. (2001). A bear voice from Turkey. In L. Wright (Ed.), *The bear book II: Further readings in the history and evolution of a gay male subculture* (pp. 253–261). New York: Harrington Park Press.

Smith, T., & Bale, C. (2012). *Guide for the modern bear: A field study of bears in the wild.* Townsend, WA: Pixelita Press.

Stoltenberg, J. (1998). Learning the F words. In D. Atkins (Ed.), *Looking queer: Body image and identity in lesbian, bisexual, gay, and transgender communities* (pp. 393–411). New York: Harrington Park Press.

Suresha, R. (2002a). *Bears on bears: Interviews and discussions.* Los Angeles, CA: Alyson Books.

Suresha, R. (2002b). The birth of Girth & Mirth: An interview with Reed Wilgoren. In R. Suresha (Ed.), *Bears on bears: Interviews and discussions* (pp. 63–76). Los Angeles, CA: Alyson Books.

Suresha, R. (2002c). International bear brotherhood. In R. Suresha (Ed.), *Bears on bears: Interviews and discussions* (pp. 318–340). Los Angeles, CA: Alyson Books.

Suresha, R. (2014). Genderfuzz, or, how I learned to stop worrying and love bisexuality. In R. Ochs, & H. Williams (Eds.), *Recognize: The voices of bisexual men* (pp. 23–28). Boston, MA: Bisexual Resource Center.

Tan, C. (2016). Gaydar: Using skilled vision to spot gay "bears" in Taipei. *Anthropological Quarterly, 89*(3), 841–864.

Tan, C. (2019). Taipei gay "bear" culture as a sexual field, or, why did Nanbu bear fail? *Journal of Contemporary Ethnography, 48*(4), 563–585.

Textor, A. (1999). Organization, specialization, and desires in the big men's movement: Preliminary research in the study of subculture-formation. *International Journal of Sexuality and Gender Studies, 4*(3), 217–239.

Wann, M. (2009). Foreword. In E. Rothblum, & S. Solovay (Eds.), *The fat studies reader* (pp. ix–xxv). New York: New York University Press.

Warner, M. (2005). *Publics and counterpublics.* New York: Zone Books.

Webster, J. (1997). Kiwi bears. In L. Wright (Ed.), *The bear book: Readings in the history and evolution of a gay male subculture* (pp. 239–250). New York: Haworth Press.

Whitesel, J. (2010). Gay men's use of online pictures in fat-affirming groups. In C. Pullen, & M. Cooper (Eds.), *LGBT identity and online new media* (pp. 215–229). New York: Routledge.

Whitesel, J. (2014). *Fat gay men: Girth, mirth, and the politics of stigma.* New York: New York University Press.

Whitesel, J. (2015, Sept 15). Chubby guy swag. *From the Square.* https://www.fromthesquare.org/chubby-guy-swag.

Whitesel, J. (2017a). *James Unsworth: Girth and Mirth* [Exhibition catalogue]. Tel Aviv, Israel: Raw Art Gallery. https://rawartmedia.s3-eu-west-2.amazonaws.com/exhibitions_catalogues/2017-12-04/James_Unsworth_catalog_girth_and_mirth-_final.pdf

Whitesel, J. (2017b, Jun 30). Same-gender-loving big men of color. *From the Square.* https://www.fromthesquare.org/same-gender-loving-big-men-color.

Whitesel, J. (2019). Big gay men's performative protest against body shaming: The case of Girth and Mirth. In C. Bobel, & S. Kwan (Eds.), *Body battlegrounds: Transgressions, tensions, and transformations* (pp. 129–143). Nashville, TN: Vanderbilt University Press.

Whitesel, J., & Shuman, A. (2013). Normalizing desire: Stigma and the carnivalesque in gay bigmen's cultural practices. *Men and Masculinities, 16*(4), 478–496.

Whitesel, J., & Shuman, A. (2016). Discursive entanglements, diffractive readings: Weight-loss-surgery narratives of girth & mirthers. *Fat Studies, 5*(1), 32–56.

Wright, L. (1997). *The bear book: Readings in the history and evolution of a gay male subculture.* New York: The Haworth Press.

Wright, L. (2001). *The bear book II: Further readings in the history and evolution of a gay male subculture.* New York: Harrington Park Press.

PART 5

Fat disruptions

Part 5 rattles the foundations of Fat Studies as a discourse that has been shaped primarily by fat, cis, white, straight able-bodied perspectives. "Fat disruptions" seeks to complicate many of the commonly held notions of fatness and fat studies by investigating the ontological merits of aspects of the existing framework. Using the critical lens of other inter-disciplinary theories and by denouncing limiting narratives currently used to frame the fat experience, this part complicates, expands, and upends current discourse forcing us to question what we know about fatness and how we came to know it.

Athia Choudhury opens with a chapter asking how the fat body has come to be racialized and classed in a modern Western context and how decolonial fat studies might destabilize such a narrative. She begins the chapter leading a classroom discussion on Junot Diaz's book, *The brief wondrous life of Oscar Wao,* in which the protagonist's fatness is meant to symbolize the historical trauma of colonial and sexual violence. Her students struggle to engage and it is clear, even in this dialogue, her body is a disruption in the space. She asks, "How can we talk about this obvious metaphor of dysfunctional and racialized fat in the novel when such a body – in flesh and bone – interrupts the classroom space?" (p. 239). She continues, "The image of the poor, fat Latino child makes sense of our modern racial discourse on obesity – one that uncritically recasts and flattens the fat body as a problem of imperial foodways, diaspora/displacement, and settler colonialism" (p. 240). Choudhury offers that our current discourse around fatness centers white, Western womanhood and in that it either problematizes or erases the fat body that exists outside the circumference of a white Western female framework of Fat Studies. She posits decoloniality offers a non-linear, non-hierarchical methodology by which to disturb current fat frameworks offering,

> Rather than simply map "correctives" to the current literature or offer a monolithic genealogy that can seamlessly stitch together the unified theory of fat, I urge scholars to move horizontally across multiply layered temporalities and histories. Let us linger in the fissures of possibilities, pause in the gaps, and grasp at the questions that might get us closer to finding the body in Empire.
>
> *(p. 241)*

In Hunter Ashleigh Shackleford's chapter "When you are already dead: Black fat being as afrofuturism", they propose that against the backdrop of a white supremacist history and present, the black body is already presumed dead, thereby rendering any and all acts of embodiment as a sort of super-human, super natural feat. They sets the context of this superhuman act of "Being" by inviting us to explore the definition of abundance. Shackleford states, "Abundance crosses borders and breaks chains and disrupts binaries" (p. 253). They propose that Black fat as a politic of abundance is consequently inherently disobedient to a world of anti-Blackness which is a world that expects and invites Black death. Hunter asks the reader to consider, "What if instead of believing that Blackness and fatness are separate embodiments, that we connect the shrinking and active killing of Blackness as the same violence that asks us to shrink and disappear all fat bodies?" (p. 254). In this framing, Shackleford invites us to explore how the violent treatment of fat bodies exists on a spectrum whose only logical conclusion would be anti-Blackness, while subsequently suggesting, "Black fat being, of all genders and those who are none-of-the-above, is the ground and embodiment of resistance. Black fat being is a literal geography of abundance, illegibility, and audacity" (p. 254). In this, they offer us a way forward in fat Black bodies, "creating a new world that was never imagined or expected" (p. 257).

Using a comic strip format, Sam Orchard explores how fatness is policed on trans people's bodies and used by medical professionals to deny gender affirming treatments and procedures. The subject of the comic, a trans man, contends with fatphobic physicians, economic barriers and a pervasive narrative that to truly be a trans man, he must be unhappy with his fat curvy body. This piece disrupts normative assumptions about fatness and trans identity while also challenging the health narratives that treat fatness as causal to negative health outcomes and conditions. Utilizing a popular media format Orchard challenges the prevailing narratives of fat trans bodies and demands better from the systems that serve them.

In Esther Rothblum's chapter "Lesbians and fat", her review of the literature illuminates the disruptive nature of fat lesbian body image and identity. Through an exploration of methodological critiques, Rothblum raises the complex contradictions in the findings regarding lesbians' ideas about weight and size for themselves and their partners. For example, Esther offers, "Studies have found that lesbians diet frequently, even while aware that the lesbian community may consider dieting oppressive to women" (p. 264). This is true even while women who participated in research focus groups reported "women agreed that lesbians are more accepting of higher weight and wished for a focus on health rather than weight" (p. 266). Rothblum ultimately concludes that the early contradictory research and subsequent decades of additional research prove primarily that Lesbians experience a spectrum of ideas, beliefs and behaviours about weight as a result of being privy to the same systems of structures of weight related beliefs as heterosexual women citing, "Lesbians, like heterosexual women, are socialized by their families, the workplace, the media, and the general community to focus on their own weight and appearance" (p. 269). However, many studies also show that "lesbians focus less on their weight and appearance" and to that end may be a group to look to for fresh ways to disrupt fatphobia (p. 269).

Lastly, Allison Taylor explores how the discipline of queer studies could be and has been used to expand the field of vision for Fat Studies while concurrently being used to disrupt and critique existing narratives within the field. Taylor offers five categorizations for a queer fat studies framework. She opens the chapter offering a guiding question, "What is the queer potential of fatness?" but goes on, using the work of queer fat scholars to posit, "that, rather than an appropriation of queer narratives, strategies, or theories, scholarly efforts to queer fatness result from the fact that queers are 'woven into the history of fat liberation'" (p. 273). Exploring the existing literature of both Fat Studies and Queer Studies scholars, Taylor puts these theoretical frameworks in conversation with each other. The result is a more expansive perspective on both fields. Taylor writes of one such example, "Cooper uses queer theory to provide a more nuanced understanding of fat studies and activist practices, demonstrating the utility of queer theory for conceptualizing the complex 'both/and' instead of a simplistic 'either/or': the fundamental ambiguity of fatness" (p. 277). Ultimately, Taylor puts forth a conversation between fat and queer studies that has the power to disrupt either disciplines leanings toward mainstream ideals of fatness and ultimately serve as a tool for dismantling fat oppression.

25

GENEALOGIES OF EXCESS
Towards a decolonial Fat Studies

Athia N. Choudhury

On finding the fat body

I am leading a discussion section for a course titled *Peoples and Cultures of the Americas*. The professor has assigned Junot Díaz's (2008) novel *The brief wondrous life of Oscar Wao*. My students are unusually hesitant, stumbling over their words. The protagonist, Oscar, is fat – nerdy, ugly, unable to get with the ladies – his fatness is a central metaphor for the destructive, recursive, and generational legacies of colonial and sexual violence explored throughout the novel.[1] Not one person has mentioned the word *fat*. Big. Fluffy. Rotund. Obese. They skirt around *fat* at whatever cost; their tongues stuck to the roof of their mouths, glued tight by civility and decorum. I can sense how my fat body in the classroom, as instructor, unsettles them. How can we talk about this obvious metaphor of dysfunctional and racialized fat in the novel when such a body – in flesh and bone – interrupts the classroom space? Despite thinking through flesh and race throughout the course, we are now struggling to articulate how empire is viscerally embodied in the characters.

The complex, submerged renderings of fatness and race that press into the novel and our everyday lives tightly bind us, shut. Oscar and my body are swallowed whole by the visual and visceral logics of fatness and neither I nor our discussion can move forward until I break off a piece of myself as offering. My body stiffens – I ask, *can we talk about fat and racial formation and landedness? What do we think about fatness being made to represent the trauma of 400 years of conquest, rape culture, and state violence?*

I am unsure of the thickness that hangs between us – if I have exposed too much of my own body and what is at stake in who and what gets leftover by internalizing fat as colonial loss and dysfunction against the backdrop of modernity. I feel vulnerable to the scrutiny.

Finally, someone pipes up: *It's fucked up.*

I cannot help but erupt into laughter: *Isn't it, though?*

Prelude

I think of this encounter now as I consider: is there room in the decolonial horizon for fat matters?[2] As a decolonial feminist scholar invested in questions of excess, aesthetics, and viscerality as felt structures of coloniality/modernity (Quijano, 2000), my work often begins by asking, quite simply, how did we arrive at a narrative of fatness *as* colonial dysfunction? What are the fat origin stories we share, whose experiences do they annunciate, and what are their racial logics? Díaz, like other artists working to illuminate a decolonial epistemic turn, makes sense of fat as a story of colonial loss, difference, and effeminization (Fresno-Calleja, 2017; Perez, 2010; Griff, 2016; Inness, 2005; Saldaña-Tejeda & Wade, 2018). Oscar's life is ultimately an inescapable tragedy wrought on by the twin valences of hypermasculine and fat-antagonistic publics condensed through centuries of colonial violence made bare across the body.[3] The image of the poor, fat Latino child makes sense of our modern racial discourse on obesity – one that uncritically recasts and flattens the fat body as a problem of imperial foodways, diaspora/displacement, and settler colonialism. Fatness, then, *is* the destructive, recursive, and ongoing force of colonial damage and trauma manifested onto the body. Yet, how did this image of the fat, poor, racialized child come to proliferate with meaning?

We know this story of fat racialization. It appears along the golden arches of McDonalds in Chile, India, Sri Lanka, Los Angeles – the impact of Western-industrial foods felt on added poundage, deteriorating health, and disappearing local foodways. In a world populated with the specter of a global obesity epidemic (Boero, 2012), the visual drama (and multinational-corporate manufacturing) of the malnourished versus the overfed, and the realities of North/South currents of extractivism (Gómez-Barris, 2017) – what could possibly be decolonial about fat? I stretch my unruly body into this question, finding myself in spaces of deep fracture, blame, and shame. Where does the fat body fit within the decolonial? As problem? As victim? As something else entirely?

To move us towards decolonizing Fat Studies and a decolonial fat methodology, I first piece together the story of fat and race as we understand it in our contemporary epoch and reach for ways to complicate such theorization. First, I map how an onto-epistemology of race and fatness has been conceptualized through Fat Studies and obesogenic research by discreet (but overlapping) methodological and critical approaches to the study of fat that continue to center on white womanhood.[4] In the following sections, I untangle how Fat Studies historical materialist projects and obesogenic sociological frameworks – operating as distinct tendencies at enmeshed rhetorical frequencies – codify, consolidate, and narrate a unidimensional paradigm of fat liberation or health re-education that continues to foreground white colonial subjecthood.[5]

I argue that Fat Studies projects deploying historical materialist and cultural critiques of the socialities, textualities, and visual economies of fat perpetuate the center of fatness as being white, Western, and female. I meditate on what is discarded through such a rendering and offer a racial capitalist framework for teasing out the racial logics of body-making as they are grounded in ontologies of colonialism and capital. Obesogenic research, in turn, renders fatness as a form of risk/race coding where systemic poverty and ecological crisis are the environmental conditions that innately produce (poor) fat populations (of color). This section explores how public health rhetoric around racialized "obesity-fat" – and the *war on obesity* – consolidates state powers contingent on framing poor communities of color as at-risk populations in need of proper management and governance. Moreover, I examine how our study of "obesity-fat" would shift when we consider how body-sovereignty and land-sovereignty are deeply intertwined.

This chapter is capacious in that it makes room for different approaches to dreaming and doing decolonial Fat Studies and argues that the current tendencies in the field sediment a shorthand for the study of fat and race that must be both provincialized and proliferated from global and social peripheries. Often, decolonizing fatness (or, decolonizing body-love) comes to stand in for *undoing Euro-centric beauty standards*. These soul-body-healing projects of examining and dismantling beauty standards, desirability politics, internalized fatphobia, food and eating disorders, body dysmorphia, and colonial body traumas are absolutely crucial for us to get free.

However, we must press for a decolonial fat methodology that expands our theorization of flesh and the body beyond questions of representation and recognition within the white supremacist settler state when such a regime sustains itself through the disappearance, exploitation, and death of Indigenous, black, migrant, disabled, and chronically ill peoples.

Moving through the world as a diasporic fat femme, I am acutely aware of the ways in which body-size, ability, and perceived dis-ability aggregate conceptions of race, nation, gender, and sexuality not adequately reflected or explored in critical race, postcolonial, and transnational feminist discourses. Fat Studies, as a critical intra-discipline that has grappled with how bodies become naturalized through state and self-governance is uniquely positioned to interrogate how the body acts as archive and index for race and empire across disciplinary fields, geopolitical locations, and political solidarities. Rather than simply map "correctives" to the current literature or offer a monolithic genealogy that can seamlessly stitch together *the* unified theory of fat, I urge scholars to move horizontally across multiply layered temporalities and histories. Let us linger in the fissures of possibilities, pause in the gaps, and grasp at the questions that might get us closer to finding the body in Empire.

Decolonial fat methodology or stiffening as method

This decolonial fat methodology begins with the body, registering the aftermath of colonial encounter and the sticky impressions left-behind and carried over which become sediment as everyday thought. Impressions – *marks produced by pressure* – weigh psycho-affectively and materially on the body *as* and *in* formation, to be made bare through moments of bodily tension and resonance. The anecdotes I share throughout are attendant to moments of fat bodily stiffening, an anxious pause, a widening gap, that oscillates between an anticipatory reaction to mechanisms of punitive discipline and breaking oneself open as vulnerable to those technologies of control. As in my opening anecdote, my fat presence as instructor in the classroom complicates theorizing fatness as a metaphor for colonial dysfunction for my students. My own stiffening measures the anticipatory pause before I break open an invisible seal that calls attention to my body and subsequently all the bodies in the room that drastically shapes and informs the kinds of conversations we can have.

It is in these moments of tension and tensing, of contact between flesh and episteme, touch and ontology, that the fat body of color grazes uncomfortably against what Frantz Fanon calls a *colonial vocabulary*, and it is here that I trace a genealogy of excess. In *Wretched of the earth*, Fanon (1963) writes about the native's encounters with European values (the zoological, colonial vocabulary that marks the native as beastly, savage, less than) as producing a kind of bodily *stiffening* or *muscular lockjaw*. As he grounds the phenomenology of encounter within his own black, colonial, Martinique flesh, he details a bodily and visceral reaction that demonstrates the distance between what he feels and knows about himself versus what he is told about his body and appetites (Fanon, 1963). Building off of this work, I consider moments of fat bodily stiffening as breaking open the seal around a colonial vocabulary of fleshy propriety – oscillating between what we feel and know about ourselves versus what we are told about our bodies. How we break open and offer up parts of our flesh is indicative of the distance we must travel to decolonize Fat Studies and fatten decolonial theory.[6]

A decolonial fat methodology is a tender look at the bodies – waiting – stiffened through fat origin stories and fleshy myths and asks us to interrogate "clichéd and shorthand forms in some everyday habits of thought" (Chakrabarty, 2000, p. 4) that sediment fat and race over time. The following sections interrogate the shorthand histories of fat and race that press into our skin – the stories we intuitively share, inherit, and perpetuate.

De-mythologizing fat

Fat Studies has asked crucial and important questions about embodiment, governance, medicalization, gender, and sexuality (Boero, 2009; Harjunen, 2016; LeBesco, 2011; Mollow, 2017; Usiekniewicz, 2016). Through a myriad of approaches to the cultural study of fat, scholars have examined the force of fatness in Western societies to organize and re-arrange intimate domains of life and zones of contact both mediated and unmediated by the state and globalization (Boero, 2012; Cooper, 2010; Farrell, 2011; Greenhalgh, 2012; Murray, 2008, 2009). In this section, I examine a recurring shorthand in our everyday thought: the evolutionary trajectory of fat – or, in other words, the story of how fatness was once a desirable corporeal form (a sign of good health, access to food/wealth, and strong reproductive capacities) and has now shifted into a symbol for excess, poor choices, lack of self-governance, and moral/health decay. When deployed by cultural critiques, this shorthand for our shifting orientations towards fat is meant to demonstrate its malleability and social constructiveness. Feminist theorists and cultural critiques often deploy such logics in order to complicate the morality of thinness and call for an end to fat-based discriminatory practices. I consider this motif an evolutionary trajectory, however, because of the ways in which this very same narrative is utilized by social scientists to map the social, political, and material terrain in which fat bodies are no longer *needed* in our modern society and should therefore be eradicated. I interrogate the logics of this shorthand not as a means of disproving fatness's malleability or social construction, but instead to ask: how is this evolutionary timeline enmeshed in racial taxonomies and capitalist time? What does it tell us of the story of perversity/inclusion, white colonial health aesthetics, and systems of governance?

Fat history, whiteness, and the modern savage

A dominant Western history of fatness often begins with the figure of the *portly European* settler who sought factory work in industrialized cities, signaling to the American public a crisis of class and migrant contagion (Bordo, 2004; Schwartz,1986). Fat Studies historians detail the malleability of fatness from desirable to derisive by tracking the historical influx of new settlers which caused the American public to fixate on food, appetite, and stature/body size at the height of hygiene reform. Such a fixation was meant to ideologically consolidate an ethno-national identity that could still fit within the cultural vernacular of the savage versus the civilized – a vocabulary inherited through colonial[7] and American Nativist ideologies (Higham, 2002). As the category of whiteness became bound and unbound through class lines, the *cult of slenderness* emerged as a fleshy marker of bodily propriety. For example, Peter Stearns traces American diets and eating cultures in the nineteenth to twentieth centuries, following the winding history of a fear of fat grounded in class discourses where early Americans transposed French and British sensibilities around slenderness as a form of class distinction from the new flood of *hefty* working-class settlers (Stearns, 2002). The story that is told, then, foregrounds and yet disappears race and landedness from fat history, a sleight of hand necessitated by the ongoing process of consolidating the boundaries of whiteness in the US. However, this is also a moment of productive tension, that can help us read, horizontally, the intimacies between fat, racialism, and capital.

Cedric Robinson's theorizing on racial capitalism allows us to sit within this tension. Robinson defines racial capitalism as a system of dispossession, primitive accumulation, and the manufacturing of uneven life chances that sutures around racialism/racialization to produce the conditions of capitalism and economies of attraction (Robinson, 2000). He argues that racial taxonomies have always been foundational to capitalist origins and pushes back against Marxist frameworks that mark capitalism as a distinct break from European feudalism. Such a break from the social and economic world order would suggest that capitalism was "racial" only insofar as the ruling class needed to separate laborers to discourage uprisings or provide justification for slavery and dispossession. Rather, Robinson argues that capitalism is not a breaking point, but an extension of a Western ontoepistemology of differentiation, or, racialism embedded in the common-sensing, economy, and political fashioning of everyday life. Part of the fabric of early European society was the process of marking the racial other *within* Europe, where the first proletariats were already racial subjects and victims of captivity, criminalization, dispossession, and death. A Cultural Studies reading of fat and class must therefore attend to racial formation as the bedrock of body-hierarchies.

In thinking about how the fear of the ethnic other creeping into the cities manifested itself through fatphobic images and rhetoric, Amy Farrell (2011) details how it was during the 1900s that the fat (female) body acted as the staging ground for public speculation over the repercussions of industrialization and modernization by marking fat as a racial stain that was no longer racial. The xenophobic body-anxiety of the twentieth century was grounded in ideas of criminality and underdevelopment that was linked not only as a mental disability, but as a genetically predisposed condition of newly arrived not-yet-white European settlers that could be tracked onto the body. Farrell gestures to Cesare Lombroso's *The Female Offender* – a critical text that has informed modern penal reform – to understand how these public sentiments came to be. As I think alongside Farrell and Lombroso through penal and eugenicist transnational knowledge formations that permeated public discourse (Mitchell & Snyder, 2003), the connectivity between fatphobia, shifting conditions of whiteness, and race science which pinpoint the collisions between American Nativism (the project of consolidating settler identity to the land) and the colonial body (the process of curating the nation through the body) becomes apparent. Lombroso and Ferrero (2004) defined white criminals as exhibiting behaviors similar to those amongst the *lower levels of civilization* writing that:

> Female criminals are shorter than normal women and in proportion to their stature, prostitutes and female murderers weigh more than honest women .... Prostitutes' greater weight is confirmed by the notorious obesity of those who grow old in their unfortunate trade and gradually become positive monsters of fatty tissue.
>
> *(p. 74)*

The fatty, monstrous, excessive sexual and consumptive appetites of the criminal woman set the stage for the distrustful lens in which we view the fat (female) body (of color), and connects contemporary biopedagogies of state and self-surveillance to the much older desire to contain and manage the criminal ethnic other. The impetus to define and delineate fat origin stories is a confrontation in class, whiteness, criminality, labor, and modernity – where the culturally saturated fat body takes on fluctuating meanings through shifting ideas of health and punitive disciplinary technologies of the body (a claim I interrogate more closely in the next section).[8]

Where fat historical materialists and cultural studies projects interrogate fat through a locus of annunciation within Western genealogies of white desirability, sexual desire, and performing proper gender/citizenship roles as a more recent phenomenon of the nineteenth and twentieth century, I turn to the site of racialized fat to consider how the perimeters of who is considered human have always included questions of body size, appetites, and excess. *Fat, desire, and disgust in the colonial imagination* (Forth, 2012) traces the colonial anxiety felt by British and French imperialists in the eighteenth century over Indigenous fattening practices, documenting them as body disorders and marking the difference between civilized (and therefore populations who could regulate and manage themselves) versus savage behavior. Forth notes how much of this colonial anxiety around body size was predicated on the ways in which women's bodies and sexualities were a speculative terrain read through fat, diet-regulation, economy, and reproductive viability. I gesture to these works to excavate how coloniality ideologically limits the scope and scale of bodily possibility while framing health within very narrow perimeters of whiteness, able-bodiedness, and thin functionality. By orienting ourselves in partial histories and incomplete archives, Fat Studies scholars can ask different kinds of questions about the specters that haunt our modern medical system, carceral state, ecologies, and public spaces and architecture.

On being "at-risk"/on being fat, poor, and brown

I'm sitting in the audience at the *Edible feminisms: On discard, waste, and metabolism* conference at UCLA. I am engrossed by and impressed with the panel of speakers – a mix of academics, cultural workers, and activists who have generously shared their stories about sustainability and food justice work. Progressivism, decolonization, and radical ways of caring for one another have been evoked several times throughout. It feels life-giving. I am particularly taken by a food justice activist from the Bronx. She is an exuberant public speaker – a fat, black femme mother who has planted herself in her neighborhood and found ways to connect and grow power in her community.

She tells us a story about food education and literacy. I am listening intently – happy to hear her talk about her relationship to food, her stories of cooking with kin, and the stakes of eating together. The mere act of a fat person talking openly about food in such a public way feels powerful and vulnerable. But I catch a change in her demeanor. The ease in which she occupied the stage makes way for a stiffness that is all too familiar. I ready myself. While she shares about a program she created to utilize the produce from the community garden by starting cooking classes in her predominantly black, low-income community, she pauses. Her eyes dart across the room, body stiffened, as she quickly offers: *I mean, I'm working on my weight. I want to be healthy for my kid.*

My stomach drops. *Did I imagine that she looked at me?* I feel the wind knocked out of me as I survey the room of over a hundred (mostly thin, mostly white) academics. It was only a moment and I'm sure not many noticed how her body changed, how even her voice strained – as though to shrink her thickness in anticipation of breaking open, offering herself, purifying her fat at the pyre of *health*. What does it mean for a fat, black femme food justice activist to proffer her own weight-loss intentions to this room of thin, (white) feminist scholars? How many times have I offered up my own body in a similar way? What are the ways health becomes a rhetorical dead-end that binds the body to racialized-thinness?

Where Fat Studies cultural critiques might have neglected to tell a thicker story of race and fat outside of the West and whiteness, obesogenic research has taken to undertheorizing and over-representing the vulnerabilities of women, children, and communities of color as highly susceptible to "obesity-fat." Public health crisis, medicalization, and environmental catastrophe narratives become saturated with overlapping fat-racial-contamination. Obesogenic researchers speculate risk, harm, and economy through genealogies of becoming fat (and subsequently losing fat) to consider the forces both inside and outside of the body that produce fleshy responses to food, environment, and economy. I contend that this literature often results in risk-coding as race-coding – where fat embodiment comes to symbolize symptoms of minoritized and marginalized social conditions produced by industrial harm, an account that often relies on old colonial, classist, and white supremacist tropes of the savage brown other.

While discursive feminist critiques of fat/ness and the body attempt to situate the shifting meanings of fat across whiteness, womanhood, the civilized and (un)governable body through

Euro-American Enlightenment and beyond, obesogenic research has been more interested in determining the environmental factors that produce *at-risk* populations susceptible to the "obesity epidemic" or advocating for a study of fat outside of its social symbolism. Obesogenic projects offer what they assume is a corrective to what Megan Warin (2015) notes as an over-investment in representations of fat life. Warin contends that the "celebrations of 'fat flesh' do not engage with material or biological bodies, but squarely sit within a social constructivist frame … [as they present] important debates about identity, not about the materiality of flesh" (p. 48). Warin is speaking to the ways in which Fat Feminist theory and activism has been scaffolded around and against the "globesity crisis" and is, therefore, weary of how biology, human nature, and nutritional science has been leveraged as disciplinary mechanisms from inclusion into full citizenship, human rights, and dignity.

Scholars such as Lauren Berlant (2011), Rebecca Yoshizawa (2012), and Elspeth Probyn (2009), Samantha Murray (2008, 2009), Edward Norman and Fiona Moola (2019), have all argued that the discursive turns in feminist theories of the body make it difficult to engage with biological matter and the very real negative consequences of capitalism run amok on public health, while highlighting how a refusal to look at the *facts* of "obesity-fat" reproduce Cartesian logics as well as theories on the body that are overly invested in recuperating and re-centering the human.[9] Oftentimes employing an ecological Marxist analysis of over-industrial foodways, an alienation of labor to land to mouth, and modern populations' shift to sedentary lifestyles as the (chrono)logical trajectory of the obesity epidemic, much of the work centers around framing target populations as vulnerable to state and corporate violence, particularly amongst poor, working class women and children (of color). However, in doing so, these feminist scholars recast race, gender, and fatness through ideas of risk-coding – what Anna Ward (2013) describes as a process by which "subjects are fixed in a setting, installed in a field that nurtures a particular appetitive response, a response that produces not just fat, but also a particular racialized and classed embodiment of fat" (p. 5). As Ward suggests, risk-coding and race-coding are conflated within obesogenic research, often deployed by white feminists advocating for particular forms of environmental and health conservation and redress that results in the hyper-surveillance of communities of color through state nutritional and health programs.

Obesogenic researchers argue that a focus on representations of fat life and liberation politics deflects from the very real harm done onto vulnerable populations by multinational agribusinesses and other forms of environmental degradation, noting that the fat body represents the scale of environmental collapse – the yellow canary in the poisoned mines.[10] Such claims only serve to justify further punitive measures for fat people, whether manifested in psycho-affective or material consequences. Ultimately, as Ward and Anna Kirkland (2011) argue, obesogenic studies fail to recognize the inherently classist (white supremacist) logics that are invisible to many of these researchers, as the fat-poor body is perceived as more susceptible to its environments than the elite bodies who manage to stay thin and healthy despite environmental conditions. Though many of these feminist scholars claim to be sympathetic to, aware of, and even in agreement with Fat Studies critiques of the stigmatized fat body, the work often reflects an inability to grapple with the murkiness of fat as both material stuff and symbolic order due to an uncritical optimistic investment in health.

Where scholars of foodscapes and food deserts utilize a neoliberal framework of global capitalism to analyze why at-risk populations are more susceptible to food-related chronic illness (obesity always listed amongst them), the reigning logic says that issues of obesity and illness are created by lack of access, fast food franchising, and lack of nutritional education. Though there is an extreme urgency for food justice and sovereignty, movements which challenge state-corporate interests and environmental degradation of our water and foodways, I must call for a closer examination of the rhetoric around obesity-fat as it targets *at-risk* populations, a strategy that often serves to deepen divides between the Global North/South and to further stigmatize fat racialized bodies. What does it mean, then, to be an at-risk body working towards shrinking yourself? Where Fanon and W. E. B. Du Bois have asked what it feels like to be a problem – of being black in a world built on anti-blackness – or what does it feel like to live with the double-consciousness as colonial subject that must move through colonial spaces, I turn these questions to racialized fat. How does it feel to be a bodily problem and product of modernity as fat bodies of color move through a world that has already marked them for dead?

One possible entry into this question is through critical race scholarship that has engaged the question of health and contamination as one rhetorically bound within notions of race science and medicalization (Ahuja, 2016; Shah, 2001; Shaw, 2006). Sabrina Strings (2015) traces a history of racialized "obesity-fat" through black female sensualism, mediating between health/contamination narratives of the black female body. She writes:

> Ideologies of black female sensualism have historically revolved around black women's presumed sexual abandon during an era in which sexually transmitted diseases were major killers. However, the most recent iteration of chronic diseases employs the (equally old) stereotype of black women as gluttonous. I argue that this has resulted in a novel reconfiguration of the trope in which sensualized African American women are converted from "deadly" into "social dead weight."
>
> *(p. 2)*

Strings asks us to consider how the rhetoric around the dangers of black women's bodies shifts from infectious diseases (syphilis and tuberculosis) to chronic illness (obesity). This is one example of how following the racial history of science contextualizes the rising fascination and fabulation of the obesity epidemic in black communities without relying on classist and white supremacist tropes to define those populations.

Neglecting the ways in which risk/race coding operate within obesity-fat discourses allows for the manifestation of public health programs and initiatives that not only vilify fat people, but render fat communities of color as inept, infantile, and irresponsible. Expanding outside of the US and returning to my earlier contention that body sovereignty and land sovereignty are intrinsically bound, I consider the universalization of risk/race-coding applied to Indigenous communities in the Pacific. In "The burden of brown bodies," Jaleh V. McCormack and Lisette Burrows (2015) take up obesity research in New Zealand that frame Pasifika as homogenous, problem populations. Their analysis of sociological and public health studies demonstrates how healthcare practitioners and researchers not only ask leading questions (weighted down by Western perceptions of the Pasifika body), but also flatten Pasifika histories, cultures, and futures into an imaginary monolithic *Indigenous* figure. Further, McCormack and Burrows argue that this homogenized Pasifika (crafted by researchers, foundations, and politicians) is typecast as ignorant of true and valuable health standards, citing that the backwards culture of the Pasifika people allows for the valorization of obesity, and therefore the death of their people. They note:

> Glover, another public health researcher based in New Zealand, is quoted in a national daily newspaper in Feb 2013 stating "quit-smoking and other health promotion campaigns need to be long-term, backed by support and take account of cultural differences. For instance, Pacific people's beliefs around beauty and body image are a challenge for obesity campaigns.
>
> *(p. 375)*

Here, a monolithic Pasifika belief system needs to be re-educated because they do not perform an accurate enough depiction of fat shame and hatred. In such an order of things, these "backwards" views of fatness (that have yet to catch up with the evolutionary timeline of fat I mentioned several sections ago) is then leveraged by the settler state as a benevolent reason for continued occupation and surveillance. Further, such a narrative fails to grapple with alternate body-cosmologies, body-diversity, and the enmeshed histories of establishing a colonial politic in opposition to fleshy corporeal figures.

I use these two articles as examples in how moving towards a decolonial Fat Studies requires us to interrogate how obesogenic research – that can find itself in progressive, radical, and anti-capitalist movements and ideologies – actually recast old prejudices of racial contamination into more palatable discourses through health and wellness.[11] We must consider how these discourses are weaponized against black, Indigenous, and communities of color as people advocate for better living/work conditions, anti-capitalist organizing, sovereignty and self-governance, and structural representation that can unwittingly paint said communities as incompetent and complicit in their own self-destruction.

Both, neither, all and none; towards a genealogy of excess

A rumor was immediately circulated that Sojourner was an impostor; that she was, indeed, a man disguised in women's clothing … Sojourner told them that her breasts had suckled many a white babe, to the exclusion of her own offspring; that some of those white babies had grown to man's estate; that, although they had sucked her colored breasts, they were, in her estimation, far more manly than they (her persecutors) appeared to be; and she quietly asked them, as she disrobed her bosom, if they, too, wished to suck! In vindication of her truthfulness, she told them that she would show her breast to the whole congregation; that it was not to her shame that she uncovered her breast before them, but to their shame. Two young men (A. Badgely and J. Horner) stepped forward while Sojourner exposed her naked breast to the audience. I heard a democrat say, as we were returning home from meeting, that Dr. Strain had, previous to the examination, offered to bet forty dollars that Sojourner was a man! So much for the physiological acumen of a western physician.

(Truth, 2018)

The above is an excerpt from a letter written in October of 1858 detailing the events that transpired at an anti-slavery meeting in Northern Indiana. Sojourner Truth, abolitionist and prototypical black feminist, was accused by the crowd she was speaking to (regarding abolition and women's rights) of being a man disguised as a woman. Personal letters described her physical appearance, often calling her elderly, dark, *ugly* – not at all up to the sensibilities of white female beauty and fragility. The crowd began demanding that she *bare her bosom* to medical doctors for inspection.

I begin with this scene to demonstrate how histories of enslavement complicate understandings of gender, and further how Truth's fat flesh marks what her objectors sensed as an alarming ambiguity in relation to her sex. Though feminist scholars have taken up this scene as a means of tracing the impossibility of black female enfleshment, what would a decolonial Fat Studies reading have to offer such an analysis? How does fat interrupt clear delineations of sex and gender? This is where the work gets messy, where the citations require a coaxing, and the theorizing is more flirtation than fact. In connecting a Fat Studies analysis to Women of Color Feminist theorizing on the body, we are better able to engage with how race, gender, and fatness are codified under the same system of racial capitalism – a system of black, migrant, and Indigenous denigration of life, land, and labor under the rubric of progress and extractivism. Black feminist scholars and activists have deeply shaped the ideological and political terms within which Women Of Color Feminisms theorize the body. Anti-blackness and coloniality have sutured the imperial body as two sides of the same coin, and much of our vocabulary for understanding racialized fat is indebted to black feminist/femme theorizing (Lorde, 1984; Shaw, 2006). The racialized (fat) femme body has been a historic site of speculation, surveillance, social/state policing; she is at once visually captured and fugitively outside of the boundaries of the human (Crenshaw, 1990; Da Silva, 2007; Wynter, 2003).

Truth's performance layers across intersecting gazes – of nineteenth century medical science, of white supremacy, and modes of gender performance and regulation. Nineteenth century medical science and Enlightenment philosophy were co-constitutive: formalizing objects as knowable, truth as empirical, and rationality and reason as the highest capacity of Man (Wynter, 2003). The codification of European epistemologies as truth, as the singular way of being human, foreclosed *infinite and extraordinary possibilities* (Césaire, 1972) through colonial technologies that solidified racial taxonomies and gendered/sexual difference. Truth forces us to reckon with how the enslaved female flesh escapes the category of woman – her blackness, her age, her undesired-but-hypersexualized body. Black flesh, fat fleshy commodity, at once is excluded from categories of nation and gender and at the same time, remain the very bedrock of politics. In *Mama's baby, Papa's maybe: An American grammar book*, Hortense Spillers (1987) offers critical interventions into gender and racial formation in the US by thinking through flesh, black kinship, histories of containment, and dispossession. She argues that the Middle Passage and enslavement represent "zero degree of social conceptualization" in which flesh accrues a more fundamental level of meaning that is, over time, subject to different discursive feats. Spillers posits that the *symbolic integrity* of "male" and "female" as two subject positions lose validity and differentiation within a regime of captivity and dispossession, only to be rearticulated as dichotomous positionalities through white supremacist patriarchy.

There has been much theorizing on Spiller's groundbreaking work, and I wade further into murky waters to connect how fatness produces a problem of gender that is reified through racial logics, collected impressions of power and unfreedoms, bending us towards the white settler body. I turn to Performance Studies scholar Caleb Luna (2018) to connect how racialized fatness continues to produce gender in specific ways, writing:

> I have a big, soft belly and what might be called breasts on a different body. This is a feminized fatness that is different from the hard, muscular guts found on athletes and those in masculinized spaces like the bear community. I have very little body hair that follows the patterns of my father and other Indigenous men I see who look like him. This is another marker of masculinity that my body fails, that, along with my fatness, locates me in a kind of gender purgatory—both, neither, all and none.
>
> *(para. 9)*

Both, neither, all and none. Fat, race, and gender are inseparable to the categories of the human – of who is authentic, real, and worthy. Decolonial fat widens – it pushes through, appears where things don't fit, and reminds us of the radically different ways in which bodies can/must occupy space, ways that are not neatly contained and inevitably contaminated. I offer this reading not to exceptionalize the fat body as the ultimate site of liberation or resistance or denigration, but rather to mark how punishing bodily difference marks the affect of capital: where moving to the site of racialized fat layers multiple histories of (un)freedom, desire, and possibility – from enslaved black women, portly European settlers, Pasifika bodies, and diasporic subjects.

In the tradition of a Woman of Color Feminism that calls for an unwillingness to seek easy resolutions – refusing the production of knowledge that demands positivist answers – this piece instead sits in the muck of tension/tensing. This chapter reckons with a deep fracture in the world as our fat, brown, femme bodies experience it versus the world as it has been historicized and contextualized through a colonial vocabulary. This fracture is the distance between what we inherit and learn about our bodies through our great grandmother's traumas and the indexing of risk/race-coding as a new racial formation in the 21st century. Decolonizing Fat Studies means wanting more than anyone is willing to give you, being stuck between worlds that can't contain all of you and moving about those spaces without asking permission or forgiveness. It is a patchwork of incomplete archives, cross-disciplinary methodologies, and partial histories that are felt onto our bodies and into our spaces. It is uncovering a looking at and after ourselves despite all the ways scholars, doctors, and kin have already defined us. Decolonizing Fat Studies is the healing work we do for ourselves and each other – even when we aren't ready, even when there are no citations.

Notes

1 Diaz has stated in interviews that Oscar's fatness symbolizes the trauma of colonial domination and a legacy of rape – that the fukú, the intergenerational curse, becomes embedded into Oscar's flesh through fatness as a response to the trauma of rape culture. For example, in an interview with the Boston Review (Moya, 2012), Diaz says: "Oscar isn't fat just to be fat – at least not in my head. His fatness was partially a product of what's going on in the family in regards to their bodies, in regards to the rape trauma." In Diaz's conceptualizing of race, fat, gender, and coloniality, Oscar's body symbolizes the dysfunction of 400 years of conquest, of a rape culture that begins with la Malinche, and reappears in the violence of Trujillo's regime.

2 My use of the decolonial horizon considers how becoming cannot be decoupled from colonialism, global capitalism, and white supremacy; there are no clear divides between post/colonial, premodern/(post)modern, human/nonhuman. As Sylvia Rivera Cusicanqui (1991) and Laura Lomas (2008) argue: there are alternative, decolonial histories that are always already *here*. Where there is power and surveillance and regulation by the settler colonial state, there is always resistance and this resistance does not rupture time and place (Rivera Cusicanqui, 1991). This re-imagined temporality, instead, constitutes an animated decolonial horizon where struggle and resistance are not thought of as events or fleeting moments, but the conditions of possibility and becoming.

3 There are other interpretations of Oscar's life – that he was the only character to defeat the fukú by experiencing true love and intimacy. However, if we are to look at the structural and systemic ways in which his life was discarded and laid bare, I believe my analysis of the dead-end of fat continues to ring true (see Kunze, 2013; Mitchell, 2013).

4 I delineate between Fat Studies projects and obesogenic projects partly through their disciplinary methods and whether they study fat/ness or obesity-fat. Obesogenic research is often framed through Science and Technology Studies, New Materialisms, Feminist Science Studies to interrogate multiple forms of governance, and is interested in understanding: *what in our society produces fat? How might we then manage the various disorders that, amongst other things, produce fat populations?* The Fat Studies projects I name here are cultural studies, historical materialist, or media studies projects engaged with questions of representation (less so about aesthetics), but deeply grounded in fat activism.

5 Following the tradition of postcolonial and decolonial scholars who put pressure on the figure of the human in western discourses, this chapter asks us to consider how ideas of individualism, enlightenment, personhood, and cohesive-subjecthood are contingent upon labor, racialization, and the body. For an interdisciplinary reading of western liberalism as it has informed/been informed by Empire in Europe, Asia, Africa, and the Americas, see Lisa Lowe's *Intimacies of four continents* (2015).

6 Much of my reading of muscular tension and Fanon is indebted to and deepened by Neetu Khanna's life-affirming graduate seminar "Colonial Affect" at USC and her forthcoming book *The visceral logics of decolonization*.

7 I name this as colonial because as Rebecca Earle (2012) notes, Spaniards in the Americas fixated on diet and food as a means by which early settlers maintained racial and class difference in contact zones where flesh and fluid were in constant interchange and flux, dissolving the boundaries between self and other.

8 Farrell's (2011) discussion on the matter of race/gender/fatness is more centered on white suffragist's desire for legibility within white male-publics but does meditate on the slippages between racialization and racialism.

9 Though I agree that Fat Studies has certain limitations in theorizing alongside the human, I route my critiques through Sylvia Wynter (2003) and Denise Da Silva's (2007) work on race, science, and embodiment in order to think through an urgency in decolonizing conceptualizations of health and fatness. That discussion remains outside the scope of this chapter, but also complicates how the Feminist Science Studies scholars I have listed above have taken up the question of fatness, materiality, and humanness.

10 Despite the move to depoliticize fat and to materialize fat outside of cultural critique, the fat body remains an ideological and representational force that furthers public policy recommendations around agriculture, city ordinances around fast food and soda, child services, welfare and healthcare, and environmental policies – many of which are central points of focus for obesogenic research. For further discussion on how fat and environmental apocalypse are collapsed categories, see Russell & Semenko (2016); White (2013).

11 In a similar vein, Lucas Crawford's (2017) *Slender trouble: From Berlant's cruel figuring of figure to Sedgwick's fat presence* offers a strong analysis of how even queer theory overdetermines the stagnation and dead ends of fatness.

References

Ahuja, N. (2016). *Bioinsecurities: Disease interventions, empire, and the government of species.* Durham, NC: Duke University Press.

Berlant, L. (2011). *Cruel optimism.* Durham, NC: Duke University Press.

Boero, N. (2009). Fat kids, working moms, and the "epidemic of obesity": Race, class, and mother blame. In E. Rothblum, & S. Solovay (Eds.), *The fat studies reader* (pp. 113–119). New York: New York University Press.

Boero, N. (2012). *Killer fat: Media, medicine, and morals in the American "obesity epidemic."* New Brunswick: Rutgers University Press.

Bordo, S. (2004). *Unbearable weight: Feminism, western culture, and the body.* Oakland: University of California Press.

Césaire, A. (1972). *Discourse on colonialism.* Trans. Joan Pinkham. New York: Monthly Review Press. (Original work published 1955).

Chakrabarty, D. (2000). *Provincializing Europe: Postcolonial thought and historical difference.* Princeton: Princeton University Press.

Cooper, C. (2010). Fat studies: Mapping the field. *Sociology Compass, 4*(12), 1020–1034.

Crawford, L. (2017). Slender trouble: From Berlant's cruel figuring of figure to Sedgwick's fat presence. *GLQ: A Journal of Lesbian and Gay Studies, 23*(4), 447–472.

Crenshaw, K. (1990). Mapping the margins: Intersectionality, identity politics, and violence against women of color. *Stanford Law Review, 43*(6), 1241–1299.

Da Silva, D. F. (2007). *Toward a global idea of race* (Vol. 27). Minneapolis, MN: University of Minnesota Press.

Díaz, J. (2008). *The brief wondrous life of Oscar Wao.* New York: Penguin.

Earle, R. (2012). *The body of the conquistador: Food, race and the colonial experience in Spanish America, 1492–1700.* Cambridge: Cambridge University Press.

Fanon, F. (1963) *The wretched of the earth.* New York: Grove Press.

Farrell, A. E. (2011). *Fat shame: Stigma and the fat body in American culture.* New York: New York University Press.

Forth, C. E. (2012). Fat, desire and disgust in the colonial imagination. *History Workshop Journal, 73*(1), 211–239.

Fresno-Calleja, P. (2017). Fighting gastrocolonialism in Indigenous Pacific writing. *Interventions, 19*(7), 1041–1055.

Gómez-Barris, M. (2017). *The extractive zone: Social ecologies and decolonial perspectives.* Durham, NC: Duke University Press.

Greenhalgh, S. (2012). Weighty subjects: The biopolitics of the US war on fat. *American Ethnologist, 39*(3), 471–487.

Griff, E. C. (2016). *Too much to belong: Latina/o racialization, obesity epidemic discourse, and unassimilable corporeal excess* (unpublished doctoral dissertation). College Park, MD: University of Maryland.

Harjunen, H. (2016). *Neoliberal bodies and the gendered fat body: The fat body in focus.* London: Routledge.

Higham, J. (2002). *Strangers in the land: Patterns of American nativism, 1860–1925.* New Brunswick: Rutgers University Press.

Inness, S. (2005). *Secret ingredients: Race, gender, and class at the dinner table.* New York: Springer.

Kirkland, A. (2011). The environmental account of obesity: A case for feminist skepticism. *Signs: Journal of Women in Culture and Society, 36*(2), 463–485.

Kunze, P. C. (2013). Send in the clowns: Extraordinary male protagonists in contemporary American fiction. *Fat Studies, 2*(1), 17–29.

LeBesco, K. (2011). Neoliberalism, public health, and the moral perils of fatness. *Critical Public Health, 21*(2), 153–164.

Lomas, L. (2008). *Translating empire: José Marti, migrant Latino subjects, and American modernities.* Durham, NC: Duke University Press.

Lombroso, C., & Ferrero, G. (2004). *Criminal woman, the prostitute, and the normal woman.* Durham, NC: Duke University Press.

Lorde, A. (1984). *Sister outsider: Essays and speeches.* Trumansburg, NY: The Crossing Press.

Lowe, L. (2015). *The intimacies of four continents.* Durham, NC: Duke University Press.

Luna, C. (2018). In the gender non-conformity of my fat body. *The Body is Not an Apology.* https://thebodyisnotanapology.com/magazine/the-gender-nonconformity-of-my-fatness/

McCormack, J. V., & Burrows, L. (2015). The burden of brown bodies: Teachings about Pasifika within public health obesity research in Aotearoa/New Zealand. *Cultural Studies? Critical Methodologies, 15*(5), 371–378.

Mitchell, D., & Snyder, S. (2003). The eugenic Atlantic: Race, disability, and the making of an international eugenic science, 1800–1945. *Disability & Society, 18*(7), 843–864.

Mitchell, K. I. (2013). *Narrating resistance through failure: Queer temporality and reevaluations of success in Junot Díaz's* The brief wondrous life of Oscar Wao (unpublished doctoral dissertation). Boulder, CO: University of Colorado.

Mollow, A. (2017). Unvictimizable: Toward a fat black Disability Studies. *African American Review, 50*(2), 105–121.

Moya, P. M. (2012). The search for decolonial love: An interview with Junot Díaz. *Boston Review, 26.*

Murray, S. (2008). Pathologizing "fatness": Medical authority and popular culture. *Sociology of Sport Journal, 25*(1), 7–21.

Murray, S. (2009). Marked as "pathological": "Fat" bodies as virtual confessors. In J. Wright, & V. Harwood (Eds.), *Biopolitics and the "obesity epidemic"* (pp. 78–90). New York: Routledge.

Norman, M. E., & Moola, F. J. (2019). The weight of (the) matter: A new material feminist account of thin and fat oppressions. *Health, 23*(5), 497–515.

Perez, C. S. (2010). *From unincorporated territory [Saina].* Oakland, CA: Omnidawn.

Probyn, E. (2009). Fat, feelings, bodies: A critical approach to obesity. In M. Burns, & H. Malson (Eds.), *Critical feminist approaches to eating dis/orders* (pp. 113–123). Hove: Routledge.

Quijano, A. (2000). Coloniality of power and eurocentrism in Latin America. *International Sociology, 15*(2), 215–232.

Rivera Cusicanqui, S. (1991). The historical horizons of internal colonialism. *Report on the Americas, 25*(3), 18–45.

Robinson, C. J. (2000). *Black Marxism: The making of the black radical tradition.* Chapel Hill, NC: University of North Carolina Press.

Russell, C., & Semenko, K. (2016). We take "Cow" as a compliment: Fattening humane, environmental, and social justice education. In E. Cameron, & C. Russell (Eds.), *The fat pedagogy reader: Challenging weight-based oppression through critical education* (pp. 211–220). New York: Peter Lang Publishing.

Saldaña-Tejeda, A., & Wade, P. (2018). Obesity, race and the Indigenous origins of health risks among Mexican Mestizos. *Ethnic and Racial Studies, 41*(15), 2731–2749.

Schwartz, H. (1986). *Never satisfied: A cultural history of diets, fantasies, and fat.* New York: Free Press.

Shah, N. (2001). *Contagious divides: Epidemics and race in San Francisco's Chinatown* (Vol. 7). Oakland, CA: University of California Press.

Shaw, A. E. (2006). *The embodiment of disobedience: Fat black women's unruly political bodies.* Lanham: Lexington Books.

Spillers, H. J. (1987). Mama's baby, Papa's maybe: An American grammar book. *Diacritics, 17*(2), 65–81.

Stearns, P. N. (2002). *Fat history: Bodies and beauty in the modern west*. New York: New York University Press.

Strings, S. (2015). Obese black women as "Social dead weight": Reinventing the "Diseased black woman". *Signs: Journal of Women in Culture and Society, 41*(1), 107–130.

Truth, S. (2018). *Narrative of Sojourner Truth: A northern slave*. Boston, MA: Squid Ink Classics.

Usiekniewicz, M. (2016). Dangerous bodies: Blackness, fatness, and the masculinity dividend. *A Journal of Queer Studies*, 11a, 19–45.

Ward, A. (2013). Fat bodies/Thin critique: Animating and absorbing fat embodiments. *The Scholar and Feminist Online*. Issue 11.3. https://sfonline.barnard.edu/life-un-ltd-feminism-bioscience-race/fat-bodiesthin-critique-animating-and-absorbing-fat-embodiments/

Warin, M. (2015). Material feminism, obesity science and the limits of discursive critique. *Body & Society, 21*(4), 48–76.

White, F. R. (2013). "We're kind of devolving": Visual tropes of evolution in obesity discourse. *Critical Public Health, 23*(3), 320–330.

Wynter, S. (2003). Unsettling the coloniality of being/power/truth/freedom: Towards the Human, after man, its overrepresentation—An argument. *CR: The New Centennial Review, 3*(3), 257–337.

Yoshizawa, R. S. (2012). The Barker hypothesis and obesity: Connections for transdisciplinarity and social justice. *Social Theory & Health, 10*(4), 348–367.

26

WHEN YOU ARE ALREADY DEAD

Black fat being as afrofuturism

Hunter Ashleigh Shackelford

Abundance is insurrection. Abundance swallows the known whole. Abundance crosses borders and breaks chains and disrupts binaries. Abundance is the elephant in the room. Abundance is a eulogy and a baptism. Abundance is erratic and fugitive and not. Abundance is monstrosity and viciously unhumble. Abundance rolls deep, like the ocean, like my niggas. Abundance is always Black.

Blackness is always abundant

Alexis Pauline Gumbs (2012) writes in '*Black feminism be(yond)*', "Measure love. Measure the universe. Measure God. Black Feminism cannot be quantified" (para 1). In that same vein, Blackness cannot be quantified. Blackness can be hunted, surveilled, preyed upon, microscopically studied, caged, and will never be fully accounted for. It is an ever present, ubiquitous integer where limit and fracture do not exist. Mathematical theorem will always come after niggas because abundance has no equation. *Abundance is always Black.*

The quantifiable, the logical, the controllable variable, and the knowable are derivatives of the un-imagination and the toolbox of white supremacy. The expectation that Black bodies should shrink, be quiet, fit within the (color) lines, to lighten, to become the cage, to erase the "sin" that is attached to our very essence, to always be seen and always be out of sight, is to demand that we embody nothingness as being. Become *no*-thing. Do not take space because it is not yours. Do not spill over the armrest because your very being is the assault. Your existence does not afford you the right to be too much, too loud, too full, too human, too living, too free, too abundant…

Black fats are cyborgs, and human, and otherwise

Cyborg, as explained by Vargas and James (2012), was to acknowledge the 'Black Cyborg' who takes on different characteristics of superhumanistic traits to subvert and survive the violences of anti-blackness beyond the "ordinary negro" and sometimes embody rebellion. *Cyborg*, as I define it for Black fats, is ontological being beyond the humanist grammars of antiblackness (Vargas & James, 2012). The definition of human most referenced and embedded within our antiblack subconscious is defined and caged to the carceral imaginations of non-Blackness. Defying the confinement of the overestimation of demonic white cisgender heterosexual nonvalue and illogic, Black fatness never qualified because non-Black humanist grammars are designed to fail *everyone* who applies. Black fat bodies, Black fat being, will always exist out of bounds and will always be uncapturable. We occupy a reality and a space of being, life, death, other, imagination, extravagance, and abundant-nigga-galactica. If the prescribed expectation is that we're dead, then every breath we take, every chair we break, and every map we make is radically illegible and beyond this iteration of time.

The police union lawyer Stuart London pronounced in court, "He died from being morbidly obese. He was a ticking time bomb that resisted arrest. If he was put in a bear hug, it would have been the same outcome" (Cheney-Rice, 2019, para 1). Eric Garner was put in a chokehold that crushed his throat, cut off his body's access to air and freedom, and restricted his ability to breathe. He said, "I can't breathe" 11 times.

Eric Garner was murdered. London's need to argue that Eric's body, his literal numerical weight, his dimensions, the calculations and mathematics of a Black fat dark skin body was the reason for his death – that he was already dead – is the cyborgic multidimensionality of Black fat being. What does it mean when you are already dead, yet there is a warrant to assure the death of your flesh? If Eric was a "ticking time bomb," who sets the countdown? How do we hold the mathematical projections anti-Blackness cages our Black fat bodies within, knowing the entire system is a zero-sum game? If he is already presumed dead, why did his loitering call for an escalated public death? What does it mean to say you cannot breathe if breath never belonged to you?

Vargas and James (2012) state, "Antiblackness depends on impossible time that has no beginning because it has no end" (pp. 193–205) Blackness, in this system, exists on borrowed time, surviving an ontological atomic bomb that has no chronological countdown because this un/liveability is the radiation, the aftermath of a nonmathematical and nonlinear trauma. Black fat being means surviving mutating time-altering forms of violence, it means literally defying presumed and prescribed death while surviving more versions of fatality. The afrofuturistic multidimensionality that is required of the Black fat consciousness and Black fat being is a rubric of cyborg divergence, beyond "human" grammar, beyond the cages of thinness and whiteness.

What if instead of believing that Blackness and fatness are separate embodiments that we connect the shrinking and active killing of Blackness as the same violence that asks us to shrink and disappear all fat bodies? What if being dead is not the worst or the final thing you can be when anti-Blackness is a system designed to be unlivable? What if being seen or identified as a Black "death-fat"[1] is actually the poetic and geographical resistance of existing beyond, before, and after projected-death? How has the prescribed and presumed death of fat being not been epistemologically identified as the derivative of Blackness?

In *Demonic grounds*, Katherine McKittrick (2006) elaborates, "The real and imaginary geographic processes important to Black women are not just about limitations, captivities, and erasures; they are also about everyday contestations, philosophical demands, and the possibilities the production of space can engender for subaltern subjects" (p. 121). McKittrick breaks down the nontraditional being and mapping of Black women's geographies as sites/cites of resistance.

Black fat being, of all genders and those who are none-of-the-above, is the ground and embodiment of resistance. Black fat being is a literal geography of abundance, illegibility, and audacity. The space we embody, the space we take up, and the space we swallow whole is the ontological syllabus of abundance, of Black fat being.

The dispossession of space is the ontological terror of Black fat being. The contention with Eric Garner is that of the demand that he no longer exist, that his Black fat dark skin body no longer swallow space that is not his; the demand for Eric to stop consuming, to stop swallowing, to stop breathing, to stop overindulging on what does not belong to him or his body in this time and space. For Black fat being, the site of disruption is not the lack of land to ground our bodies, it is the demand for *fullness as being* – the room in our jeans and the space on street corners to breathe deep, the release of our folded arms from shrinking our latitude, the freedom to be niggas unbound and unchained, the liberty to eat and be nourished and be full and otherwise, to move without surveillance, to experience architecture that holds every pound of our Blackness, to spill out without punishment, to run without fugitivity, to imagine new geographies of safety, to be deep as dark and dark as deep, to embody oceans, to be limitless like the archive of the Black Atlantic, to personify uncapturable abundance.

The *Politics of Black Abundance* is that of recognizing that the hunting and preying upon abundance, gluttony, extravagance, darkness, queerness, fullness, deep breathing, and space is that of the hunter seeking to shrink what is unshrinkable, to capture what is uncapturable – Blackness. Our flesh that cannot be captured, that is never one-size-fits-all, is always surviving the attempt of capture – resisting the psychic and physical carcerality of anti-Blackness. Black fat being cannot be killed, cannot explode, cannot be dieted, cannot be erased. Black fat being is tangible and not; Black fat being is that of energy, which cannot be created or destroyed, only change form. We know that the un-imagination and illogicalness of anti-Blackness is to find new ways to destroy Blackness, that which is abundance, yet require Blackness to exist to siphon its power and labor. Anti-Blackness requires the abundance, the largeness, the immeasurableness of Blackness to seek an ontological identity. Blackness cannot die, and anti-Blackness depends on it to live. Abundance cannot die, because nothing exists without it.

Amy Erdman Farrell writes,

The articles and advertisements within African American periodicals rarely focused on fat as a significant problem. Instead, concern about the excessiveness of fatness showed up primarily in publications geared toward white, middle-class audiences, marking a key instance in which we see how deeply racialized the concerns of the modern period were.

(2011, p. 39)

The historical cartographies of fatness and excess lead us back to the fact that white fat-flight, the politics of scarcity and shrinkage, and the systemic shift to not wanting to embody abundance explicitly, is that of the continual plague of anti-Blackness.

Blackness births the abundances, the freedoms, the otherness we seek to protect. Fatness, queerness, darkness, disability, gender expansiveness are epistemologies of Black lexicons. The "other" within white supremacy is always rooted in the power and expansiveness of Blackness. Fat is a marker of Blackness and that of a failure of no-Blackness because that box is too small. Beyonce says in 'Ego', "It's too big, it's too wide, it's too strong, it won't fit, it's too much" (Williams et al., 2008). Blackness is egotistical, and abundance is viciously unhumble. Whiteness, and specifically all non-Blackness, must be forewarned of fatness because abundance, largeness, Rubenesqueness is that of sin, of nigger, of the uncontrollable and unruly slave. Therefore, any and everyone who navigates and exists within fatness as a spectrum is by proxy experiencing the violence of anti-Blackness (the hunt to kill Blackness/abundance).

Fatness as Blackness means that the spectrum of punishment and violence for fat people across identities is layered, yet always in direct relationship with anti-Blackness. The implication is raced, and always derivative of the non-Black imaginary. The difference in non-Black people being fat means that there is still a humanization and legibility that comes with that embodiment. You have failed whiteness/the non-Black, but you are not an embodied slave/Black, so there is always space (or shrinkage) to negotiate and integrate within the non-Black imagination. Within Blackness, intersections of identities and privileges broaden the spectrum for how you navigate death/the non-Black imaginary, but you are still read and presumed as dead. These same spectrums and manifestations also construct the mapping and mobilization through social and liberatory movements to maintain the cage around abundance (read: Blackness).

The "Body Positivity" movement has consistently removed fatness (read: Blackness) from the center and the origin, and it continues to thrust those who are closer to thinness, whiteness, lightskinness, non-Blackness, and able-bodied-ness to the performative and the visible. "Body positivity" is a co-optation of struggle to create new mutations of the same anti-Black systems and to cosplay the slave. Charlotte Cooper's (2016) work in *Fat activism* maps fat activism through a timeline that begins between 1967 and 1989, specifically with Steve Post who led a "Fat-In" in New York City in 1967.

The very title of "Fat-In" already uses Blackness as the framework in which to mimic "sit-in"'s done within the beginning of the Civil Rights Movement. "The Greensboro sit-in was a civil rights protest that started in 1960, when young African-American students staged a sit-in at a segregated Woolworth's lunch counter in Greensboro, North Carolina, and refused to leave after being denied service" (History.com Editors, 2010, para 1). The demand to be seen, to be accommodated, to eat, to have space is the demand to exist. Blackness serves as the very model of protest and struggle non-Black fatness seeks to usurp and siphon from.

The ventriloquism of body politic movements that fail to viciously assert and center niggas only reifies the minstrelsy of White Feminism. The mutations of both "body positivity" and "fat activism" are the same because the villain is the same – Blackness. Hence why anti-Black propaganda of self-love such as Aerie's "Real" campaign or Dove's "#MyBeautyMySay" campaign makes this a performance of mannequining freedom (#AerieREAL Life!, 2019; Dove, n.d.). This particular tactic maintains the false representation of "self-love" as the goal, or as the purpose of existing unapologetically in your body as a means to be free. "Self-love" or "positivity" do not dismantle systems of violence that tell us we need to be closer to thinness and whiteness to be worthy, that tell us we must be non-Black to be human, and that we must perform through our trauma and shame in order for our ontological being to evolve into a knowable and legible grammar.

The best performing slave does not get to freedom quicker. A good nigga is still a nigga. Loving yourself is not required. Loving yourself is not mandatory to demand your right to exist. Love is not a neutral or linear concept. Autonomy is before the flesh, and consent is before love. This formula around using love as a weapon, as a way to control our emotional navigation around our trauma, puts the onus of liveability and humanity on Black people – as something we have failed to achieve for ourselves. *Loving ourselves is not required.* Self-love can never be the contingency for freedom and humanity. Love is immeasurable but these cages have dimensions.

If Black fat being cannot represent or embody life, because the fat body is seen as a representation of the death that which is abundance, that which is Blackness, then we are already twice over dead here. Our continued resistance, existence, and persistence is not only a metaphysical anomaly of anti-Blackness, but also a glitch within the non-Black imaginary every time we breathe. If Blackness is the original sin, the villain of white supremacy's bedtime stories, the basis for why everyone under white supremacy (read: anti-Blackness) struggles with access to liveability, then fatness cannot exist without Blackness. There is nothing to be *positive* about if our bodies are deemed as enslaved, as unruly flesh, as dead. There is no freedom if we are implicit in ignoring who the cages were built for and that the chains are still very much intact. There is no activism to actualize if the deathly hollows of anti-Blackness go ignored, erased, and avoided in the cartographies of abundance. Freeing fatness is freeing Blackness is freeing abundance. As proclaimed by Audre Lorde (1988), "I am writing these words as a route map – an artifact for survival – a chronicle of buried treasure – a mourning" (p. 448).

Black fat being. Being is abundance. Any future we create and name for ourselves, any future we embody and demand in real time, and any future that we dream and imagine for ourselves is a *conjuring* from the dead, the un/living, and the beyond. This space of *concurrent afrofuturism* is the positionality of inhabiting multiple realities and periods of time at once. Black fat being is the literal embodiment of occupation of space, abundance, and unbound time dimensionality.

We exist concurrently as we exist in the present while embodying futuristic narratives and realities, while holding the legacies and storytelling of our pasts. Every inch we acquire, every breath we inhale and demand like Eric Garner, we are maintaining abundance and being through the death marked upon our bodies, while also creating a new world that was never imagined or expected.

Note

1   'Death-Fat' is a term to define those who are fat beyond "acceptable" standards, specifically those who exceed a size 26 in US sizes and/or do not fit within clothing that is readily accessible in stores.

References

#AerieREAL Life! (2019, Apr 4). Welcome to your #AerieREAL life! *#AerieREAL Life!* https://www. ae.com/aerie-real-life/2019/04/04/welcome-to-your-aeriereal-life/

Cheney-Rice, Z. (2019, Jun 14). NYPD union lawyers claim Eric Garner would've died anyway because he was obese. *New York Magazine.* http://nymag.com/intelligencer/2019/06/eric-garner-death-inev-itable-says-lawyer.html

Cooper, C. (2016). *Fat activism: A radical social movement.* Bristol: HammerOn Press.

Dove (n.d.) My beauty my say. *Dove.* https://www.dove.com/us/en/stories/campaigns/my-beauty-my-say.html

Farrell, A. (2011). *Fat shame.* New York: New York University Press.

Gumbs, A. P. (2012, Mar 27). Black feminism be(yond): Abundance (Part 4 of Can black feminism be quantified). *The Feminist Wire.* https://thefeministwire.com/2012/03/black-feminism-beyond-abundance-part-4-of-can-black-feminism-be-quantified/

History.com Editors (2010, Feb 4). Greensboro sit-in. *History.com.* https://www.history.com/topics/black-history/the-greensboro-sit-in

Lorde, A. (1988). On my way out I passed over you and the Verrazano bridge. *Feminist Studies, 14*(3), 446–449.

McKittrick, K. (2006). *Demonic grounds.* Minneapolis, MN: University of Minnesota Press.

Vargas, J. C., & James, J. A. (2012). Refusing Blackness-as-victimization: Trayvon Martin and the Black cyborgs. In G. Yancy, & J. Jones (Eds.), *Pursuing Trayvon Martin: Historical contexts and contemporary manifestations of racial dynamics* (pp. 193–204). Plymouth: Lexington Books.

Williams, E., Lilly, H. & Carter-Knowles, B. (2008). Ego [Recorded by B. Carter-Knowles]. On *I am... Sascha Fierce* [CD]. Atlanta, GA: Tree Sound Studies.

27
TRANSFAT

Sam Orchard

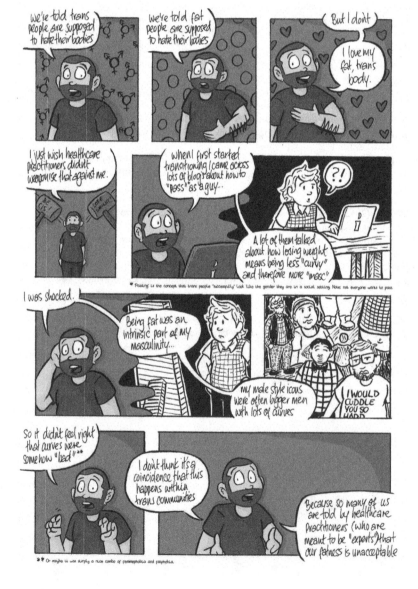

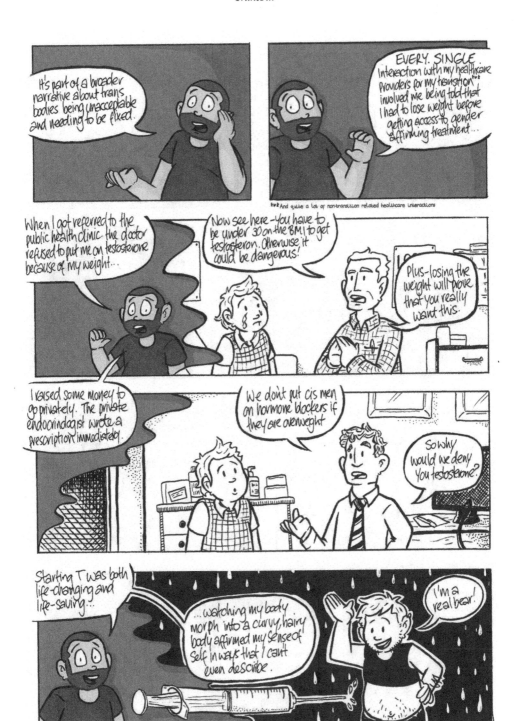

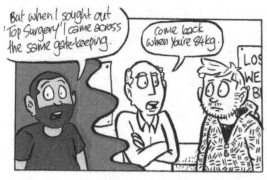

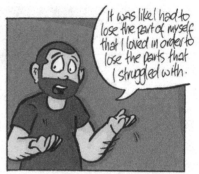

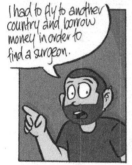

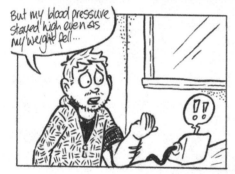

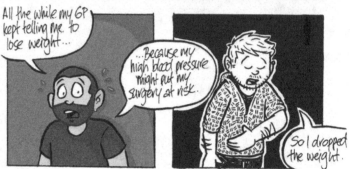

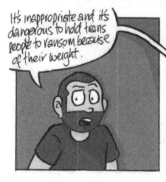

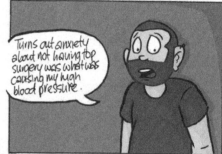

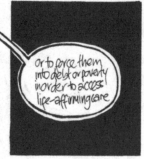

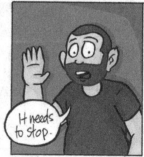

28

LESBIANS AND FAT

Esther D. Rothblum

I am a lucky fat woman.
If I lie in bed and have a fantasy
about eating six chocolate cakes
of being fed six chocolate cakes
by six fat womyn
who are admiring my six new rolls of flesh
I can get pleasure from my fantasy
and know that it's resistance
to this ridiculous persistence of shame
thrown at me.

Elana Dykewomon, *the real fat womon poems*
(copyright 1987, reprinted with permission)

Lesbians have been part of the fat activist movements from the outset. There were lesbians in the Fat Underground, formed by a group of fat women in Los Angeles in the 1970s to organize against the medical profession's discrimination of fat people (Fishman, 1998). One of its members, lesbian Judy Freespirit, co-authored the Fat Liberation Manifesto in 1983, which demanded respect and equal rights for fat people. The work singled out the false claims of the dieting industries, and, paraphrasing Karl Marx, ended with the statement "Fat people of the world, unite! You have nothing to lose" (Freespirit & Aldebaran, 1983, p. 53). That Manifesto was published in the anthology book *Shadow on a tightrope: Writings by women on fat oppression* (Schoenfielder & Wieser, 1983) that included chapters by other lesbians, and was published by Spinsters/Aunt Lute, a feminist lesbian publishing company. In 1981, the fat performance group Fat Lip Readers Theatre was started by nine lesbians and one bisexual woman (Bock & Squires, 2019). Around that same time, Laura Brown (1987, p. 5) wrote: "Lesbians appear to be over-represented among fat activists, that is, people who define fatness as a normative variation and the stigmatization of fat people as political oppression." She went on to draw a parallel between loving women as lesbians and consequently loving themselves as women.

Lesbians have also been represented in fat studies scholarship, including Elana Dykewomon whose poem begins this chapter. There were lesbian authors in *The fat studies reader* (Rothblum & Solovay, 2009), *Fat studies in the UK* (Tomrley & Naylor, 2009) and *The fat pedagogy reader*

(Cameron & Russell, 2016), among many other books. The past and present editorial boards and authors of *Fat Studies: An Interdisciplinary Journal of Body Weight and Society* include many lesbians, as does scholarship published by lesbians in other academic books and journals.

Are these lesbian activists and scholars representative of lesbians in the general community? If so, what is it about being a lesbian that serves as a preventive factor for society's obsession with weight and dieting? On the other hand, is it true, as Dworkin (1989, p. 33) wrote: "The rejection of men for sexual partners and the critical analysis of patriarchal oppression of women has not helped lesbians escape from attempting to mold their bodies into the male image of women"? This chapter will review social science research on lesbians, fat and body weight.

Is weight less of an issue for lesbians?

Some of the earliest convenience studies found that lesbians are less concerned with their weight than heterosexual women. For example, Herzog et al. (1992) reported that lesbians weighed more than heterosexual women, but lesbians were less concerned about their weight, less concerned about their appearance, and chose higher ideal weights than did heterosexual women. Carpenter's (2003) analyses of population-based data indicate that 66.8 percent of women in same-sex couples reported a desire to weigh less, compared with 68.4 percent of women in different-sex couples and 74.4 percent of women in heterosexual married couples. Studies of body image have found lesbians to have a more positive body image, despite weighing more than heterosexual women (Owens et al., 2003). In a more recent study (Alvy, 2013), lesbians weighed more, reported a larger ideal figure size, were more satisfied with their body, and had less discrepancy between their real and ideal weight than did heterosexual women.

On the other hand, several studies have found lesbian and heterosexual women to be similar in body image measures. Peplau et al. (2009) did not find a significant difference in body image between lesbians and heterosexual women. Heffernan (1996) similarly found lesbians and heterosexual women not to differ in attitudes about weight and appearance, or frequency of dieting. In a study by Striegel-Moore, Tucker and Hsu (1990), lesbians and heterosexual female college students were comparable on body esteem. Koff, Lucas and Grossmith (2010) found lesbian, bisexual and heterosexual women to have similar attitudes about body satisfaction, their ideal body, and what they perceived as the cultural ideal for women's bodies.

Is weight less of an issue for people in relationships with women instead of men?

Brand, Rothblum and Solomon (1992) as well as Siever (1994) have speculated that people sexually involved with women, that is to say heterosexual men and lesbians, are less concerned with weight and body image than people sexually involved with men that is, heterosexual women and gay men. This speculation is based on research showing that personal ads placed by men show a strong preference for physical attractiveness in their partner. Both studies found some evidence for this. Lesbians and heterosexual men reported higher ideal weights and were less preoccupied with weight than were heterosexual women and gay men (Brand et al., 1992). In Siever's study, lesbians had the highest Body Mass Index (BMI) of the four groups but were least concerned with physical appearance. Both lesbians and heterosexual men had higher scores on body satisfaction than did gay men or heterosexual women.

A number of other studies have provided evidence for this. Strong, Williamson, Netemeyer and Geer (2000) found that heterosexual men had less concern with body shape and size compared with gay men and lesbians had less concern than did heterosexual women.

In that study, lesbians and heterosexual men also reported less influence from the media about ideal body shape than did gay men or heterosexual women. Lakkis, Ricciardelli and Williams (1999) found gay men to score higher on body dissatisfaction and restrained eating than heterosexual men, whereas lesbians scored lower on these measures than did heterosexual women. In a study by Engeln-Maddox, Miller and Doyle (2011), lesbians and heterosexual men perceived less "body surveillance" (p. 524) than did heterosexual women or gay men.

On the other hand, studies have also found areas in which gender is more salient than sexual orientation. Brand et al. (1992) found that both lesbians and heterosexual women reported lower body satisfaction, greater concern with weight, and greater frequency of dieting than did gay or heterosexual men. Similarly, Beren, Hayden, Wilfley and Grilo (1996) found that gay men reported more body dissatisfaction and distress than did heterosexual men, but lesbians did not differ significantly from heterosexual women.

Morrison, Morrison and Sager (2004) conducted a meta-analysis of 27 studies on body satisfaction among lesbians, gay men, and heterosexual women and men. Overall, heterosexual men were slightly more satisfied with their body than gay men. The difference between lesbians and heterosexual women was not significant. However, lesbians tended to weigh more, and when that was taken into account, lesbians were slightly more satisfied with their body than heterosexual women.

Which other factors relate to weight and body image among lesbians?

If lesbians have more positive attitudes about their weight than heterosexual women, why is this so? The number of studies that find lesbians to be less focused on weight than heterosexual women has led researchers to examine possible reasons for this.

Connection to the lesbian community

Given Brown's (1987) theory that lesbian communities view the focus on women's appearance, weight and dieting as political oppression, a number of researchers have focused on the connection between lesbians' attitudes about weight and membership in the lesbian communities. Heffernan (1996) found that women who were more involved in lesbian communities had lower concerns about weight and were less likely to diet. Ludwig and Brownell noted that lesbian and bisexual women who had mostly heterosexual female friends had more negative body image than those who had mostly lesbian or bisexual friends. In a study by Mason, Lewis and Heron (2017), lesbians who experienced weight discrimination reported less social support from friends.

Hanley and McLaren (2015) examined three senses of belonging that were key components of the lesbian community: a sense of belonging to the broader lesbian community, to the organizational lesbian community in terms of specific interest or social groups, and to a personal network of lesbian friends. Their results indicated that all three components buffered depression due to body dissatisfaction, and that this relationship was strongest for the organizational and personal network components.

Other studies have not found this association between lesbian community participation and attitudes about the body. Beren et al. (1996) did not find an association between body satisfaction and connection with the lesbian community. Alvy (2013) also did not find participation in or connection to the lesbian community to be related to body satisfaction.

Coming out

If lesbian communities are less focused on weight, then women who are in the process of coming out may change their attitudes about weight. Krakauer and Rose (2002) asked women about changes in their physical appearance after coming out as lesbian. Women mentioned a number of changes, including dressing for comfort and having less concerns about weight. Lesbians who had been out longer were older and also had fewer concerns about weight. Similarly, Cogan (1999) found that lesbians dressed for comfort and gave up some traditional appearance practices such as wearing make-up after coming out. On the other hand, lesbians interviewed in a study by Huxley, Clarke and Halliwell (2011) also felt pressure from the lesbian communities to lose weight.

Masculine, feminine and androgynous gender roles

Given Dworkin's (1989) theory that women in general are expected to adhere to standards of physical attractiveness, it is possible that femme-identified women may experience this pressure more so than butch-identified women. Ludwig and Brownell (1999) assessed lesbian and bisexual women's perceived gender roles as masculine, feminine or androgynous. Feminine women had more body dissatisfaction than did masculine or androgynous women. Similarly, Heinrichs-Beck and Szymanski (2016) investigated butch/femme gender expression among lesbians. Lesbians who reported a more masculine appearance as well as behaviors and characteristics of masculinity had greater body satisfaction and were less likely than femmes to idealize thinness. However, masculine emotional expression (i.e., emotional restriction) was related to lower body satisfaction than feminine emotional expression (i.e., emotional communication).

Minority stress, perceived discrimination and internalized homophobia

A number of studies have found that lesbians are considered unattractive and masculine by the general public, and are liked most when they conform to ideal standards of heterosexual female appearance (c.f. Rothblum, 2002, for a review). Consequently, it is possible that lesbians may internalize these negative attitudes about themselves. To examine this, Alvy (2013) included measures of perceived discrimination and internalized heterosexism in her study of lesbians and body image, but these factors were not related to body dissatisfaction.

How does weight affect intimate partner relationships?

Given that men place greater focus on the physical attractiveness of their sexual and romantic partners (Sprecher et al., 1994), does this imply that women involved in intimate relationships with women are less focused on weight? The American Couples Study (Blumstein & Schwartz, 1983), compared heterosexual married, heterosexual cohabiting, gay male and lesbian couples in the 1970s (p. 250). Among their findings was the following:

> Of the four types of couples, only lesbians have triumphed over looks. Whether a lesbian is physically beautiful or not, her partner's sexual fulfillment, her happiness, and her belief that the relationship will last are equally unaffected. Time and again gay women have told us that conventional standards of female beauty ultimately do not matter to them, and when we examine the way their relationships work, we find this is generally true.

One way that researchers have examined the role of weight in sexual or romantic relationships is to ask participants to rate the attractiveness of women in photographs. Swami and Tovée (2006) asked feminist and non-feminist lesbians and heterosexual women, respectively, to rate photographs of women. BMI was a strong predictor of attractiveness ratings by all four groups, but lesbians found heavier women to be more attractive than did heterosexual women. These findings correspond to those of Cohen and Tannenbaum (2001), who compared lesbian and bisexual women's ratings of female figure drawings that varied in weight, waist-to-hip ratio, and breast size (this study did not include heterosexual women). Lesbians and bisexual women preferred the heavier figure with large breasts. Participants' own gender conformity or non-conformity did not affect the results. Legenbauer et al. (2009) assessed body dissatisfaction and internalization of society's ideals of thinness among heterosexual women and men, lesbians, and gay men. They also asked participants about characteristics of their preferred partner. Both gay and heterosexual men preferred physically attractive partners, weight and body shape dissatisfaction was related to partner weight and appearance for heterosexual women and men, but these effects were not found for lesbians.

Another way to study what lesbians want in partners is to examine the content of personal ads. Smith and Stillman (2002) examined the content of 357 personal ads of lesbians, 334 ads of heterosexual women, and 135 ads of bisexual women seeking female partners. Lesbians were less likely to indicate their weight than were bisexual women, and lesbians offered the least physical descriptions of themselves compared to the other groups.

Other research has asked participants directly about their own partnered relationships. Whereas Carpenter (2003) found that heavier gay men were less likely to be in a partnered relationship, the opposite was true for lesbians. He states (p. 73):

> This pattern suggests that obesity—which is more prevalent in the lesbian community compared to their heterosexual female counterparts—is generally associated with an *increased* likelihood of being in a partnership for lesbians relative to heterosexual women, even after controlling for the overall lower likelihood of partnership among lesbians.

In a rare study that surveyed both members of lesbian and heterosexual romantic couples (Markey & Markey, 2014), lesbians tended to desire heavier bodies than did heterosexual women. But both lesbians and heterosexual women perceived themselves as heavier when they were in relationships with thinner romantic partners. Heffernan (1999) found that about two-thirds of lesbians in her study reported that the physical attractiveness of their partner was important to them. However, the lesbians tended to focus more on physical conditions such as fitness, rather than weight or physical attractiveness.

Some qualitative research has focused on a more in-depth analysis of factors affecting weight in lesbian and bisexual women's romantic relationships. Lesbians interviewed by Huxley et al. (2011) indicated that physical appearance was less salient in lesbian relationships, that partners understood and shared experiences related to appearance, and that feeling attracted to women had a positive effect on their appreciation of their own body. On the other hand, lesbians compared themselves to their partner's physical appearance and weight, and were influenced by their partner's attitudes about her own body.

What about dieting and exercise?

Extensive research since the 1950s has shown over and over again that permanent weight loss is not possible. Both commercial and research weight loss programs have high drop-out rates, rarely result in BMIs in the "normal" weight range, and participants who lose even 5–10 percent of weight regain it a year later (c.f. Rothblum, 2018, for a review). Nevertheless, attempts at dieting continue, including programs aimed at minority consumers often referred to as "culturally sensitive" (Roberts et al., 2010). Thus Fogel, Young, Dietrick and Blakemore (2012) reported on a weight-loss program for 31 lesbians; only 64.5 percent of the participants returned for the six-month follow-up session. The average weight loss from the beginning of the program to the six-month follow-up was less than one pound.

Studies have found that lesbians diet frequently, even while aware that the lesbian community may consider dieting oppressive to women (Heffernan, 1999). Roberts et al. (2010) ran focus groups to ask lesbians about weight reduction. The women agreed that lesbians are more accepting of higher weight and wished for a focus on health rather than weight. This would serve as support for the arguments of the Health at Every Size (*HAES*) movement for lesbians (Bacon, 2008; Burgard, 2009). HAES is a movement which focuses on improving health of all people without a focus on weight.

It is extremely difficult to get an accurate account of exercise via self-report. Not everyone defines "light," "moderate" or "extreme" exercise the same way. Surveys often ask respondents about how many minutes or hours they exercise each day (Carpenter, 2003). This makes it difficult for people to estimate who may exercise different amounts on different days or weeks. For example, Owens et al. (2003) asked about exercise via only one item, ranging from exercising *never* (0) to *daily* (4).

Carpenter's (2003) analysis of US population-based data found that 80.7 percent of women in a same-sex couple reported that they were "exercising more" compared with 72.6 percent of women in different-sex couples and 72.7 percent of women in heterosexual married couples. When he focused on the 2001 California Health Interview Survey, 61.6 percent of lesbians reported engaging in "vigorous exercise" compared with 48.7 percent of heterosexual women. Similarly, the Epidemiologic Study of Health Risk in Lesbians (Aaron et al., 2001) found 63.2 percent of lesbians to report *no exercise* compared with 86.3 percent of women in the Behavioral Risk Factor Surveillance System survey.

What about health?

There has been no longitudinal research assessing the health of lesbians across the lifespan. Yet it is very common for researchers to speculate that lesbians are at increased risk of mortality due to their higher weight.

A review by Eliason (2014) searched scholarly databases for empirical studies on lesbians and chronic physical health problems. Overall, lesbians and heterosexual women did not differ on prevalence of diabetes, including a study that used laboratory data (Hatzenbuehler et al., 2013) and one that compared Latina, African American and Asian American lesbian and heterosexual women (Mays et al., 2002). Similarly, population-based studies have found no differences between lesbians and heterosexual women on hypertension or cholesterol levels, including those that measured these levels directly. Eliason compares studies that regard lesbians at higher *risk* for cardiovascular disease (for example, based on their BMI), yet the vast majority of studies of actual prevalence have not found differences between lesbians and heterosexual women on heart disease. Similarly, many researchers have reported that lesbians are at higher *risk* for breast and reproductive systems cancer, yet studies generally find no differences from heterosexual women. Given these findings, longitudinal studies of lesbians would be important in order to determine factors that are related to health and mortality.

Do lesbians weigh more than heterosexual women?

A number of studies have compared lesbians with heterosexual women on weight using population-based samples. Data from the 2002 National Survey of Family Growth (Boehmer et al., 2007) found that lesbians were more likely to have BMIs in the "overweight" and "obese" categories than heterosexual women. Analyses from the 2001–2008 Massachusetts Behavioral Risk Factor Surveillance surveys (Conron et al., 2010) indicated that 47.8 percent of lesbians versus 53.5 percent of heterosexual women reported BMIs in the "normal weight" category; the corresponding percentages were 23.9 percent for lesbians and 26.3 percent for "overweight" BMIs (indicating that lesbians were less likely to be "overweight"), and 26.4 percent for lesbians and 17.4 percent for heterosexual women for "obese" BMIs. Carpenter (2003) used data from the 1996–2002 Behavioral Risk Factor Surveillance System, a survey focused on couples. The results indicated that 20.2 percent of women in same-sex couples were "obese" compared with 15.3 percent of women in different-sex couples and 16.1 percent of women in heterosexual married couples. Carpenter (2003) also used data from the 2001 California Health Interview Survey (not focused on couples) and found that 36.9 percent of lesbians were "obese" compared with 24.7 percent of heterosexual women. An analysis of the 2006 National College Health Assessment (Struble et al., 2010) found the BMIs of lesbians (24.77) and bisexual women (24.53) to be higher than those of heterosexual women (23.12).

Other population-based studies have not found lesbians and heterosexual women to differ significantly on weight. Bogaert and Friesen (2002) analyzed data from a probability sample of households in the United Kingdom and did not find a significant effect between sexual orientation and weight for women. Cochran et al. (2001) examined the results of seven lesbian health surveys for risk indicators. Across the surveys, 28 percent of lesbians were "obese," which was comparable to surveys of adult women in the general US population, but higher than expected given the demographics of the lesbian samples (e.g., higher level of education, etc.). The most recent population-based study, the National Health Interview Survey 2013 conducted by the Centers of Disease Control, found no difference between lesbian and heterosexual female respondents on reported weight (Ward et al., 2014).

Not all of these studies are cited by other researchers to the same extent. When researchers want to argue for the need for weight loss programs for lesbians, they tend to cite the studies showing the greatest discrepancies.

How is weight reported?

Unfortunately, many researchers do not report the actual BMIs of their lesbian and heterosexual female samples. For example, Carpenter reports only the percentage of each group that was "obese." Bogeart and Friesen (2002) indicate that weight was recorded in kilograms, but do not report weights in their text or tables.

On the few occasions when researchers report BMI, the difference between lesbians and heterosexual women is statistically significant, but slight. For example, Owens et al. (2003) collected data from women in several US cities and found that the BMI of lesbians was 29.6 versus 28.2 for heterosexual women. In a large sample of over 50,000 respondents from MSNBC.com (Peplau et al., 2009) lesbians had a mean BMI of 25.4, compared with 24.2 for heterosexual women.

The analysis of Struble et al. (2010) is particularly noteworthy because the authors include *both* average BMIs and the percent of each group in the "underweight," "healthy weight" and "overweight or obese" categories (p. 53). Thus, the average BMIs indicate a slight but significant difference (24.77 for lesbians, 24.53 for bisexual women, and 23.12 for heterosexual women). Yet the percentages of "healthy weight" indicate 58.1 percent for lesbians, 60.1 percent for bisexual women, and 71.8 percent for heterosexual women, and the percentages of "overweight and obese" indicate 35.2 percent for lesbians, 35.1 percent for bisexual women, and 22.8 percent for heterosexual women. Had the authors included only the weight category results, this would give the impression that the group differences are larger than the mean BMIs would indicate.

Do lesbians report their weight more accurately?

All community and population-based studies of weight are based on participants' self-reporting. How accurate are these reports? In studies of the general population where researchers have actually weighed participants after asking them to self-report their weight, the researchers find that women tend to somewhat under-report their weight (e.g., Krul et al., 2009; Stommel & Schoenborn, 2009). Is it possible that lesbians report their weight more accurately because they are less concerned about their weight? In fact, some studies do find that lesbians have a smaller discrepancy than heterosexual women between their actual weight and the weight they would ideally like to have (e.g., Alvy, 2013; Brand et al., 1992; Herzog et al., 1992).

Which comparison groups are used for lesbians?

Researchers often have access to hundreds of college student participants, who may receive course credit or extra credit for being part of a study. However, only a very small percentage of these students identify as lesbian, gay or bisexual (LGB) so researchers then recruit LGB samples from community organizations. This is confounding, since college students are younger than community residents, and weight increases with age. Also, college students are generally more economically privileged than the community at large, an important factor, as weight is inversely related to income.

In a study about body satisfaction (Strong et al., 2000), over 90 percent of the heterosexual women and men were recruited from psychology classes whereas the majority of lesbian and gay men were recruited from university and community organizations. Similarly, Brand et al. (1992) obtained heterosexual student participants from psychology classes and lesbians and gay men from community events. As a result of these recruiting methods, in a study by Beren, Hayden, Wilfley and Grilo (1996), the mean age of lesbians was 34.9 years compared with 18.4 years for heterosexual women.

What are the limitations of this research?

Although the research on lesbians and weight has proliferated since the 1970s, it is still limited. The overwhelming majority of studies are focused on White lesbians in the US, with a few on lesbians in the UK and Australia. This is a significant limitation, since research indicates that African American and Latina women are less focused on weight and have more positive body image than White women (Owens et al., 2003).

Furthermore, most of the research has focused on adults, given that parents and school personnel, as well as institutional review boards, are reluctant to approve studies asking children and adolescents about their sexual orientation. Yet this is an important area, given that attitudes about weight and dieting begin at early ages. French, Story, Remafedi, Resnick and Blum (1996) compared LGB students in grades 7 to 12 on body image and dieting. Lesbian students had a more positive body image than heterosexual female students, but the two groups were comparable in rates of dieting. Hadland, Austin, Goodenow and Calzo (2014) used data from the Massachusetts Youth Risk Behavior Survey that is administered in high schools. Lesbian and bisexual female students weighed more than heterosexual female students but were more than twice as likely as heterosexual female students to view themselves as having a healthy weight. Much more research on lesbian youth is needed.

Whereas the early studies typically compared lesbians to heterosexual women, and then also to gay and heterosexual men, more recent research tends to focus on women who are sexual minorities or non-heterosexual (Huxley et al., 2011; Koff et al., 2010). Although these categories are now inclusive of the variety of sexual and gender identities (e.g., genderqueer, pansexual, asexual), the results no longer allow researchers to focus specifically on lesbians. Thus, bisexual women who are currently in relationships with men, for example, may have different attitudes about their weight and appearance than lesbians.

In conclusion, what is the future of lesbians and Fat Studies?

When Laura Brown and Sari Dworkin's theoretical articles appeared in the late 1980s, their contrasting views about lesbians and weight spurred a decade of research to see who was correct. As this chapter has shown, they were both right. Lesbians, like heterosexual women, are socialized by their families, the workplace, the media, and the general community to focus on their own weight and appearance.

Members of minority groups straddle two or more communities, and lesbians are no exception. Kelly (2007, p. 876) has referred to this phenomenon in two ways: "(a) the dominant culture (outsider expectations), and (b) lesbian cultural norms (insider expectations)". For lesbians this can present dilemmas when negotiating these two different worlds. Interviews conducted in a study by Beren et al. (1997) indicate a variety of lesbian appearance ideals: being fit and strong as well as thin, not appearing too feminine, and influence of the mainstream media's focus on women's appearance. Both this study and one by Cogan (1999) imply that lesbians know what they are *supposed* to feel about their bodies but are conflicted based on how the dominant culture objectifies women.

But many studies show that lesbians are less focused on weight and appearance. Engeln-Maddox et al. (2011) refer to the salience of the male gaze in the dominant culture: "Women are subjected to sexualized gazes from both men and women more often than men are. However, men are most frequently the ones doing the gazing" (p. 519). A study by Share and Mintz (2002) found lesbians to have "lower levels of internalization of cultural attitudes about appearance" (p. 99). In regard to that great phrase, lesbians could serve as a model of weight and body acceptance for heterosexual women.

References

Aaron, D. J., Markovic, N., Danielson, M. E., Honnold, J. A., Janosky, J. E., & Schmidt, N. J. (2001). Behavioral risk factors for disease and preventive health practices among lesbians. *American Journal of Public Health, 91*(6), 972–975.

Alvy, L. M. (2013). Do lesbian women have a better body image? Comparisons with heterosexual women and model of lesbian-specific factors. *Body Image, 10*(4), 524–534.

Bacon, L. (2008). *Health at Every Size: The surprising truth about your weight.* Dallas, TX: Benbella Books.

Beren, S. E., Hayden, H. A., Wilfley, D. E., & Grilo, C. M. (1996). The influence of sexual orientation on body dissatisfaction in adult men and women. *International Journal of Eating Disorders, 20*(2), 135–141.

Beren, S. E., Hayden, H. A., Wilfley, D. E., & Striegel-Moore, R. H. (1997). Body dissatisfaction among lesbian college students: The conflict of straddling mainstream and lesbian cultures. *Psychology of Women Quarterly, 21*(3), 431–445.

Blumstein, P., & Schwartz, P. (1983). *American couples: Money, work, sex.* New York: Pocket Books.

Bock, L., & Squires, C. (2019). Fat Lip Readers Theatre: A recollection in two voices. *Fat Studies, 8*(3), 219–239.

Boehmer, U., Bowen, D. J., & Bauer, G. R. (2007). Overweight and obesity in sexual-minority women: Evidence from population-based data. *American Journal of Public Health, 97*(6), 1134–1140.

Bogaert, A. F., & Friesen, C. (2002). Sexual orientation and height, weight, and age of puberty: New tests from a British national probability sample. *Biological Psychology, 59*(2), 135–145.

Brand, P. A., Rothblum, E. D., & Solomon, L. J. (1992). A comparison of lesbians, gay men, and heterosexuals on weight and restrained eating. *International Journal of Eating Disorders, 11*(3), 253–259.

Brown, L. S. (1987). Lesbians, weight, and eating: New analyses and perspectives. In the Boston Lesbian Psychologies Collective (Eds.) *Lesbian psychologies* (pp. 294–309). Urbana, IL: University of Illinois Press.

Burgard, D. (2009). What is "Health at Every Size"? In E. D. Rothblum, and S. Solovay (Eds.), *The fat studies reader* (pp. 42–53). New York: New York University Press.

Cameron, E., & Russell, C. (2016). *The fat pedagogy reader: Challenging weight-based oppression in education.* Bern: Peter Lang.

Carpenter, C. (2003). Sexual orientation and body weight: Evidence from multiple surveys. *Gender Issues, 21*, 60–74.

Cochran, S. D., Mays, V. M., Bowen, D., Gage, S., Bybee, D., Roberts, S. J., Goldstein, R. S., Robison, A., Rankow, E. J., & White, J. (2001). Cancer-related risk indicators and preventive screening behaviors among lesbians and bisexual women. *American Journal of Public Health, 91*(4), 591–597.

Cogan, J. C. (1999). Lesbians walk the tightrope of beauty: Thin is in but femme is out. *Journal of Lesbian Studies, 3*(4), 77–89.

Cohen, A. B., & Tannenbaum, I. J. (2001). Lesbian and bisexual women's judgments of the attractiveness of different body types. *The Journal of Sex Research, 38*(3), 226–232.

Conron, K. J., Mimiaga, M. J., & Landers, S. J. (2010). A population-based study of sexual orientation identity and gender differences in adult health. *American Journal of Public Health, 100*(10), 1953–1960.

Dworkin, S. H. (1989). Not in man's image: Lesbians and the cultural oppression of body image. *Women & Therapy, 8*(1/2), 27–39.

Dykewomon, E. (1987/2015). real fat womon poems. In E. Dykewomon *What can I ask—New and selected poems 1975–2014.* New York: Midsummer Night's Press.

Eliason, M. J. (2014). Chronic physical health problems in sexual minority women: Review of the literature. *LGBT Health, 1*(4), 259–268.

Engeln-Maddox, R., Miller, S. A., & Doyle, D. M. (2011). Tests of objectification theory in gay, lesbian, and heterosexual community samples: Mixed evidence for proposed pathways. *Sex Roles, 65*(7–8), 518–532.

Fishman, S. (1998). Life in the Fat Underground. *Radiance.* http://www.radiancemagazine.com/issues/1998/winter_98/fat_underground.html

Fogel, S., Young, L., Dietrich, M., & Blakemore, D. (2012). Weight loss and related behavior changes among lesbians. *Journal of Homosexuality, 59*(5), 689–702.

Freespirit, J., & Aldebaran (1983). Fat Liberation Manifesto. In L. Schoenfielder, and B. Wieser (Eds.), *Shadow on a tightrope: Writings by women on fat oppression* (pp. 52–53). San Francisco: Spinsters/Aunt Lute.

French, S. A., Story, M., Remafedi, G., Resnick, M. D., & Blum, R. W. (1996). Sexual orientation and prevalence of body dissatisfaction and eating disordered behaviors: A population-based study of adolescents. *International Journal of Eating Disorders, 19*(2), 119–126.

Hadland, S. E., Austin, S. B., Goodenow, C. S., & Calzo, J. P. (2014). Weight misperception and unhealthy weight control behaviors among sexual minorities in the general adolescent population. *Journal of Adolescent Health, 54*(3), 296–303.

Hanley, S., & McLaren, S. (2015). Sense of belonging to layers of lesbian community weakens the link between body image dissatisfaction and depressive symptoms. *Psychology of Women Quarterly, 39*(1), 85–94.

Hatzenbuehler, M. L., McLaughlin, K. A., & Slopen, N. (2013). Sexual orientation disparities in cardiovascular biomarkers among young adults. *American Journal of Preventive Medicine, 44*(6), 612–621.

Heffernan, K. (1996). Eating disorders and weight concern among lesbians. *International Journal of Eating Disorders, 19*(2), 127–138.

Heffernan, K. (1999). Lesbians and the internalization of societal standards of weight and appearance. *Journal of Lesbian Studies, 3*(4), 121–127.

Heinrichs-Beck, C. L., & Szymanski, D. M. (2016). Gender expression, body-gender identity incongruence, thin ideal internalization, and lesbian body dissatisfaction. *Psychology of Sexual Orientation and Gender Diversity, 4*(1), 23–33.

Herzog, D. B., Newman, K. L., Yeh, C. J., & Warshaw, M. (1992). Body image satisfaction in homosexual and heterosexual women. *International Journal of Eating Disorders, 11*(4), 391–396.

Huxley, C. J., Clarke, V., & Halliwell, E. (2011). "It's a comparison thing, isn't it?" Lesbian and bisexual women's accounts of how partner relationships shape their feelings about their body and appearance. *Psychology of Women Quarterly, 35*(3), 415–427.

Kelly, L. (2007). Lesbian body image perceptions: The context of body silence. *Qualitative Health Research, 17*(7), 873–883.

Koff, E., Lucas, M., & Grossmith, S. (2010). Women and body dissatisfaction: Does sexual orientation make a difference? *Body Image*, 7(3), 255–258.

Krakauer, I. D., & Rose, S. M. (2002). The impact of group membership on lesbians' physical appearance. *Journal of Lesbian Studies*, 6(1), 31–43.

Krul, A. J., Daanen, H. A. M., & Choi, H. (2009). Self-reported and measured weight, height and body mass index (BMI) in Italy, the Netherlands and North America. *European Journal of Public Health*, 21(4), 414–419.

Lakkis, J., Ricciardelli, L. A., & Williams, R. J. (1999). Role of sexual orientation and gender-related traits in disordered eating. *Sex Roles*, 41(1–2), 1–16.

Legenbauer, T., Vocks, S., Schäfer, C., Schütt-Strömel, S., Hiller, W., Wagner, C., & Vögele, C. (2009). Preference for attractiveness and thinness in a partner: Influence of internalization of the thin ideal and shape/weight dissatisfaction in heterosexual women, heterosexual men, lesbians, and gay men. *Body Image*, 6(3), 228–234.

Ludwig, M. R., & Brownell, K. D. (1999). Lesbians, bisexual women, and body image: An investigation of gender roles and social group affiliation. *International Journal of Eating Disorders*, 25(1), 89–97.

Markey, C. N., & Markey, P. M. (2014). Gender, sexual orientation, and romantic partner influence on body image: An examination of heterosexual and lesbian women and their partners. *Journal of Social and Personal Relationships*, 31(2), 162–177.

Mason, T. B., Lewis, R. J., & Heron, K. E. (2017). Indirect pathways connecting sexual orientation and weight discrimination to disordered eating among young adult lesbians. *Psychology of Sexual Orientation and Gender Diversity*, 4(2), 193–204.

Mays, V. M., Yancey, A. K., Cochran, S. D., Weber, M., & Fielding, J. E. (2002). Heterogeneity of health disparities among African American, Hispanic, and Asian American women: Unrecognized influences of sexual orientation. *American Journal of Public Health*, 92(4), 632–639.

Morrison, M. A., Morrison, T. G., & Sager, C. (2004). Does body satisfaction differ between gay men and lesbian women and heterosexual men and women? A meta-analytic review. *Body Image*, 1(2), 127–138.

Owens, L. K., Hughes, T. L., & Owens-Nicholson, D. (2003). The effects of sexual orientation on body image and attitudes about eating and weight. *Journal of Lesbian Studies*, 7(1), 15–33.

Peplau, L. A., Frederick, D. A., Yee, C., Maisel, N., Lever, J., & Ghavami, N. (2009). Body image satisfaction in heterosexual, gay, and lesbian adults. *Archives of Sexual Behavior*, 38(5), 713–725.

Roberts, S. J., Stuart-Shore, E. M., & Oppenheimer, R. A. (2010). Lesbians' attitudes and beliefs regarding overweight and weight reduction. *Journal of Clinical Nursing*, 19(13–14), 1986–1994.

Rothblum, E. D. (2002). Gay and lesbian body images. In T. F. Cash, and T. Pruzinsky (Eds.), *Body images: A handbook of theory, research, and clinical practice* (pp. 257–265). New York: Guilford Press.

Rothblum, E. D. (2018). Slim chance for permanent weight loss. *Archives of Scientific Psychology*, 6(1), 63–69.

Rothblum, E. D., & Solovay, S. (Eds.) (2009). *The fat studies reader*. New York: New York University Press.

Schoenfielder, L., & Wieser, B. (Eds.) (1983). *Shadow on a tightrope: Writings by women on fat oppression*. San Francisco: Spinsters/Aunt Lute.

Share, T. L., & Mintz, L. B. (2002). Differences between lesbians and heterosexual women in disordered eating and related attitudes. *Journal of Homosexuality*, 42(4), 89–106.

Siever, M. D. (1994). Sexual orientation and gender as factors in socioculturally acquired vulnerability to body dissatisfaction and eating disorders. *Journal of Consulting and Clinical Psychology*, 62(2), 252–260.

Smith, C. A., & Stillman, S. (2002). What do women want? The effects of gender and sexual orientation on the desirability of physical attributes in the personal ads of women. *Sex Roles*, 46(9), 337–342.

Sprecher, S., Sullivan, Q., & Hatfield, E. (1994). Mate selection preferences: Gender differences examined in a national sample. *Journal of Personality and Social Psychology*, 66(6), 1074–1080.

Stommel, M., & Schoenborn, C. A. (2009). Accuracy and usefulness of BMI measures based on self-reported weight and height: Findings from the NHANES and NHIS 2001–2006. *BMC Public Health*, 9(1), 421.

Striegel-Moore, R. H., Tucker, N., & Hsu, J. (1990). Body image dissatisfaction and disordered eating in lesbian college students. *International Journal of Eating Disorders*, 9(5), 493–500.

Strong, S. M., Williamson, D. A., Netemeyer, R. G., & Geer, J. H. (2000). Eating disorder symptoms and concerns about body differ as a function of gender and sexual orientation. *Journal of Social and Clinical Psychology*, 19(2), 240–255.

Struble, C. B., Lindley, L. L., Montgomery, K., Hardin, J., & Burcin, M. (2010). Overweight and obesity in lesbian and bisexual college women. *Journal of American College Health*, 59(1), 51–56.

Swami, V., & Tovée, M. J. (2006). The influence of Body Mass Index on the physical attractiveness preference of feminist and nonfeminist heterosexual women and lesbians. *Psychology of Women Quarterly, 30*(3), 252–257.

Tomrley, C., & Naylor, R. K. (2009). *Fat studies in the UK*. York: Raw Nerve Books.

Ward, B. W., Dahlhamer, J. M., Galinsky, A. M. & Joestl, S. S. (2014). Sexual orientation and health among U.S. adults: National Health Interview Survey, 2013. *National Health Statistics Reports, 77*, 1–10.

29

WHAT'S QUEER ABOUT FAT STUDIES NOW?

A critical exploration of queer/ing fatness

Allison Taylor

Introduction

In this chapter I explore the Fat Studies sub-field of queer Fat Studies. Queer Fat Studies ana-lyzes the parallels in queer and fat identities and experiences, alongside the utility of queer the-ory for conceptualizing and challenging fat oppression.[1] I contend that queer/ing (the studying of) fatness offers both a means of expanding normative conceptions of fatness and a critique of the broader field of Fat Studies. Accordingly, the following three questions guide this chapter: What is the queer potential of fatness? How might queer theory help scholars generate richer accounts of fatness? What queer theories are useful for Fat Studies scholars to draw upon for identifying, negotiating, and eradicating fat oppression? I divide the queer Fat Studies literature into five branches to show how the ideas, debates, and methods in the sub-field have devel-oped thus far. Overall, with this chapter I demonstrate the importance of queer/ing fatness by analyzing the utility of bringing queer theory and Fat Studies together to resist fat oppression.

Contextualizing queer Fat Studies: Queer/ing fat activisms

Elena Levy-Navarro (2009) asserts that, rather than an appropriation of queer narratives, strat-egies, or theories, scholarly efforts to queer fatness result from the fact that queers are "woven into the history of fat liberation" (p. 63). Indeed, Charlotte Cooper (2016) states that "queering fat activism involves acknowledging the foundational presence and contributions of queers to the movement. It is fat activism done by queers" (p. 192). In tracing the history of the fat activist movement, the intricate ties between queer and fat people are evident and significant. The Fat Underground, *FaT GiRL: The zine for fat dykes and the women who want them*, LG5 (Lesbiennes Grosse Cinq or Five Fat Lesbians), Pretty, Porky, and Pissed Off, and The Chubsters are all examples of important queer fat activist groups influenced by queer activisms, experiences, and theories. Because queers have played an integral role in developing, critiquing, and expanding conceptions of fat activism since its beginnings, it could be argued that fat activism has queer roots. Moreover, as scholars have noted (Luckett, 2017), because the academic discipline of Fat Studies grew out of fat activist movements, it would follow that Fat Studies shares fat activism's queer roots. Accordingly, the intersection of queer and fat, or queer theory and Fat Studies, is important to acknowledge and explore.

Branches of queer Fat Studies

Fat and/as queer

The first branch of queer Fat Studies literature is comprised of earlier works on queer/ing fatness. This literature analyzes similarities and differences between queer and fat identities and activisms and explores how queer theories and methods might be useful for Fat Studies and activisms. Of primary interest to the literature in this branch are the insights that queer identity, theory, and activism might have for resisting fat oppression.

Michael Moon's and Eve Kosofsky Sedgwick's (1990) meditation on the convergences in fat women's and gay men's lived experiences is a seminal text in queer Fat Studies, and queer fat scholars often argue that Moon and Sedgwick (1990) were the first academics in a Western context to seriously consider how queerness and fatness intersect from a fat-affirmative perspective (LeBesco, 2001; Murray, 2008). Moon and Sedgwick (1990) posit three dis/similarities in experience between these two groups: the closet, coming out, and identity politics. First, Moon and Sedgwick (1990) explore whether a "closet of size" exists alongside a "closet of sexuality" asking, "what kind of secret can the body of a fat woman keep?" (pp. 26–27). Their answer: none, because fatness "is the stigma of visibility" (p. 26). Second, Moon and Sedgwick (1990) analyze the role of the coming out process in gay men's and fat women's lives, arguing that coming out as fat can be a meaningful way for fat women to politicize their fatness by claiming space for their own fat-affirming conceptions of fatness. Finally, Moon and Sedgwick (1990) find that the fat liberation movement owes "a profound and unacknowledged historical debt" to the gay liberation movement for challenging conceptions of queerness and thereby, fatness, as "problems" with "causes" (p. 31). In charting these dis/similarities between queerness and fatness, Moon and Sedgwick emphasize the political need for anti-essentialist theories and politics of fatness that move conceptions of fatness from the realm of science into the realm of culture. Kathleen LeBesco (2001) distinguishes essentialist theories of fatness – which posit fatness as the necessary result of a biological or sociocultural "failure" – from anti-essentialist theories of fatness. The latter focus on how people ascribe different, competing meanings to fatness through communication and politics. Moon and Sedgwick's (1990) discussion of the closet, coming out, and fat identity politics offers conceptual and political tools for fat scholars and activists – queer and otherwise – to challenge fat oppression.

LeBesco (2001) responds to Moon and Sedgwick's (1990) call for an anti-essentialist theory of fatness. LeBesco (2001) draws on queer theory to conceptualize fat identities and bodies as discursively re/produced and, thus, situated within the realm of culture, power, and language. Specifically, LeBesco (2001) posits fatness as performative using Judith Butler's (1990) theory of gender performativity. Butler's (1990) theory of gender performativity argues that gender is not natural or inherent to individuals but, rather, is re/produced through the repetition of gendered acts and behaviors. Positing fatness as performative enables LeBesco (2001) to explore how subjects might re-work and resist norms of fatness, creating space to theorize and embody fatness in non-pathologizing and non-essentialist ways.

LeBesco (2001) also takes up the idea of fat identity politics, arguing that "we must inquire into the political construction and regulation of fat identity, rather than trying to make shared identity a foundation for fat politics" (p. 80). In this way, LeBesco (2001) expands upon Moon and Sedgwick's (1990) articulation of a fat identity politics, challenging the idea that a shared fat identity should be the foundation of such a politics. LeBesco (2001) suggests that, when groups are "organized by a desire to work or play together, rather than a shared identity … individuals can inscribe themselves with meanings over against dominant inscriptions" (p. 82). With this statement, LeBesco (2001) gestures towards the radical potential of "fat play" (p. 83), whereby performances of fatness have the potential to destabilize or resignify dominant constructions of fatness. Examples of fat play include scale smashings, ice cream eat-ins, and fat bikini swim meets (LeBesco, 2001). Ultimately, LeBesco (2001) uses Butler's (1990) work on bodies, gender, and language to begin to theorize how subjects can resist dominant constructions of fatness, and to offer new and playful ways of re/conceptualizing fatness.

In a subsequent piece, LeBesco (2004) argues that fatness is a "subset of queerness" (p. 88). LeBesco (2004) posits fatness as *like* queerness because both have been constructed as "problems" needing to be explained away. For example, both fatness and queerness have been posited as the result of "genes, hormones, [a] fear of being sexually attractive," and/or "lifestyle preferences over which individuals have considerable control" (p. 85). Moreover, fat and queer individuals "share a reputation for sexual deviance" insofar as queers have been posited as predators or publicly "flaunting" their sexuality, and fats have been posited as simultaneously hypersexual and asexual (LeBesco, 2004, p. 86).

For LeBesco (2004), fatness *is* queer in two principal ways. First, because fatness is desexualized in dominant framings of fatness, fat sex – sex involving a fat person – is queer. Second, fatness affects the ways in which subjects are read as gendered – by "accentuat[ing] the size and shape of certain sexualized body parts," for example – and can queer the genders of fat subjects (LeBesco, 2004, p. 89). These parallels in discursive framings of queerness and fatness, and the queerness of fatness, make clear why queering fatness is an appropriate and useful theoretical and political project.

Of particular interest to LeBesco (2004) in this piece are discourses of the closet and outing. LeBesco (2004) challenges Moon and Sedgwick's (1990) argument that fatness cannot be closeted by conceptualizing the shame or repentance fat subjects may feel about their bodies as forming a metaphorical closet for fat people. LeBesco (2004) discusses the "internal contradictions" fat subjects may experience – such as simultaneous feelings of shame and pride – around their fatness. Accordingly, LeBesco argues that fat politics needs to recognize the "depressing aspects of oppression" (p. 96).

Complicating Moon and Sedgwick's (1990) and LeBesco's (2001, 2004) analyses of the productive relationships between queer and fat politics and queerness and fatness is the fatphobia that is deeply entrenched within contemporary queer communities (Taylor, 2018). For example, the slur "no fats/no femmes" is pervasive in Western gay men's sexual cultures and is often employed in tandem with racist ideologies (Han, 2008; Pyle & Klein, 2011). Even though Fat Studies owes a "historical debt" (Moon & Sedgwick, 1990, p. 31) to queer politics, and despite similarities between fatness and queerness, queer communities can be complicit in the (re)production of the marginalization of fatness.

Overall, Moon and Sedgwick (1990) and LeBesco (2001, 2004) offer foundational insights and approaches to queer/ing fatness. Examining how fatness is un/like queerness, and how queer theory can challenge and offer alternatives to dominant and oppressive conceptions of fatness, these scholars identify the significant role queer theory can play in negotiating fat oppression. Moon and Sedgwick (1990) and LeBesco (2001, 2004) make the important first step of theorizing the possibility for less oppressive ways of embodying fatness.

Queer/ing Fat Studies as critique

The second branch of queer Fat Studies follows Samantha Murray's (2008) criticisms of some strains of fat studies and activisms for refiguring fat as "normal" or "beautiful" and thus, sustaining dominant structures of power. Responding to these criticisms, this branch of queer Fat

Studies scholarship argues for ambiguity and multiplicity in relation to fatness, recognizing the impossibility of removing oneself fully from dominant discourses of fatness. This branch of queer Fat Studies poses a critique of some trends within the broader fields of Fat Studies and activism, demonstrating how queer theory is useful as a critical tool for Fat Studies.

Murray (2008) develops a rigorous critique of three key problems she identifies with some fat pride strains of Fat Studies and activisms. Murray (2008) characterizes these strains of fat pride as following Marilyn Wann's (1998) call for fat women to "turn fat hatred back on itself" (p. 28), discard dominant, negative notions of fatness, and find self-empowerment by taking pride in their fat. Murray's (2008) first point of contention with this brand of fat activism is that it assumes that individuals have the power to define themselves and control how others read their bodies. For Murray (2008), this brand of fat activism is also predicated on the notion that individuals can fully embrace fat pride without retaining feelings of doubt, shame, or ambiguity about their bodies. Second, Murray (2008) argues that this type of fat activism relies on and reproduces a split between the mind and the body. This split occurs insofar as Wann (1998) contends that individuals can exercise the power of their minds over their bodies by changing how they perceive their fat bodies. For Murray (2008), this splitting is problematic because it neglects the central role that bodies play in how individuals experience their identities and the world, thus obscuring the potential for individuals to truly embody their fatness. Finally, Murray (2008) finds that this strain of fat pride rhetoric engages in "an uncritical re-hierarchising of a 'fat' aesthetic over a normative 'thin' one" (p. 90). Here, Murray (2008) suggests that in simply reversing current logic about body size to posit fat as beautiful and desirable reproduces heteronormative "visual regimes" (p. 117) that measure a woman's value by how closely she conforms to normative beauty ideals.

On one hand Murray's (2008) arguments respond to LeBesco's (2001) call for Fat Studies not to overlook the more depressing aspects of fat lived experience. On the other hand, Murray's argument is a critique of LeBesco's (2004) and Moon and Sedgwick's (1990) arguments. For Murray, LeBesco's (2004) and Moon and Sedgwick's (1990) calls for subjects to come out as fat assume both that a person's fatness constitutes a stable or essential truth about that person, and that individuals can intentionally decide to reject the discourses that constitute them as subjects. Both assumptions run counter to the queer theory that Murray (2008) draws on, specifically Moon and Sedgwick's (1990) "epistemology of the closet," which argues that there is no "one" who "comes out," because subjects are produced, preceded, and constrained by discourse. Murray (2008) problematizes the idea of "coming out" as fat as a singularly radical and liberating act.

Moreover, analyzing LeBesco's (2001) discussion of "fat play," Murray (2008) finds that the activist groups LeBesco (2001, 2004) analyzes posit individuals as able to intentionally take up, parody, and thus subvert norms of gender, sexuality, and/or fatness. Murry (2008) asserts that this understanding of subjectivity relies on a mis-reading of Butler's (1990) theory of gender performativity. The appeal of this mis-reading of Butler's (1990) theory of performativity is that it allows for "the possibility of acting at will" (Murray, 2008, p. 112) and having control over how one defines oneself. However, Murray (2008) argues that, because processes of meaning-making and identity re/production are intersubjective processes, parody is not always inherently subversive nor are parodic performances always read by others as such. Accordingly, Murray (2008) calls for Fat Studies scholars and activists to re-conceptualize their understandings of agency by interrogating "how, why, and under what conditions the reiteration of gender norms is necessarily complex, unpredictable and open to change" (Murray, 2008, p. 112). Murray (2008) thus engages with Butler's (1990) theory of gender performativity to provide a queer critique of Fat Studies scholarship and fat activisms. Murray's (2008) argument is nuanced in that she acknowledges the importance of coming out as fat and/or fat play for fat individuals themselves, while also recognizing the limitations inherent in these acts.

Cooper (2016), who follows Murray (2008) in calling for space for a multiplicity of fat experiences and embodiments in Fat Studies and activisms, takes issue with Murray's assertion that fat individuals' attempts to resignify the meanings of fatness through performance are doomed to fail. Instead, Cooper (2016) argues that queer theory allows for both the resignification of fat and, thus, alternative conceptions of fatness, *and* the reproduction of dominant, oppressive notions of fat. Cooper (2016), following Butler (1990), argues that subversion is context-dependent and cannot be predicted ahead of time. In this way, Cooper (2016) uses queer theory to provide a more nuanced understanding of Fat Studies and activist practices, demonstrating the utility of queer theory for conceptualizing the complex "both/and" instead of a simplistic "either/or": the fundamental ambiguity of fatness.

Murray's (2008) work marks an important turn in queer Fat Studies towards using queer theory as a tool to interrogate both mainstream Fat Studies and activist notions of fatness. This branch of queer Fat Studies demonstrates how queer theory can be applied to Fat Studies to critique the ways in which Fat Studies and activisms may unintentionally re/produce dominant structures of power. Therefore, queer/ing fatness helps to create space for multiple, ambiguous, and contradictory fat embodiments, making for a more inclusive movement.

Intersectional theories of queer/ing fatness

The third branch of queer Fat Studies posits reciprocal relationships between Fat Studies and queer theory, as well as other sites of critical inquiry, principally trans studies and critical disability studies. This scholarship examines commonalities, tensions, and contradictions between fields by bringing them to bear on one another. This branch demonstrates the potential of examining how Fat Studies and queer theory intersect with other critical disciplines.

Zoë Meleo-Erwin (2012) brings Fat Studies, queer theory, and critical disability studies together to trouble oppressive norms of health and embodiment that are re/produced by some Fat Studies and activist works. Specifically, Meleo-Erwin (2012) argues

> that rather than basing fat politics on the assertion of 'proper' health behaviour [ie. 'healthy' eating and exercise habits], thereby defining fat activism as inclusive only of those who are most palatable to and reflective of the mainstream world, fat politics should take as a core mission the troubling of normative ideas and ideals of health … and argue for a more complex, multidimensional and nuanced framing [of health].
>
> *(p. 393)*

Drawing on both queer theory as a critical tool to interrogate the concept of "normal" and to analyze how it re/produces dominant structures of power and control, and critical disability studies to challenge mainstream understandings of health, illness, normalcy, pathology, and cure, Meleo-Erwin (2012) can offer a more comprehensive approach to fat politics that disrupts some of the foundations of fat oppression. Meleo-Erwin (2012) gestures towards a queer/ed fat politics that includes fat people with disabilities and "unhealthy" or "bad" "fatties." Therefore, Meleo-Erwin (2012) demonstrates how queer theory, Fat Studies, and critical disability studies can reveal each other's limitations, oversights, and exclusions.

Francis Ray White (2014) performs a similar task by theorizing upon the experiences of individuals who are both fat and trans to "disrupt some of the dominant tropes of fat and trans narratives" (p. 87) and to reveal similarities and tensions in fat and trans theories and experiences. In doing so, White (2014) finds that fatness "contributes to producing a reading of bodies as legibly gendered in the first place," and that "fatness is not only read culturally as undermining gender, but as enhancing and magnifying it," producing an ambiguous relationship between fatness and gender (p. 91). White (2014) also finds that trans and fat activists have different approaches to body malleability. While trans studies embraces the malleability of bodies via gender affirming technologies, Fat Studies tends to insist on the fixity of the fat body to resist fatphobia. LeBesco (2014), too, interrogates the intersection of fat and trans, drawing on notions of gender fluidity to question why bodily fluidity – specifically the fluidity of fatness – is often resisted within fat communities. This contradiction leaves subjects who are fat and trans in a difficult position, especially when access to gender affirming surgeries is dependent upon weight loss, requiring fat, trans subjects to choose between their political commitments to fat or trans activisms (White, 2014). To address this conflict, White (2014) turns to queer theory and argues that "queering the intersection of fat and (trans)gender" reveals how fatness shifts gender away from binary categorization, makes room for a wider spectrum of legible fat, trans bodies, and deconstructs the binary of malleable/fixed-body (p. 97). In showing how fatness queers – troubles or challenges – normative, binary notions of gender, White's (2014) argument opens space for discussions and analyses of gender non-normativity in Fat Studies, contributes to including trans individuals and experiences in Fat Studies, and offers a nuanced analysis of the complex relationships between fat, queer, and (trans)gender subjectivities, politics, and theories.

Cat Pausé, Jackie Wykes, and Samantha Murray (2014) also make an important contribution to this branch of queer Fat Studies with their edited collection *Queering fat embodiment*. They argue that heteronormativity regulates (fat) bodies, and that fat bodies have potential "to disrupt normative imperatives and stable categories," particularly "ideas about health, sexuality, desire, and embodiment" (Wykes, 2014, p. 10). Pausé, Wykes and Murray define queer as "a mode of political and critical inquiry which seeks to expose taken-for-granted assumptions, trouble neat categories, and unfix the supposedly fixed alignment of bodies, gender, desire and identities" (Wykes, 2014, p. 4). With this notion of queer as a critique of normativity, they create conceptual space to explore the disruptive potential of fatness, and the ways in which queer theory and Fat Studies can be mutually informing (Pausé et al., 2014). Moreover, Pausé, Wykes and Murray's edited collection addresses numerous intersections between queer/ing fatness and, for example, transgender and genderqueer theories and experiences (Burford & Orchard, 2014; LeBesco, 2014), critical disability studies (Meleo-Erwin, 2014), and race and class (Jones, 2014). *Queering fat embodiment* thus begins to thicken theories of queer/ing fatness by exploring how queerness, fatness, and other axes of identity and critical theory are mutually informing.

This branch of queer Fat Studies demonstrates how bringing queer theory, Fat Studies and other fields of critical inquiry together is important for the broader field of Fat Studies. By analyzing how these fields speak to, contradict, support and challenge one another, this branch of queer Fat Studies rigorously explores and poses critiques of dominant aspects of Fat Studies and politics. Queer/ing fatness highlights exclusions in Fat Studies, contributing to more inclusive conceptions of fatness and fat oppression.

Anti-social theories of queer/ing fat

The fourth branch of queer Fat Studies literature takes up anti-social queer theory. Anti-social queer theory advocates against a liberal politics of inclusion or tolerance in favor of an embrace of negativity, failure, unruliness, and the disruptive or disturbing potential of queerness (Halberstam, 2008). Anti-social theories of queer/ing fatness emphasize the productive potential of rejecting attempts to redeem fatness within dominant frameworks of value, and of reveling in the ways that fatness deviates from social norms.

White (2012, 2013) inspired the turn to the anti-social in queer/ing fatness with their argument for the productive potential of reading dominant "obesity epidemic" discourse as a "manifestation of the logic of reproductive futurism," (White, 2012, p. 3) as theorized by Lee Edelman (2004). Reproductive futurism describes the current political and social order wherein the focus is on securing a future for the figure of "the child" (Edelman, 2004). For White (2013), reproductive futurism offers a useful framework for understanding fatness in contemporary Western societies insofar as "obesity epidemic" discourses "position fat as a queer, future-negating force" (p. 28) by framing fatness in terms of disease, disintegration, and death. Drawing on Edelman's (2004) notion of queer "not as a fixed identity, but as that which queers [i.e. disturbs or disrupts] the social order," (p. 5) White (2012) argues that fatness can be theorized as queer. For White (2012, 2013), fat subjects are queer/ed because of the ways in which fatness transgresses "normative standards of gender and sexuality, health and morality" (2012, p. 5) as well as "the very foundations of heteronormative binary gender that reproductive futurism is built on" (2013, p. 28).

White's (2012, 2013) turn to Edelman (2004) responds to Murray's (2008) criticism of Fat Studies and politics for re/producing the systems of power/knowledge they seek to deconstruct. White (2012) is not interested in resignifying fatness in more "positive" ways, fitting into the current social order, or appealing to the general public as means of challenging fat oppression. Instead, White (2012) uses Edelman (2004) to locate the queer potential of fatness in its ability to disrupt normativity. For White (2012), queer/ing fatness involves embracing the ways in which fatness is discursively constructed as non-normative: in doing so, fat subjects may find more livable ways of embodying fatness.

In their most recent work, White (2016) turns to an alternative theorization of queer anti-sociality by Jack Halberstam (2011) to address the limitations of Edelman's (2004) theory as a framework for Fat Studies and activisms – principally that it offers no "blueprint for political action" (p. 13). Specifically, White (2016) draws on Halberstam's (2011) concept of queer failure, which posits failure as offering a social location from which subjects might resist hegemonic norms and structures by critiquing them and re-imagining more inclusive alternatives. For White (2016), a framework of queer/ing fat failure creates space for resisting, refusing, critiquing, and forging alternatives to dominant structures of power without disavowing the negativity attached to fatness. White analyzes how medical literature posits fat sex as "failing" insofar as it is un-reproductive and/or does not embody heteronormative sexual ideals, such as the prioritizing of penetrative, vaginal intercourse. Further, White (2016) draws on queer failure to theorize how emphasizing the ways in which fat sex "fails" offers more creative, livable ways of imagining fat sex and models of sexuality.

Vikki Chalklin (2016) expands upon White's (2012, 2013) work by drawing on broader notions of queer anti-sociality, specifically the productive potential of shame and trauma, to theorize queer fat subjectivities, activisms, and futures. Chalklin (2016) argues that queer anti-sociality offers a theoretical lens through which to examine "the complex ways in which an engagement with negativity, pathologization, trauma and shame might pave the way for a mode of fat activism that … could work towards a radically different understanding of the fat (and queer) subject" (p. 108). In taking up the "negative" conceptions of fatness re/produced by dominant obesity discourse, Chalklin (2016) suggests that fat subjects can re-work these conceptions of fatness to articulate more livable and queer/ed fat subjectivities. With her argument, Chalklin (2016) challenges the privileging of redemptive models of fat subjectivity, where fat subjects work to fit into "dominant frameworks of value and legitimacy" (p. 110). For Chalklin (2016), queer/ed fat subjectivities can disrupt dominant, normative conceptions of fat subjectivity. Chalklin (2016) thus seeks to create space for the proliferation of a multitude of fat embodied subjectivities.

Cooper (2016) also emphasizes queer anti-sociality in her fat activism. Cooper (2016) discusses "the delights of anti-social behaviour and fat activism," arguing that "refusing to observe the rules of obesity discourse unlocks creative, non-conformist and unruly spaces for revolting fat bodies" (p. 89). Characterizing her former fat activist group The Chubsters as anti-social fat activism in action, Cooper (2016) contends that using anti-social queer theory to queer fatness enabled them to challenge dominant obesity discourses by reveling in being unintelligibly, bizarrely, grotesquely, and happily fat on their own terms.

Anti-social queer theory offers a means of queer/ing fatness by positing "queer" as a critical tool or framework to interrogate normativity. An anti-social queer/ing of fatness finds potential in embracing the "negative" aspects of fatness and emphasizing the ways in which fatness challenges mainstream norms of gender, health, and embodiment, among other things. Such approaches to queer/ing fatness imagine ways of conceiving and embodying fatness that lie beyond current social framings of fat.

Queer/ing fat temporalities

The fifth branch of queer Fat Studies applies queer theories of time – a sub-field of queer theory called queer temporalities – to fatness. Analyzing how mainstream narratives and discourses of "obesity" use notions of time to re/produce fat oppression, queer Fat Studies scholarship that takes up queer temporalities queers fatness by imagining other ways of thinking about fat bodies in relation to time. In this way, queer Fat Studies scholars use queer theories of time to posit alternative fat temporalities.

Elena Levy- Navarro (2009) first approaches the idea of queer/ing fat time by arguing that, within "obesity" discourses, "the fat are history itself—that is, they are the past that must be dispensed with as we move toward … future progress" (p. 18). For Levy-Navarro (2009) fat individuals are queer because – within "obesity" discourses – they disobey the current Western cultural imperative to "cultivate maximum longevity" (p. 17). "Obesity" discourses marginalize fat people by constructing fatness as a necessary part of the past, and as antithetical to a "successful" future.

Lucas Crawford (2017) argues that fat people are compelled towards a thin future, which they can achieve through weight-loss, while at the same time they are told that there is no future for them if they remain fat because of associations between "obesity", disease, and early death. Crawford (2017) contends that "there is, rhetorically, no such thing as a fat present—or, therefore, fat presence" (p. 448). To address this marginalizing temporal logic of "obesity" discourse, Crawford (2017) calls for a theory of fat presents or presence by figuring "a mode of temporality that refuses to be pulled between traumatic pasts and slender futures" (p. 466).

A 2018 special issue of *Fat Studies: An Interdisciplinary Journal of Body Weight and Society* devoted to the topic of fat temporalities solidifies theories of fat time as an important part of both the broader field of Fat Studies and the sub-field of queer Fat Studies. The pieces in this issue draw on a range of queer theories of time to consider how fat individuals are marginalized by social constructs of time that re/produce "obesity" discourse, and how fat individuals can chart alternative, less oppressive ways of existing in time. For example, Jami McFarland, Vanessa Slothouber, and Allison Taylor (2017) draw on Elizabeth Freeman (2010) and Jack Halberstam (2005, 2011) to analyze how "fat women are bound, disciplined, and regulated by heteronormative time," and conclude that "queer/ed fat temporalities offer opportunities for reimagining ways of life and time" (p. 2).

Queer/ing the ways fat people exist in time, this branch of queer Fat Studies recuperates fat presents, and futures. Like anti-social approaches to queer/ing fatness, queer/ing fat temporalities involves positing "queer" as a critique of normativity, specifically dominant ways of conceiving of and structuring life and time. Rather than asking fat people to fit in and keep up with normative timelines, queer/ing fat temporalities suggests that there are different timelines that are possible for fat people, thereby challenging fat oppression.

A future for no future's queer Fat Studies

I contend that anti-social queer theory offers the most compelling approach to queer/ing fatness and Fat Studies thus far. I find the productive potential of anti-social queer theory for queer/ing fatness to be two-fold. First, the scholarship using anti-social queer theory to queer fatness draws on "queer" as a conceptual tool or framework to critique normative systems of power, instead of as a subject position or as pertaining solely to sexuality and/or gender, thus broadening the scope of analysis. In earlier queer Fat Studies work queer is posited as a subject position that can be compared to fatness (Moon & Sedgwick, 1990; LeBesco, 2004), or as a theory pertaining to sexuality and/or gender (LeBesco, 2001, 2004). However, following Murray's (2008) call to make space for ambiguous and multiple fat embodiments, anti-social queer theory shifts how "queer" is used in queer fat studies. White (2012, 2013, 2016) and Chalklin (2016) draw on "queer" as an un-fixed structural position, loosely defining queer as that which falls outside of, disturbs, disrupts, and reveals oppressive systems of power. In this sense, queer can be posited as a critical analytic: queer becomes a critique of normativity and oppressions more generally. This conceptualization of queer enables queer fat studies to broaden the scope of its analyses beyond the intersection of fat/sexuality/gender to, for instance, norms of embodiment (White, 2013; Chalklin, 2016), health (White, 2012, 2013, 2016), and time (Crawford, 2017; McFarland et al., 2017), as well as broader models of sexuality (White, 2016) and morality (Chalklin, 2016; White, 2012, 2013). Anti-social queer theory therefore suggests the productive potential of queer as a tool or framework of critique for queer Fat Studies.

Second, by creating space for a variety of fat embodiments, rather than privileging one "right" or "best" way to be fat, anti-social queer fat scholarship can offer greater space for theorizing (how to) queer fatness. Following Murray (2008), White (2016) states that a fat politics premised only on pride and positivity produces "new spheres of fat failure in those who, for whatever reason, cannot learn to 'love themselves' or who feel ambivalent about their bodies" (p. 26). Anti-social queer theory provides an effective means of addressing this problem by insisting on the productive potential of both the negative and positive aspects of queer and, thus, fat embodiment. In refusing the dominant, oppressive frameworks for understanding and de/re/valuing fat bodies, anti-social queer theory points towards other, multiple ways of embodying fatness. Anti-social queer theory therefore offers queer Fat Studies a theoretical framework for re/valuing a variety of fat embodiments without re/producing the dominant structures of power that work to keep fat bodies in subordinated positions. Anti-social queer theory's potential to critique broader structures of normativity and to re/value and re/imagine multiple ways of being fat position it as the most compelling approach, thus far, to queer/ing fatness.

In/conclusions: New directions for queer Fat Studies

Queer/ing the study of fatness is an important scholarly endeavor for those in Fat Studies because it has the potential to expand normative notions of fatness and challenge the re/production of fat and other oppressions within and beyond the field of Fat Studies. This does not mean, however, that this sub-field is without problems, gaps, or limitations. In this final section,

I suggest new directions queer Fat Studies scholars might pursue in developing the field that expand upon and address gaps in the existing literature.

A first direction for future queer Fat Studies scholars to explore might be the idea of queer/ing fat futurities or utopias. Within the field of queer studies, the concepts of anti-sociality and futurity provide different positions on ways to (not) imagine queerness in relation to (no) future (Caserio et al., 2006). The most recent work on queer/ing fat temporalities suggests the productive potential of imagining fat futures, and White (2013) and Chalklin (2016), in their works on queer anti-sociality and fatness, suggest that a Muñozian approach to queer futurity may offer a useful theoretical framework for theorizing queer/ing fat futures. For Muñoz (2009), "queerness is primarily about futurity. Queerness is always on the horizon" (Caserio et al., 2006, p. 825). Some questions for this scholarship might include: How might considering fat futurities or utopias offer an alternative to, or challenge, anti-social theories of queer/ing fatness? Where might we currently catch glimpses of fat futurities and utopias?

A second direction for future Fat Studies scholars to take is to continue to flesh out the relationships between queer Fat Studies and the fields of critical disability studies and trans studies. Meleo-Erwin (2012) and White (2014) demonstrate that such an endeavor is incredibly fruitful in teasing out parallels, tensions, and contradictions between fields, and for producing more inclusive and intersectional analyses of fatness. Scholars might also consider analyzing queer/ing fatness in relation to critical race theory, and other sites of critical inquiry.

Relatedly, future Fat Studies scholars might ask how they can thicken their analyses of queer/ing fatness by incorporating race, class, nationality, and other sites of oppression into their work in meaningful ways. Mecca J. Sullivan (2013) demonstrates one possible avenue for doing so by drawing on Cathy Cohen's notion of queer "as a collectivizing identifier in which sexual difference is inextricable from racial, ethnic, class, and other social nonnormativities" (p. 201). This notion of queer considers race as an axis of oppression, offering a way of conceptualizing queerness in relation to fatness that does not necessarily privilege sexuality over other sites of non-normativity, and gesturing towards how other queer fat studies scholars might center race in their engagements with queer/ing fatness.

Queer/ing fatness is a valuable project for the broader field of Fat Studies. Queer Fat Studies has the potential to explore the queer potential of fatness, generate richer accounts of fat embodiment, pose critiques of problematic aspects of Fat Studies and, ultimately, identify and eradicate fat oppression. I urge fat studies scholars to "fatten up" their work by engaging with and further developing this important sub-set of the Fat Studies literature.

Note

1   Queer is an umbrella term to describe sexual identities that diverge from social norms. Queer theory is a branch of critical theory that identifies, interrogates, and deconstructs social norms, especially norms of gender, sexuality, and desire (Jagose, 1996).

References

Burford, J., & Orchard, S. (2014). Chubby boys with strap-ons: Queering fat transmasculine embodiment. In C. Pausé, J. Wykes, & S. Murray (Eds.), *Queering fat embodiment* (pp. 61–74). Farnham: Ashgate.

Butler, J. (1990). *Gender trouble: Feminism and the subversion of identity*. New York: Routledge.

Caserio, R. L., Edelman, L., Halberstam, J., Muñoz, J. E., & Dean, T. (2006). The anti-social thesis in queer theory. *PMLA, 121*(3), 819–828.

Chalklin, V. (2016). Obstinate fatties: Fat activism, queer negativity, and the celebration of "obesity". *Critical Psychology, 9*(2), 107–125.

Cooper, C. (2016). *Fat activism: A radical social movement.* Bristol: HammerOn Press.

Crawford, L. (2017). Slender trouble: From Berlant's cruel figuring of figuring to Sedgwick's fat presence. *GLQ: A Journal of Lesbian and Gay Studies, 23*(4), 447–472.

Edelman, L. (2004). *No future: Queer theory and the death drive.* Durham, NC: Duke University Press.

Freeman, E. (2010). *Time binds: Queer temporalities, queer histories.* Durham, NC: Duke University Press.

Halberstam, J. (2005). *A queer time and Place: Transgender bodies, subcultural lives.* New York: New York University Press.

Halberstam, J. (2008). The anti-social turn in queer studies. *Graduate Journal of Social Science, 5*(2), 140–156.

Halberstam, J. (2011). *The queer art of failure.* Durham, NC: Duke University Press.

Han, C. (2008). No fats, femmes, or Asians: The utility of critical race theory in examining the role of gay stock stories in the marginalization of gay Asian men. *Contemporary Justice Review, 11*(1), 11–22.

Jagose, A. (1996). *Queer theory: An introduction.* New York: New York University Press.

Jones, S. (2014). The performance of fat: The spectre outside the house of desire. In C. Pausé, J. Wykes, & S. Murray (Eds.), *Queering fat embodiment* (pp. 31–48). Farnham: Ashgate.

LeBesco, K. (2001). Queering fat bodies/politics. In J. E. Braziel, & K. LeBesco (Eds.), *Bodies out of bounds: Fatness and transgression* (pp. 74–87). Berkeley, CA: University of California Press.

LeBesco, K. (2004). The queerness of fat. In *Revolting bodies: The struggle to redefine fat identity.* Amherst: University of Massachusetts Press.

LeBesco, K. (2014). On fatness and fluidity: A meditation. In C. Pausé, J. Wykes, & S. Murray (Eds.), *Queering fat embodiment* (pp. 49–60). Farnham: Ashgate.

Levy-Navarro, E. (2009). Fattening queer history: Where does fat history go from here? In E. Rothblum, & S. Solovay (Eds.), *The fat studies reader* (pp. 15–22). New York: New York University Press.

Longhurst, R. (2014). Queering body size and shape: Performativity, the closet, shame and orientation. In C. Pausé, J. Wykes, & S. Murray (Eds.), *Queering fat embodiment* (pp. 13–26). Farnham: Ashgate.

Luckett, S. D. (2017). *Young, gifted and fat: An autoethnography of size, sexuality and privilege.* New York: Routledge.

McFarland, J., Slothouber, V., & Taylor, A. (2017). Tempo-rarily fat: A queer exploration of fat time. *Fat Studies, 7*(2), 135–146.

Meleo-Erwin, Z. (2012). Disrupting normal: Toward the "ordinary and familiar" in fat politics. *Feminism & Psychology, 22*(3), 388–402.

Meleo-Erwin, Z. (2014). Queering the linkages and divergences: The relationship between fatness and disability and the hope for a livable world. In C. Pausé, J. Wykes, & S. Murray (Eds.), *Queering fat embodiment* (pp. 97–114). Farnham: Ashgate.

Moon, M., & Sedgwick, E. K. (1990). Divinity: A dossier, a performance piece, a little-understood emotion. *Discourse, 13*(1), 12–39.

Murray, S. (2008). *The "fat" female body.* New York: Palgrave Macmillan.

Muñoz, J. E. (2009). *Cruising utopia: The then and there of queer futurity.* New York: New York University Press.

Pausé, C., Wykes, J., & Murray, S. (Eds.). (2014). *Queering fat embodiment.* Farnham: Ashgate.

Pyle, N. C., & Klein, N. L. (2011). Fat. Hairy. Sexy: Contesting standards of beauty and sexuality in the gay community. In C. Bobel, & S. Kwan (Eds.), *Embodied resistance: Challenging the norms, breaking the rules* (pp. 78–87). Nashville, TN: Vanderbilt University Press.

Sullivan, M. J. (2013). Fat mutha: Hip hop's queer corpulent poetics. *Palimpsest: A Journal on Women, Gender, and the Black International, 2*(2), 200–213.

Taylor, A. (2018). "Flabulously" femme: Queer fat femme women's identities and experiences. *Journal of Lesbian Studies, 22*(4), 459–481.

Wann, M. (1998). *Fat!So? Because you don't have to apologize for your size.* Berkeley, CA: Ten Speed Press.

White, F. R. (2012). Fat, queer, dead: "Obesity" and the death drive. *Somatechnics, 2*(1), 1–17.

White, F. R. (2013). No fat future? The uses of anti-social queer theory for fat activism. In E. H. Yekani, E. Kilian, & B. Michaelis (Eds.), *Queer futures: Reconsidering ethics, activism, and the political* (pp. 21–36). Farnham: Ashgate.

White, F. R. (2014). Fat/Trans: Queering the activist body. *Fat Studies, 3*(4), 86–100.

White, F. R. (2016). Fucking failures: The future of fat sex. *Sexualities, 19*(8), 962–979.

Wykes, J. (2014). Introduction: Why queering fat embodiment? In C. Pausé, J. Wykes, & S. Murray (Eds.), *Queering fat embodiment* (pp. 1–13). Farnham: Ashgate.

INDEX

Printed in the United States
By Bookmasters